Medical Coding in the Real World Student Workbook

Third Edition

Elizabeth Roberts

MA Ed, CCS, CPC, CRC

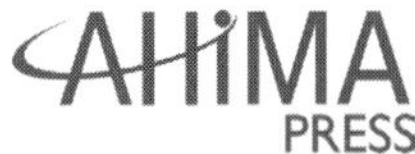

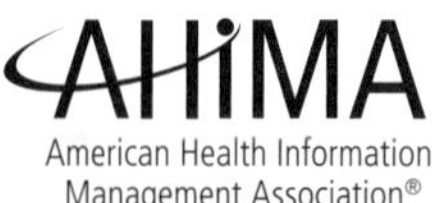

ISBN: **978-1-58426-799-7**
eISBN: **978-1-58426-838-3**
AHIMA Product No.: AC235021

AHIMA Staff:
Rachel Schratz, MA, Assistant Editor
Chelsea Brotherton, MA, Production Development Editor
Christine Scheid, Content Development Manager
Megan Grennan, Director, Content Production and AHIMA Press
James Pinnick, Vice President, Content and Product Development

Cover image: © I_Mac / iStock

For more information, including updates, about AHIMA Press publications, visit **http://www.ahima.org/education/press.**

American Health Information Management Association
233 North Michigan Avenue, 21st Floor
Chicago, Illinois 60601-5809
ahima.org

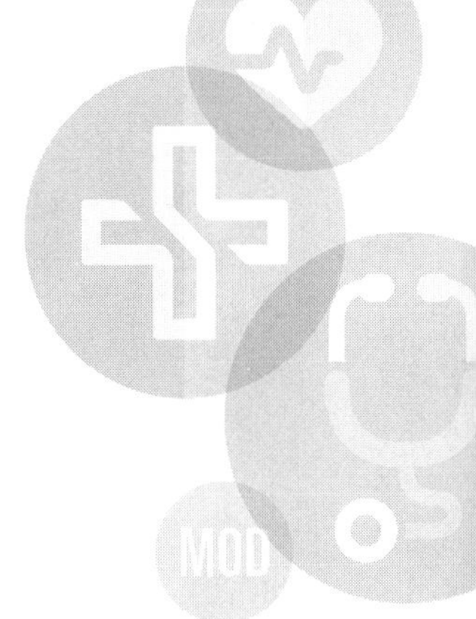

Brief Table of Contents

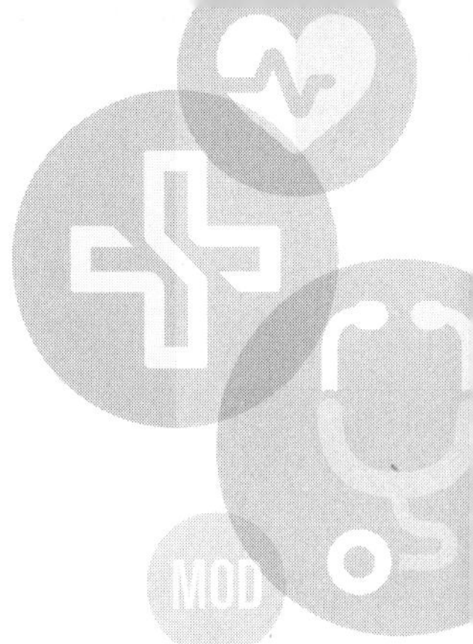

About the Author

Elizabeth Roberts, MA Ed, CCS, CPC, CRC has worked in the healthcare industry for 20 years and is an experienced coding educator. Mrs. Roberts has a master's degree in education and extensive experience in healthcare coding and reimbursement. In addition to serving as the program director for the allied health department at Vista College in Las Cruces, New Mexico, and lead instructor for the medical billing and coding department for Virginia College in Austin, Texas, she was the senior director of content for Implement HIT, a healthcare information technology company that specialized in bite-sized educational modules for medical providers and clinical staff. She now manages the medical coding department for Optum in Colorado Springs, CO, and continues to educate providers and clinical staff in fee-for-service and risk adjustment coding processes. An experienced consultant in healthcare coding and reimbursement, including practice management, HIPAA, compliance, insurance regulations, and healthcare coding (CPT, ICD-10, HCPCS), Mrs. Roberts enjoys helping billers, coders, clinical staff, and providers unweave the complicated tangle of coding and billing in order to optimize healthcare reimbursement.

How to Use This Workbook

Medical Coding in the Real World Student Workbook, Third Edition, is a comprehensive student workbook designed to enhance important information addressed in each chapter of *Medical Coding in the Real World*, and to reinforce learning through practice. This student workbook includes 20 chapters, each of which corresponds to the information presented in the textbook. Each workbook chapter includes several true/false, multiple choice, matching, short answer, coding, and case study exercises.

The student workbook is meant to be a companion to, and should be used in conjunction with, the textbook, chapter by chapter. In this manner, the workbook should be used to reinforce the information learned in each chapter of the text, and to provide practice searching for, selecting, sequencing, and reporting the appropriate ICD-10-CM, CPT, HCPCS, and ICD-10-PCS codes, as necessary.

Acknowledgments

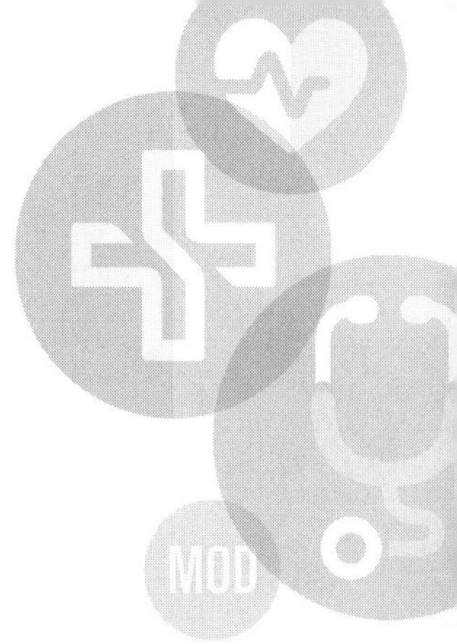

The author and AHIMA Press would like to acknowledge Dr. Aerian H. Tatum, MSHCA, RHIA, CCS, CPHIMS for her valuable contributions to this workbook.

Part I

Medical Billing and Coding Basics

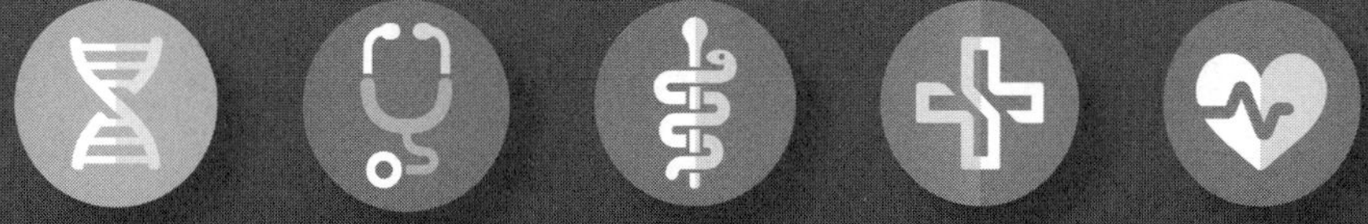

CHAPTER 1

Your Coding Career

Vocabulary

Instructions: Define each of the following key terms in the space provided.

1. Administrative personnel: ______________________________

____

____

2. Ambulatory surgical center (ASC): ______________________________

____

____

3. American Health Information Management Association (AHIMA): ______________

____

____

4. Certified Coding Specialist (CCS): ______________________________

____

____

5. Classification system: ______________________________

____

____

6. Clinical personnel: ______________________________

____

____

7. Code of ethics: ______________________________

____

____

8. Coding certification: ______________________________

____

____

9. Continuing education unit (CEU): ______________________________

____

____

10. Date of service: ______________________________

____

____

11. Diagnosis: ______________________________

____

____

12. Emergency department: ______________________________

____

____

13. Encounter: ______________________________

____

____

14. Healthcare billing: ______________________________

____

____

15. Healthcare coding: ____

____

____

16. Healthcare provider: ____

____

____

17. Healthcare specialty: ____

____

____

18. Hospital: ____

____

____

19. Inpatient: ____

____

____

20. Internal medicine provider: ____

____

____

21. Large group practice: ____

____

____

22. Mid-level provider: ____

____

____

23. Outpatient: ____

____

____

24. Physician: ______________________________

____

____

25. Primary care provider (PCP): ______________________________

____

____

26. Procedure: ______________________________

____

____

27. Professional organization: ______________________________

____

____

28. Remote coding: ______________________________

____

____

29. Small group practice: ______________________________

____

____

30. Solo practice: ______________________________

____

____

31. Surgical specialist: ______________________________

____

____

32. Urgent care facility: ______________________________

____

____

Matching

Instructions: Match the terms with the appropriate descriptions.

1. _______	Primary Care Provider (PCP)	**A.** Specializes in conditions affecting the feet
2. _______	Specialty Provider	**B.** Treats adult patients and specializes in the health of the entire body, including health maintenance and preventive care
3. _______	Pediatrician	**C.** Specializes in a particular area of medical expertise, including diagnosis, management, and treatment
4. _______	Family Practice	**D.** Treats patients from birth to elderly
5. _______	General Practitioner	**E.** Specializes in the prevention and treatment of adult internal diseases
6. _______	Internal Medicine	**F.** Specializes in disorders of the immune system
7. _______	Obstetrics and Gynecology	**G.** Treats patients ages 0 to 18
8. _______	Holistic and Integrative Specialists	**H.** Provides whole-health care, maintains patient health history, and performs preventive examinations and services
9. _______	Behavioral Health	**I.** Specializes in the diagnosis and treatment of the cardiovascular system; can be surgical, invasive, noninvasive; or specializes in treatment strategies
10. _______	Allergy/ Immunology	**J.** Specializes in conditions affecting the kidneys
11. _______	Anesthesiology and Pain Management	**K.** Specializes in women's health, pregnancy, and childbirth; includes labor and delivery, maternal fetal medicine, fertility services, and midwife services
12. _______	Cardiology	**L.** Specializes in whole-body health with an emphasis on holistic techniques, such as acupuncture

Matching continued on next page

(Continued)

13. _______	Surgical Specialist	**M.**	Specializes in anesthesia services and the treatment and management of pain
14. _______	Therapy and Rehabilitation	**N.**	Specializes in the testing or pathology and laboratory specimens
15. _______	Laboratory and Pathology	**O.**	Specializes in performing and developing therapeutic and rehabilitative services for patients
16. _______	Neurology	**P.**	Specializes in performing and developing surgical techniques for each respective body system or organ
17. _______	Orthopedics	**Q.**	Specializes in geriatric medicine for elderly patients
18. _______	Dermatology	**R.**	Specializes in the mental health of patients, includes psychiatric services and addiction medicine
19. _______	Geriatric Medicine	**S.**	Specializes in diagnosis and treatment of orthopedic conditions, such as fractures and osteoporosis
20. _______	Hematology and Oncology	**T.**	Specializes in ailments of the endocrine system, such as diabetes mellitus
21. _______	Gastroenterology	**U.**	Specializes in the detection, management, and treatment of blood conditions and malignancies
22. _______	Radiology and Imaging	**V.**	Specializes in diagnosis and treatment of conditions affecting the neurological system
23. _______	Endocrinology	**W.**	Specializes in conditions affecting the gastrointestinal system
24. _______	Hospice and Palliative Care	**X.**	Specializes in the detection, treatment, and management of infectious diseases, such as HIV
25. _______	Infectious Disease	**Y.**	Provides end-of-life treatment for terminally ill patients

26. ________ Nephrology

27. ________ Ophthalmology/Optometry

28. ________ Otolaryngology

29. ________ Podiatry

30. ________ Rheumatology

31. ________ Urology

Z. Specializes in the performance of either diagnostic or therapeutic radiology services, in addition to other types of imaging services

AA. Specializes in the dermatological system (skin)

BB. Specializes in the detection and treatment of eye conditions and vision services

CC. Specializes in the urological system and the male reproductive system

DD. Specializes in rheumatism, arthritis, and other disorders of the joints

EE. Specializes in the ears, nose, and throat

True/False

Instructions: Indicate whether the following statements are true or false (T or F). For false statements, rewrite the statement on the line below to make the statement true.

1. To be successful as an online coder, you must have a lot of self-discipline.

____

____

2. A large group practice is more likely to be multispecialty.

____

____

3. A solo group practice has only one doctor.

____

____

4. If you work in a large clinic, you are more likely to have to perform multiple responsibilities throughout the clinic.

____

____

5. If you work in a small clinic, you are likely to have a more detailed job description with fewer job responsibilities.

____

____

6. In the inpatient facility setting, ICD-10-PCS codes are used to identify diagnoses.

____

____

7. In the outpatient professional setting, ICD-10-CM codes are used to identify diagnoses.

____

____

8. HCPCS codes are used to identify supplies and services in the inpatient facility setting.

____

____

9. CPT codes are used to identify procedures in the outpatient setting.

____

____

10. A mid-level provider has a medical doctorate degree, such as an MD or a DO.

____

____

Multiple Choice

Instructions: Choose the best answer.

1. In which of the following settings can you work as a medical coder?
a. Billing and coding company
b. Outpatient practices and inpatient facilities
c. Outpatient practices only
d. All three: billing and coding companies, outpatient practices, and inpatient facilities

2. Which of the following medical practices can either be standalone or attached to a hospital, and provide services on an emergent setting?
   a. Large group practice
   b. Hospital
   c. Ambulatory surgical center (ASC)
   d. Emergency department

3. Which of the following types of medical practices would be composed of four physicians, all of whom practice the same specialty?
   a. Solo practice
   b. Small group practice
   c. Large group practice
   d. Hospital

4. National Healthcare is a group practice made up of seven physicians. Three of the doctors practice internal medicine and the other four doctors practice women's health. How would this practice be classified?
   a. Small group
   b. Multispecialty
   c. Single specialty
   d. Ambulatory surgical center (ASC)

5. Which of the following would also be referred to as an acute-care facility?
   a. Outpatient clinic
   b. Hospice and palliative care facility
   c. Inpatient facility
   d. Rehabilitation facility

6. Why is it important to understand the differences between inpatient facility reporting and outpatient professional reporting?
   a. Because the codes reported differ
   b. Because coders do not work in inpatient facilities
   c. Because some facilities are larger than others
   d. Inpatient facility and outpatient professional reporting are the same

7. Which of the following is a type of medical practice in which a provider specializes after completing medical school?
   a. A healthcare specialty
   b. Primary care
   c. A mid-level provider
   d. A solo practitioner

8. What type of medical provider specializes in diagnosing and treating the entire patient, including health maintenance and preventive health screenings?
   a. A primary care provider (PCP)
   b. A medical specialist
   c. A solo practitioner
   d. An internal medicine doctor

9. Who sends the referral or prior authorization request for patients?
a. The medical specialist
b. The primary care provider
c. The internal medicine doctor
d. The hospital or inpatient facility

10. Which of the following can be an inpatient facility?
a. Ambulatory surgical center (ASC)
b. Hospital
c. Physician office
d. Urgent care clinic

11. Which of the following *best* describes a CEU?
a. A unit of measurement for proficiency in coding
b. A unit of measurement used in continuing education programs
c. A unit of measurement required for medical providers to keep their license
d. A required professional exercise for all clinical assistants

12. Which of the following provider types is increasing in numbers across many clinical settings?
a. Medical doctors (MDs)
b. Advanced clinical psychiatrists (ACPs)
c. Mid-level providers (MLPs)
d. Doctors of Osteopathy (DOs)

13. Which of the following medical specialties treats patients suffering from conditions of the kidneys?
a. Endocrinology
b. Geriatric medicine
c. Urology
d. Nephrology

14. Which of the following medical specialties performs surgical treatments on the jaw and face?
a. Maxillofacial Surgery
b. Therapy and Rehabilitation
c. Otolaryngology (ENT)
d. Podiatry

15. Why is it important that coders understand the differences between medical specialties?
a. Because the codes billed depend on the provider specialty type
b. Because medical specialists treat patients with specific medical conditions only
c. Because some medical specialists may perform surgeries whereas others may not
d. It is not important for coders to understand the differences between medical specialties.

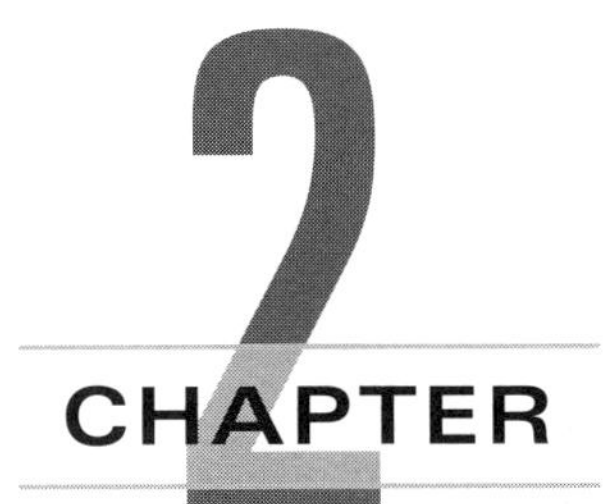

Healthcare Billing Basics

Vocabulary

Instructions: Define each of the following key terms in the space provided.

1. Accountable care organization (ACO): ____________________

____

____

2. Accreditation: ____________________

____

____

3. Administrative safeguards: ____________________

____

____

4. Advanced beneficiary notice (ABN): ____________________

____

____

5. Allowable amount: ____________________

____

____

6. Business associates (BAs): ______________________________

____

____

7. Capitation: ______________________________

____

____

8. Centers for Medicare and Medicaid Services (CMS): ______________________________

____

____

9. Charge amount: ______________________________

____

____

10. Children's Health Insurance Program (CHIP): ______________________________

____

____

11. CMS-1500: ______________________________

____

____

12. Coinsurance: ______________________________

____

____

13. Commercial insurance: ______________________________

____

____

14. Comorbidity: ______________________________

____

____

15. Complication: ______________________________

____

____

16. Computerized physician order entry (CPOE): ______________________________

____

____

17. Confidentiality agreement: ______________________________

____

____

18. Copayment: ______________________________

____

____

19. Coverage limitations: ______________________________

____

____

20. Covered entities (CEs): ______________________________

____

____

21. Data analytics: ______________________________

____

____

22. Deductible: ______________________________

____

____

23. De-identified documentation: ______________________________

____

____

24. Electronic protected health information (e-PHI): ______________________

____

____

25. Employer-sponsored insurance: ______________________

____

____

26. Encryption: ______________________

____

____

27. Enforcement Rule: ______________________

____

____

28. Entitlement health insurance: ______________________

____

____

29. Fee schedule: ______________________

____

____

30. Fee-for-service: ______________________

____

____

31. Government-sponsored insurance: ______________________

____

____

32. HCC coding: ______________________

____

____

33. Health insurance exchange: ______________________________

____

____

34. Health Insurance Marketplace: ______________________________

____

____

35. Health Insurance Portability and Accountability Act (HIPAA): ______________

____

____

36. Healthcare operations: ______________________________

____

____

37. Hierarchical Condition Categories (HCC): ______________________

____

____

38. Individual insurance: ______________________________

____

____

39. Insurance policy: ______________________________

____

____

40. Insured party: ______________________________

____

____

41. Medicaid: ______________________________

____

____

42. Medical necessity: ______________________________

____

____

43. Medicare: ______________________________

____

____

44. Medigap: ______________________________

____

____

45. Minimum necessary: ______________________________

____

____

46. Noncovered services: ______________________________

____

____

47. Notice of Privacy Practices: ______________________________

____

____

48. Out-of-pocket expense: ______________________________

____

____

49. Patient Centered Medical Home (PCMH): ______________________________

____

____

50. Payment: ______________________________

____

____

51. Performance measures: ____

____

____

52. Per member per month (PMPM): ________________________________

____

____

53. Physical safeguards: ____

____

____

54. Premium: ____

____

____

55. Prior authorization (PA): ____

____

____

56. Privacy Rule: ____

____

____

57. Prospective payment system (PPS): ____________________________

____

____

58. Protected health information (PHI): ___________________________

____

____

59. Provider contracting: ____

____

____

60. Quality improvement (QI): ______

61. Referral: ______

62. Reimbursement: ______

63. Risk adjustment: ______

64. Risk adjustment factor (RAF): ______

65. Risk analysis: ______

66. Security Rule: ______

67. Supplemental insurance: ______

68. Technical safeguards: ______

69. Third-party payer: ____

____

____

70. Treatment: ____

____

____

71. Treatment, payment, and healthcare operations (TPO): ____________________

____

____

72. TRICARE: ____

____

____

73. UB-04: ____

____

____

74. Workers' compensation insurance: ______________________________

____

____

True/False

Instructions: Indicate whether the following statements are true or false (T or F). For false statements, rewrite the statement on the line below to make the statement true.

1. HIPAA covered entities include health plans, clearinghouses, and healthcare providers.

____

____

2. PHI stands for patient health information.

____

____

3. PHI may be released for treatment, payment, and healthcare operations.

____

____

4. Administrative, technical, and physical safeguards are all components of the Privacy Rule.

____

____

5. The UB-04 claim form is used for outpatient professional billing.

____

____

6. A coinsurance is a preset amount that must be paid in full before insurance benefits will begin.

____

____

7. The total charge amount for a professional outpatient claim is entered in box 28.

____

____

8. An ABN should be issued to a patient when it is expected that Medicare will not pay for a service.

____

____

9. Capitation is a form of reimbursement that is based on an amount charged for each service performed.

____

____

10. HCC stands for Hierarchical Coding Conditions.

____

____

Multiple Choice

Instructions: Choose the best answer.

1. Which of the following HIPAA rules sets standards for the protection of personal health information by covered entities?
a. Privacy Rule
b. Security Rule
c. Enforcement Rule
d. Health Insurance Portability and Accountability Act

2. Which of the following is considered PHI?
a. Information related to the patient's educational background and history
b. Information related to the patient's credit history
c. Information related to the provision of healthcare to the patient
d. Information regarding the patient's homeowner's insurance

3. Which of the following principles states that only information that is directly related to TPO should be released?
a. Medical necessity
b. Treatment, payment, and healthcare operations (TPO)
c. Minimum necessary
d. Protected health information (PHI)

4. Which of the following evaluates the likelihood that a security breach would happen in a healthcare organization?
a. Risk adjustment
b. CPOE
c. Encryption
d. Risk analysis

5. Which of the following documents is signed by the patient to indicate that they have been made aware of the practice's policies related to patient privacy?
a. Confidentiality agreement
b. Notice of privacy practices
c. Business associate agreement
d. Covered entity agreement

6. Reimbursement is another word for which of the following?
a. The amount charged for a service
b. The write-off amount
c. The billed amount
d. The amount paid

7. Which medical claim form should be used to bill outpatient professional claims?
a. CMS-1450
b. UB-04
c. CMS-1500
d. Both the UB-04 and CMS-1500 may be used

8. In which section of the CMS-1500 form are diagnosis and procedure codes entered?
a. Carrier information
b. Physician or supplier information
c. Patient and insured information
d. Both physician or supplier information and patient and insured information

9. How many CPT or HCPCS codes may be entered on a single CMS-1500 claim form?
a. 6
b. 8
c. 12
d. 4

10. Which of the following is an amount of money that a patient must pay before they may be seen by the medical provider?
a. Deductible
b. Coinsurance
c. Copayment
d. Noncovered service fee

11. Which of the following types of insurance is purchased by a person who does attain coverage via his or her employer?
a. Employer-sponsored insurance
b. Individual insurance
c. Government-sponsored insurance
d. Entitlement health insurance

12. Which of the following is a government-sponsored insurance that provides coverage for patients who are elderly or disabled?
a. Medicare
b. Medicaid
c. Worker's compensation
d. TRICARE

13. Which of the following is an example of a supplemental insurance plan?
a. TRICARE
b. Worker's compensation
c. Medigap
d. Homeowner's insurance

14. If the patient's insurance does not authorize the services of a medical specialist via a prior authorization or referral, who is responsible for paying for the service, if provided?
   a. The patient
   b. The specialist
   c. The patient's insurance
   d. The referring provider

15. Which of the following is a group of medical providers that coordinate to provide high-quality care for their patients?
   a. CMS
   b. ACO
   c. HIPAA
   d. HCC

Case Study Performance Measure Coding

The following case study illustrates how performance measures are compiled using specific codes based on documentation in the medical record. Remember that performance measures are used to rate services provided to patients, to identify the overall performance of the providing doctor, clinic, or facility setting.

Performance measure data may be captured in several different ways, including supplemental files sent to the insurance payer, prescriptions filled by the patient, and diagnosis or procedure codes submitted on claims. Specific procedure codes, called Category II codes (discussed in chapter 5), may be reported when documentation identifies that a specific service, measurement, or other procedure has been performed. Category II codes (four-digit codes followed by the letter F) are captured by the insurance payer and then compiled into the total performance score for the provider or clinic.

In the following case study, carefully review the medical encounter documentation as well as the National Committee for Quality Assurance (NCQA) guidelines for capturing a Category II code to report completion of the performance measure. At the end of the case study, determine whether the documentation supports the Category II code(s) reported, and answer the questions that follow.

PATIENT: Pyotr Skopolov

DATE OF SERVICE: 05/01/20XX

REASON FOR VISIT: Wellness exam

HISTORY OF PRESENT ILLNESS:
Patient presents today for his wellness exam. He has been trying to eat better but has not been exercising regularly.

Timed up and go (TUG) test: Normal (30 seconds or less)
Hearing test: Right ear heard finger rub. Left ear heard finger rub.

Activities of daily living (ADLs): The patient does not need assistance with dressing, does not need assistance with feeding, does not need assistance with toileting, does not need assistance with personal hygiene, does not need assistance managing medications, does not need assistance managing money, and does not need assistance with transportation.

Documented and discussed: Patient provided with advanced care directive and medical directive power of attorney. Copy of advance care directive included in patient's electronic chart.

PHQ9: Over the past two weeks, how often have you been bothered by the following problems?

1. Little interest or pleasure in doing things? Not at all
2. Feeling down, depressed, or hopeless? Not at all
3. Trouble falling asleep or sleeping too much? Not at all
4. Feeling tired or having little energy? Not at all
5. Poor appetite or overeating? Not at all
6. Feeling bad about yourself, or that you are a failure, or have let your family down? Not at all
7. Trouble concentrating on things, such as reading a newspaper or watching television? Not at all
8. Moving or speaking so slowly that other people could have noticed, or the opposite, moving or speaking faster than usual? Not at all
9. Thoughts that you would be better off dead or hurting yourself in some way? Not at all

TOTAL SCORE: 0

There are no concerns regarding the patient's cognitive functions.

REVIEW OF SYSTEMS:
Complete review of systems, all within normal limits

PAST, FAMILY, SOCIAL HISTORY:
Allergies: No known drug allergies (NKDA)
History of: Cataract surgery, cornea transplant, bilateral eyes
Family history of COPD, severe: Father
Family history of Hypertension: Brother
Family history of Lymphoma: Mother
Patient is retired, married, enjoys volunteer work.

MEDICATION LIST:

1. Omeprazole 40 mg oral capsule delayed release. Take one capsule by mouth every day.
2. Aspirin, 81 mg tabs. Take one tablet daily.
3. Atorvastatin Calcium 20 mg oral tablet. Take one tablet by mouth at bedtime.
4. Vitamin D 2000-unit oral capsule. Take one capsule daily.

PHYSICAL EXAMINATION:
Constitutional: in no acute distress, alert

ASSESSMENT:

1. Encounter for preventive health examination. Discussed preventive care. He is up to date, but advanced directives were advised.
2. Abdominal aortic aneurysm (AAA) without rupture: 3.1 cm on US 01/20XX. Will monitor.
3. Benign essential hypertension. Improved with diet and exercise. Encourage more of the same. Monitor.
4. Mixed hyperlipidemia. Compensated with Atorvastatin. Continue same.
5. Patellofemoral syndrome of right knee. Illustrated knee exercises to increase range of motion (ROM) and decrease pain. If this does not help, I will refer to physical therapy.
6. Common wart, left foot. No treatment needed today.
7. Overweight (BMI 25.0–29.9). Goals are set and he is advised weight loss will help his hypertension.

PLAN:
Orders: 1. Colonoscopy, status—active

You have set the following goals: 1. Exercise 20 minutes per day; 2. Not eating after 6 p.m. Advised patient to create durable power of attorney and living will.

SIGNED: Dr. Ivan Foote, MD

Using the following information on performance measurement reporting, determine which, if any, Category II codes may be reported to identify aspects of the care received by the patient at this encounter. Note that in a real-world setting, these codes would be reported in addition to any other codes for procedures and diagnoses. However, for this exercise, it is necessary to identify only the proper Category II codes.

The guidelines that follow are similar to actual NCQA guidelines for performance measures but have been adapted for the purposes of this exercise (NCQA 2021).

Measures to Report Older Adult Care:

1. **Advanced Care Planning**
   - Documentation must indicate that advanced care planning was completed during the measurement year. Advanced care plan must be in the documentation.
   - Reported with code(s):
     - *1123F, Advance Care Planning discussed and documented advance care plan or surrogate decision maker documented in the medical record (DEM) (GER, Pall Cr)*
     - *1124F, Advance Care Planning discussed and documented in the medical record, patient did not wish or was not able to name a surrogate decision maker or provide an advance care plan (DEM) (GER, Pall Cr)*

2. Medication review

- Documentation must include both of the following:
  - Medication review by the provider
  - Current medication list
- Reported with code(s):
  - *1159F, Medication list documented in medical record (COA)*
  - *1160F, Review of all medications by a prescribing practitioner or clinical pharmacist (such as, prescriptions, OTCs, herbal therapies, and supplements) documented in the medical record (COA)*

3. Pain assessment

- Documentation must include a current assessment of the patient's pain, using quantifiable tool, such as scale of severity or illustrated depiction of pain status.
- Reported with code(s):
  - *1125F, Pain severity quantified; pain present (COA) (ONC)*
  - *1126F, Pain severity quantified; no pain present (COA) (ONC)*

4. Functional Status

- Documentation must include assessment of at least five of the following activities of daily living (ADLs):
  - Instrumental activities of daily living (IADLs), such as daily household chores, cleaning, cooking, driving, using public transportation, shopping, home repair and maintenance, taking prescription medications, using a telephone, and handling personal finances.
  - Activities of Daily Living (ADLs), including bathing, dressing, eating, getting up from a sitting or lying position, sitting down from a standing position, using the restroom, and walking.
- Reported with code(s):
  - *1170F, Functional status assessed (COA) (RA)*

Use the following steps to determine which, if any, of the Category II codes would be reported for the case study encounter:

1. Read through the medical encounter documentation and "Measures to Report Older Adult Care" excerpt in full.
2. Use a medical dictionary or medical terminology textbook to define any terms with which you are unfamiliar.
3. After reviewing both sections of the case study, determine which, if any, Category II codes should be reported for this encounter. Report all applicable Category II codes on the lines provided.

   Note: Do not assign additional codes, such as procedure or diagnosis codes. The purpose of this case study is only to compare the requirements for reporting a Category II code (as listed in the "Measures to Report Older Adult Care" excerpt) to the medical encounter documentation in order to determine which codes are necessary to report.

   Category II CPT code(s): ______________________________

   ____

   ____

Reference

National Committee for Quality Assurance (NCQA). 2021 (September 17). Proposed Changes to Existing Measure for HEDIS® 2020: Care for Older Adults (COA). https://www.ncqa.org/hedis/measures/care-for-older-adults/.

Resource

UnitedHealthcare. 2020. Reference Guide for Adult Health: 2020 HEDIS®, CMS Part D, CAHPS®, and HOS Measures. https://www.uhcprovider.com/content/dam/provider/docs/public/reports/path/PATH-Reference-Guide-for-Adult-Health.pdf.

Basics of Coding

Vocabulary

Instructions: Define each of the following key terms in the space provided.

1. Clinical modification (CM): ______________________________

2. Code linkage: ______________________________

3. Coding guidelines: ______________________________

4. Compliance: ______________________________

5. Current Procedural Terminology (CPT): ______________________________

6. Encoder: ______________________________

____

____

7. Evaluation and management (E/M) service: ______________________________

____

____

8. HCPCS Level I codes: ______________________________

____

____

9. HCPCS Level II codes: ______________________________

____

____

10. Healthcare Common Procedure Coding System (HCPCS): ______________________________

____

____

11. Healthcare codes: ______________________________

____

____

12. ICD-10-CM: ______________________________

____

____

13. ICD-10-PCS: ______________________________

____

____

14. ICD-11: ______________________________

____

____

15. ICD-9: ____

____

____

16. International Classification of Diseases (ICD): ______________________

____

____

17. Legacy system: ______________________________________

____

____

18. Medical necessity: ____________________________________

____

____

19. Modifier: ____

____

____

20. Procedural coding system (PCS): ___________________________

____

____

21. Reportable diagnosis: __________________________________

____

____

True/False

Instructions: Indicate whether the following statements are true or false (T or F). For false statements, rewrite the statement on the line below to make the statement true.

1. The CMS-1500 form is the numeric or alphanumeric translation of all of the services, supplies, treatments, diagnoses, conditions, and other reasons for medical treatments.

____

____

2. ICD codes are now in their tenth revision, which went into effect on October 1, 1993.

3. HCPCS Level II codes are also known simply as HCPCS codes.

4. In fee-for-service payment, CPT codes are directly attached to a charge for the procedure performed on a patient.

5. HCPCS code books are published on October 1st of each year.

6. The information compiled from the analysis of healthcare codes is also used for risk adjustment and performance measurement.

7. Code linkage is identifying the HCC score for each procedure performed on a patient.

8. If it is not documented, it never happened.

9. Coding guidelines are the rules that specify which codes to use in given situations, how to sequence them, and how much the insurance will reimburse for them.

10. A CPT modifier identifies additional information regarding the service provided.

Multiple Choice

Instructions: Choose the best answer.

1. On which date are ICD-10-CM codes updated each year?
a. October 1
b. January 1
c. Quarterly
d. Both January 1 and October 1

2. On which date are CPT codes updated each year?
a. October 1
b. January 1
c. Quarterly
d. Both January 1 and October 1

3. How often are HCPCS codes updated?
a. Annually
b. Biannually
c. Quarterly
d. Once every two years

4. Which healthcare code is used to identify procedures performed in the outpatient setting?
a. ICD-10-CM
b. ICD-10-PCS
c. CPT
d. CDT

5. Which healthcare code set is used to identify the patient's diagnosis or other reason for the encounter?
a. ICD-10-CM
b. ICD-10-PCS
c. CPT
d. CDT

6. Which of the following code sets will replace ICD-10 in the future?
a. ICD-9
b. ICD-10-PCS
c. ICD-11-PCS
d. ICD-11

7. The ICD-9 code set is important to understand because of which of the following?
   a. It is used on current claims to identify medical necessity for services provided.
   b. It is a legacy coding system that may be used by non-HIPAA covered entities.
   c. It was used on claims before October 1, 2015 to identify procedures provided to patients.
   d. The ICD-9 code set has not been in use since 1975 and it not important to understand.

8. Level II HCPCS codes are also referred to as:
   a. ICD-10-CM
   b. ICD-10-PCS
   c. CPT
   d. HCPCS

9. Medical necessity for the service performed is identified by which of the following healthcare codes?
   a. ICD-10-CM
   b. ICD-10-PCS
   c. CPT
   d. HCPCS

10. Which of the following is a two-digit code used to add additional information to a procedural description?
   a. PCS
   b. CM
   c. HCC
   d. Modifier

11. The ICD-10-PCS code set is used to report which of the following:
   a. Inpatient facility procedures
   b. Outpatient professional procedures
   c. Outpatient facility procedures
   d. Inpatient facility diagnoses

12. How many diagnosis codes may be included on the paper CMS-1500 form?
   a. 4
   b. 10
   c. 12
   d. 20

13. Annual changes in codes sets are due to which of the following?
   a. Advancements in medicine
   b. New clinical guidelines
   c. Changes in billing discourse
   d. A and B only

14. Which of the following is one of the additional uses of healthcare codes?
a. Fee-for-service reimbursement
b. Determining the reimbursement rate for provider salaries
c. Creating new diagnosis code sets
d. Public health and tracking of disease

15. Which of the following statements *best* describes the concept of code linkage?
a. Linking the procedure code with the correct fee-for-service charge
b. Linking the diagnosis code to the correct HCC category
c. Linking the procedure code with the correct diagnosis code
d. Linking the medical necessity for the procedure to the diagnosis code

Short Answer

Instructions: Using the two questions What did the doctor do? *and* Why did the doctor do it?, *identify the procedures and diagnoses from the following statements. (Only identify the diagnosis and procedure; do not look up the codes for either.)*

1. Derrick presented to the office of his gastroenterologist for a screening colonoscopy. GI doctor performed the colonoscopy, during which two colonic polyps were identified and removed with a cold knife. They were later determined to be benign.

Procedure: ______________________________

Diagnosis: ______________________________

2. Jaime presented to the emergency department with a laceration on his right arm due to a landscaping accident. ER doctor performed a simple wound repair of the 5 cm laceration.

Procedure: ______________________________

Diagnosis: ______________________________

3. Patient at 38 weeks' gestation of pregnancy presented to labor and delivery in active labor. Obstetrician vaginally delivered a newborn male infant after 4 hours of uncomplicated labor.

Procedure: ______________________________

Diagnosis: ______________________________

4. A 45-year-old male presented to the office of his primary care practitioner for a follow-up on his recent blood work. He was diagnosed with hyperlipidemia and hypertension and was started on two medications.

Procedure: ______________________________

Diagnosis: ______________________________

5. A 4-day-old infant was brought into the office of her pediatrician for a newborn well-child exam. The provider administered a complete examination and determined that the patient had neonatal jaundice. A bilirubin lab test was performed, and the patient was readmitted to the hospital for treatment.

   Procedure: ____________________

   Diagnosis: ____________________

Instructions: Answer the following question or prompt in one to three sentences.

6. Explain code linkage and how it is related to medical necessity and payment for healthcare services.

7. Explain how billing and coding are connected and why it is important for coders to understand the basics of healthcare billing.

8. Read through the additional uses of healthcare codes and identify the **two** that you believe are the most important for coders to understand. List and explain them here.

Code Linkage

Code linkage is identified on the CMS-1500 claim form by adding the letter that corresponds to each diagnosis in box 24.E for each procedure billed on the claim. For example, see the following figure that demonstrates how to link codes together. In the following figure, the diagnosis codes for swimmer's ear, H60.332—listed on line A—is linked with the first procedure code on the claim, 99213, for the office evaluation. In this case the swimmer's ear diagnosis code is linked to the office evaluation procedure code by adding the letter A to box 24.E. Similarly, the diagnosis code for the wart, B07.9—listed on line B—is linked to the procedure code for cryosurgery, 17000, the second procedure on the claim, by adding the letter B in box 24.E.

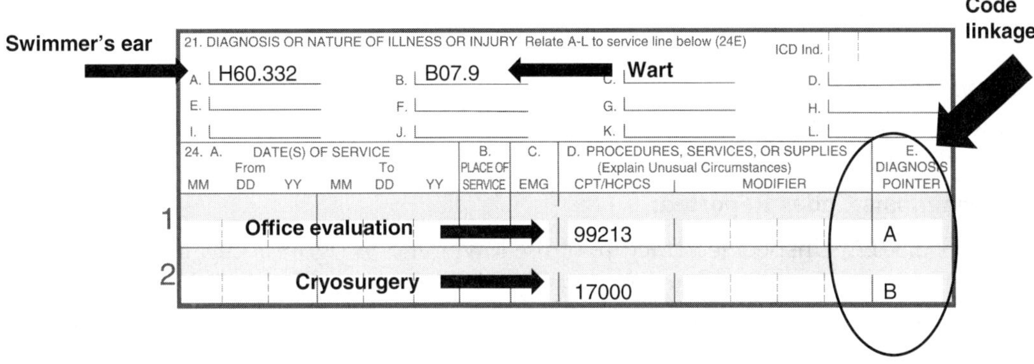

Source: CMS 2017.

In the following exercises, link the diagnosis codes to the procedure codes on the claim by adding the appropriate letter in box 24.E.

1. Clinic Note:

A 40-year-old established female presented to the office for a routine preventive exam. After performing a comprehensive physical examination with no abnormal findings, the provider also administered the annual flu vaccine to the patient.

Diagnosis Codes Reported:

- Z00.00, Encounter for general adult medical examination without abnormal findings
- Z23, Encounter for immunization

Procedure Codes Reported:

- 99396, Periodic comprehensive preventive medicine re-evaluation and management of an individual…; 40-64 years
- 90471, Immunization administration…; 1 vaccine
- 90658, Influenza virus vaccine, trivalent (IIV3), split virus, 0.5 mL dosage, for intramuscular use

Link the diagnosis codes to the appropriate procedure codes in the area below by adding the correct diagnosis pointer(s) in box 24.E for procedure codes one through three.

21. DIAGNOSIS OR NATURE OF ILLNESS OR INJURY Relate A-L to service line below (24E) ICD Ind.

A. Z00.00	B. Z23	C.	D.
E.	F.	G.	H.
I.	J.	K.	L.

	24. A. DATE(S) OF SERVICE From MM DD YY To MM DD YY	B. PLACE OF SERVICE	C. EMG	D. PROCEDURES, SERVICES, OR SUPPLIES (Explain Unusual Circumstances) CPT/HCPCS	MODIFIER	E. DIAGNOSIS POINTER
1				99396		
2				90471		
3				90658		

Source: CMS 2017.

2. Clinic Note:

A 32-year-old patient presented to the office of an orthopedist complaining of right and left wrist pain after having fallen on outstretched hands. The orthopedist completed x-rays of both wrists and diagnosed the patient with bilateral distal radius fractures, and then completed comprehensive fracture care for both fractures.

Diagnosis Codes Reported:

- S52.501A, Unspecified fracture of the lower end of right radius, initial encounter for closed fracture
- S52.502A, Unspecified fracture of the lower end of left radius, initial encounter for closed fracture

Procedure Codes Reported:

- 73100, Radiologic examination, wrist; 2 views (×2)
- 25600, Closed treatment of distal radial fracture…; without manipulation
- 25600, Closed treatment of distal radial fracture…; without manipulation

Link the diagnosis codes to the appropriate procedure codes in the area below by adding the correct diagnosis pointer(s) in box 24.E for procedure codes one through three.

21. DIAGNOSIS OR NATURE OF ILLNESS OR INJURY Relate A-L to service line below (24E) ICD Ind.

A. S52.501A	B. S52.502A	C.	D.
E.	F.	G.	H.
I.	J.	K.	L.

	24. A. DATE(S) OF SERVICE From MM	DD	YY	To MM	DD	YY	B. PLACE OF SERVICE	C. EMG	D. PROCEDURES, SERVICES, OR SUPPLIES (Explain Unusual Circumstances) CPT/HCPCS	MODIFIER	E. DIAGNOSIS POINTER
1									73100		
2									25600		
3									25600		

3. Clinic Note:

A 65-year-old patient presented to the office of his primary care provider, complaining of chronic right knee pain. He also had recent labs completed for hyperlipidemia and hypothyroidism, which were discussed with the doctor, who prescribed two medications for these conditions. The provider completed a detailed history, detailed examination, and medical decision-making of low complexity, and then performed a right knee joint injection of triamcinolone acetonide (Kenalog).

Diagnosis Codes Reported:

- E78.5, Hyperlipidemia, unspecified
- E03.9, Hypothyroidism, unspecified
- M25.561, Pain in right knee

Procedure Codes Reported:

- 99214, Office or other outpatient visit for the evaluation and management of an established patient, which requires at least 2 of these 3 key components: A detailed history; A detailed examination; Medical decision-making of moderate complexity
- 20610, Arthrocentesis, aspiration and/or injection, major joint or bursa (eg, shoulder, hip, knee, subacromial bursa); without ultrasound guidance

Link the diagnosis codes to the appropriate procedure codes in the area below by adding the correct diagnosis pointer(s) in box 24.E for procedure codes one and two.

21. DIAGNOSIS OR NATURE OF ILLNESS OR INJURY Relate A-L to service line below (24E) ICD Ind.

A. E78.5	B. E03.9	C. M25.561	D.
E.	F.	G.	H.
I.	J.	K.	L.

	24. A. DATE(S) OF SERVICE From MM	DD	YY	To MM	DD	YY	B. PLACE OF SERVICE	C. EMG	D. PROCEDURES, SERVICES, OR SUPPLIES (Explain Unusual Circumstances) CPT/HCPCS	MODIFIER	E. DIAGNOSIS POINTER
1									99214		
2									20610		
3											

4. Clinic Note:

A 42-year-old female complaining of severe vertigo was brought to the urgent care by her husband. After an expanded problem-focused history and exam, and low complexity medical decision-making, the provider diagnosed the patient with benign paroxysmal positional vertigo (BPPV) and performed the Epley canalith repositioning procedure.

Diagnosis Codes Reported:

- H81.10, Benign paroxysmal vertigo, unspecified ear

Procedure Codes Reported:

- 99213, Office or other outpatient visit for the evaluation and management of an established patient, which requires at least 2 of these 3 key components: An expanded problem focused history; An expanded problem focused examination; Medical decision-making of low complexity
- 95992, Canalith repositioning procedure(s) (eg, Epley maneuver, Semont maneuver), per day

Link the diagnosis codes to the appropriate procedure codes in the area below by adding the correct diagnosis pointer(s) in box 24.E for procedure codes one and two.

21. DIAGNOSIS OR NATURE OF ILLNESS OR INJURY Relate A-L to service line below (24E) ICD Ind.

A. H81.10	B. Z23	C.	D.
E.	F.	G.	H.
I.	J.	K.	L.

	24. A. DATE(S) OF SERVICE From MM DD YY	To MM DD YY	B. PLACE OF SERVICE	C. EMG	D. PROCEDURES, SERVICES, OR SUPPLIES (Explain Unusual Circumstances) CPT/HCPCS	MODIFIER	E. DIAGNOSIS POINTER
1					99213		
2					95992		
3							

5. Clinic Note:

A 6-month-old male was brought to the office of his pediatrician with a high fever and fussiness. Provider completed an expanded problem-focused history, a detailed examination, and low medical decision-making. Due to the patient's high fever and no other symptoms, the provider also performed a straight catheterization for urinalysis, which was negative of any findings. The patient was diagnosed with fussiness and fever of unknown origin.

Diagnosis Codes Reported:

- R50.9, Fever, unspecified
- R68.12, Fussy infant (baby)

Procedure Codes Reported:

- 99213, Office or other outpatient visit for the evaluation and management of an established patient, which requires at least 2 of these 3 key components: An expanded problem focused history; An expanded problem focused examination; Medical decision-making of low complexity
- 51701, Insertion of non-indwelling bladder catheter (eg, straight catheterization for residual urine)

Link the diagnosis codes to the appropriate procedure codes in the area below by adding the correct diagnosis pointer(s) in box 24.E for procedure codes one and two.

21. DIAGNOSIS OR NATURE OF ILLNESS OR INJURY Relate A-L to service line below (24E) ICD Ind.

A. R50.9	B. R68.12	C.	D.
E.	F.	G.	H.
I.	J.	K.	L.

	24. A. DATE(S) OF SERVICE From MM DD YY	To MM DD YY	B. PLACE OF SERVICE	C. EMG	D. PROCEDURES, SERVICES, OR SUPPLIES (Explain Unusual Circumstances) CPT/HCPCS	MODIFIER	E. DIAGNOSIS POINTER
1					99213		
2					51701		
3							

Case Study Basics of Coding—Abstracting a Medical Record

PATIENT: Pyotr Skopolov

DATE OF SERVICE: 05/01/20XX

REASON FOR VISIT: Wellness exam

HISTORY OF PRESENT ILLNESS:
Patient presents today for his wellness exam. He has been trying to eat better but has not been exercising regularly. *He has a skin spot to look at. One bump on his foot and several small spots on his face.*

Timed up and go (TUG) test: normal (30 seconds or less)
Hearing test: right ear heard finger rub. Left ear heard finger rub.

Activities of daily living (ADLs): The patient does not need assistance with dressing, does not need assistance with feeding, does not need assistance with toileting, does not need assistance with personal hygiene, does not need assistance managing medications, does not need assistance managing money, and does not need assistance with transportation.

Documented and discussed: Patient provided with advanced care directive and medical directive power of attorney. Copy of advance care directive included in patient's electronic chart.

PHQ9: Over the past two weeks, how often have you been bothered by the following problems?

1. Little interest or pleasure in doing things? Not at all
2. Feeling down, depressed, or hopeless? Not at all
3. Trouble falling asleep or sleeping too much? Not at all
4. Feeling tired or having little energy? Not at all
5. Poor appetite or overeating? Not at all
6. Feeling bad about yourself, or that you are a failure, or have let your family down? Not at all
7. Trouble concentrating on things, such as reading a newspaper or watching television? Not at all
8. Moving or speaking so slowly that other people could have noticed, or the opposite, moving or speaking faster than usual? Not at all
9. Thoughts that you would be better off dead or hurting yourself in some way? Not at all

TOTAL SCORE: 0

There are no concerns regarding the patient's cognitive functions.

REVIEW OF SYSTEMS:
Complete review of systems, all within normal limits

PAST, FAMILY, SOCIAL HISTORY:
Allergies: No known drug allergies (NKDA)
History of: Cataract surgery, cornea transplant, bilateral eyes

Family history of COPD, severe: Father
Family history of Hypertension: Brother
Family history of Lymphoma: Mother
Patient is retired, married, enjoys volunteer work.

MEDICATION LIST:

1. Omeprazole 40 mg Oral capsule delayed release. Take one capsule by mouth every day.
2. Aspirin, 81 mg tabs. Take one tablet daily.
3. Atorvastatin Calcium 20 mg oral tablet. Take one tablet by mouth at bedtime.
4. Vitamin D 2000-unit oral capsule. Take one capsule daily.

PHYSICAL EXAMINATION:
Constitutional: in no acute distress, alert.
Skin: no rash, skin was normal—dry and warm, normal skin turgor. *3-mm papule that is rough on the left foot. The right temple has some vascular engorgement but no scaling. The left temple has reddened areas similar to actinic keratosis.*

PROCEDURE:
Destruction of lesions by cryosurgery. Benefits and alternatives were discussed with the patient. Consent was obtained prior to the procedure.
Procedure note: Six actinic keratoses are treated with cryosurgery. One common wart is treated with cryosurgery. There were no complications. The patient tolerated the procedure well.

ASSESSMENT:

1. Encounter for preventive health examination. Discussed preventive care. He is up to date, but advanced directives were advised.
2. Abdominal aortic aneurysm (AAA) without rupture: 3.1 cm on US 01/20XX. Will monitor.
3. Benign essential hypertension. Improved with diet and exercise. Encourage more of the same. Monitor.
4. Mixed hyperlipidemia. Compensated with Atorvastatin. Continue same.
5. Patellofemoral syndrome of right knee. Illustrated knee exercises to increase range of motion (ROM) and decrease pain. If this does not help, I will refer to physical therapy.
6. Common wart, left foot. *Treated with cryotherapy today. May return if a second application is needed.*
7. Overweight (BMI 25.0–29.9). Goals are set, and he is advised weight loss will help his hypertension.
8. Actinic keratosis. *Six lesions are treated with cryotherapy today. May return if a second application is needed.*

PLAN:
Orders: 1. Colonoscopy, status—active

You have set the following goals: 1. Exercise 20 minutes per day; 2. Not eating after 6 p.m.
Advised patient to create durable power of attorney and living will.

SIGNED: Dr. Ivan Foote, MD

Use the following steps to identify the procedure(s) and diagnoses from the case study. Note that the medical record provided is the same documentation from the case study presented in chapter 2 of this workbook. *However, additional documentation has been added in italics to the encounter documentation.* After determining the procedure(s) and diagnoses, identify the medical necessity for the procedure(s) with code linkage.

1. Read through the case study in full, paying attention to individual details throughout the documentation. After reviewing the case study, answer the following question: *What did the doctor do?* List the procedure(s) on the lines provided:

    ____

    ____

    ____

    ____

    ____

2. Next, answer the following question: *Why did the doctor do it?* List the diagnoses individually:

    ____

    ____

    ____

    ____

    ____

3. After determining the procedure(s) and all associated diagnoses, identify the medical necessity for each procedure by linking it with the diagnosis code(s). On the lines provided, list the individual procedures and diagnoses, and link them by drawing a line from each procedure to the matching diagnosis.

    Note: In this scenario, you will have to link a procedure to multiple diagnosis codes.

Procedure	**Diagnosis**
______________	______________
______________	______________
______________	______________
______________	______________
______________	______________
______________	______________
______________	______________
______________	______________

Reference

Centers for Medicare and Medicaid Services (CMS). 2021. Details for title: CMS 1500. https://www.cms.gov/Medicare/CMS-Forms/CMS-Forms/CMS-Forms-Items/CMS1188854.html.

CHAPTER 4

Learning the ICD-10-CM Code Book

Vocabulary

Instructions: Define each of the following key terms in the space provided.

1. Accidental intent: ______________________________

____

____

2. Activity: ______________________________

____

____

3. Acute condition: ______________________________

____

____

4. Adverse effect: ______________________________

____

____

5. Assault: ______________________________

____

____

6. Benign neoplasm: ____________________

____

____

7. Bilateral: ____________________

____

____

8. Billable code: ____________________

____

____

9. Carcinoma in situ: ____________________

____

____

10. Chronic condition: ____________________

____

____

11. Code first: ____________________

____

____

12. Combination code: ____________________

____

____

13. Cross-reference: ____________________

____

____

14. Definitive diagnosis: ____________________

____

____

15. Episode of care: ______________________________

____

____

16. Essential modifier: ______________________________

____

____

17. Etiology: ______________________________

____

____

18. Excludes notes: ______________________________

____

____

19. Excludes1: ______________________________

____

____

20. Excludes2: ______________________________

____

____

21. External cause codes: ______________________________

____

____

22. External Causes of Injury Index: ______________________________

____

____

23. First-listed diagnosis: ______________________________

____

____

24. Histologic type: ______________________________

____

____

25. Includes notes: ______________________________

____

____

26. Inclusion terms: ______________________________

____

____

27. Index to Diseases and Injury: ______________________________

____

____

28. Initial encounter: ______________________________

____

____

29. Injury mechanism: ______________________________

____

____

30. Intent: ______________________________

____

____

31. Intentional self-harm: ______________________________

____

____

32. Invalid code: ______________________________

____

____

33. Laterality: ____________________

____

____

34. Main term: ____________________

____

____

35. Malignant neoplasm: ____________________

____

____

36. Manifestation: ____________________

____

____

37. Metastasis: ____________________

____

____

38. Morphology: ____________________

____

____

39. Neoplasm: ____________________

____

____

40. Neoplasm of uncertain behavior: ____________________

____

____

41. Nonessential modifier: ____________________

____

____

42. Not elsewhere classifiable (NEC): ______________________________

____

____

43. Not otherwise specified (NOS): ______________________________

____

____

44. Official Guidelines for Coding and Reporting (OGCR): ______________________________

____

____

45. Patient status: ______________________________

____

____

46. Place of occurrence: ______________________________

____

____

47. Placeholder X: ______________________________

____

____

48. Primary neoplasm: ______________________________

____

____

49. Secondary neoplasm: ______________________________

____

____

50. See also: ______________________________

____

____

51. See condition: ______________________________

____

____

52. Sequela: ______________________________

____

____

53. Sequencing: ______________________________

____

____

54. Seventh character extension: ______________________________

____

____

55. Signs: ______________________________

____

____

56. Specificity: ______________________________

____

____

57. Subsequent encounter: ______________________________

____

____

58. Subterm: ______________________________

____

____

59. Symptoms: ______________________________

____

____

60. Table of Drugs and Chemicals: ______________________________

____

____

61. Table of Neoplasms: ______________________________

____

____

62. Tabular List: ______________________________

____

____

63. Toxic effect: ______________________________

____

____

64. Underdosing: ______________________________

____

____

65. Undetermined intent: ______________________________

____

____

66. Use additional code: ______________________________

____

____

Fill in the Blank

Instructions: Complete the following statements.

1. The ______________________ is the cause of a disease.

2. A ______________________ is the sign or symptom of a disease.

3. A ______________________ code is a single code that identifies both the cause and the signs and symptoms of a disease.

4. The abbreviation NEC stands for ____

____

____

and is commonly identified as the "other" option in the ICD-10-CM code book.

5. The abbreviation NOS stands for ____

____

____

and is commonly identified as the "unspecified" option in the ICD-10-CM code book.

6. The Index that lists extenuating circumstances surrounding an injury or other medical condition is called the ____

____

____

7. The Index that lists codes that identify toxic effects of chemicals, medicinals, and other substances is called the ____

____

____

8. The Index that lists the majority of medical conditions is called the ____________

____

____

9. The ____ lists codes for neoplastic conditions.

10. A(n) ______________________________ modifier in the Index is listed in parentheses and does not impact code selection.

11. A(n) ______________________________ modifier in the Index is listed as a subterm under the main term and does impact code selection.

12. The ________________________________ note in the Tabular List note is a pure Excludes note and indicates that two conditions are mutually exclusive and should not be coded together.

13. The ________________________________ note in the Tabular List identifies conditions "not coded here" and indicates that two conditions should be coded separately if both codes exist.

14. The ____________________________ notes appear directly beneath a three-character category in the Tabular List to further define and give examples of the content that is included within the category.

15. When reporting both acute and chronic conditions, sequence the code for the

____

____

condition first.

16. List the four steps for looking up a code in the Main Index.

a. ____

b. ____

c. ____

d. ____

17. When reporting external cause codes, report a code for the

____

____

(2 words), which describes the way an injury happened.

18. The ____ (3 words) is where the patient was when an injury occurred.

19. The ________________________________ is what the patient was doing when the injury occurred.

20. The ____________________________________ (2 words) identifies the patient's work context when the injury occurred.

21. The ________________________________ (2 words) is the structured list of ICD-10-CM codes, organized alphanumerically.

Matching

Instructions: Match the terms with the appropriate descriptions.

1. _______	Index to Diseases and Injury	**A.** Noncancerous growth of tissue
2. _______	Carcinoma in situ	**B.** Deliberately acting to injure one's self

3. ________ Benign neoplasm

4. ________ Subterm

5. ________ Secondary neoplasm

6. ________ Main term

7. ________ Intentional self-harm

8. ________ Assault

9. ________ *See also*

10. ________ Underdosing

11. ________ Malignant neoplasm

12. ________ Primary neoplasm

13. ________ Accidental intent

14. ________ Adverse effect

C. The noun that describes the patient's diagnosis or reason for encounter

D. Also referred to as a metastasis, this is the site to which a neoplasm has spread

E. Indented under the main term in the Index, gives variations of the main term

F. Unintentional effect as a result of an accident or unintentional overdose

G. The main index to the ICD-10-CM code book

H. This cross-reference instructs the coder to look elsewhere for a code

I. Growth of tissue that can invade other tissues and destroy them

J. The original neoplastic growth

K. Unintended effect of a medical substance that has been correctly prescribed and correctly taken

L. Neoplastic growth that is potentially cancerous, currently not invasive

M. An act of harm purposefully inflicted upon another person

N. Occurs when a patient takes too little of a prescribed medication

Coding

Instructions: Main Term: Using the ICD-10-CM code book, identify the main terms for the following diagnostic statements.

1. Senile cataract

Main term: ____

2. Late-onset Alzheimer's Disease

Main term: ____

3. Bladder hypotonicity

Main term: ____

4. Back strain

Main term: ____

5. Third-degree burn of left thigh

Main term: ____

Instructions: Essential versus nonessential modifiers: Look up the following terms in the Main Index and identify if the modifier listed is either essential or nonessential.

	Main term	**Modifier**	**Essential or nonessential**
6.	Xanthelasma	Eyelid	*essential*
7.	Contusion	Arm	*essential*
8.	Hyperthyroid	Recurrent	*nonessential*
9.	Hyperthyroidism	with goiter	*essential*
10.	Hyperthyroidism with goiter	Diffuse	*nonessential*

Instructions: Read the following diagnostic statements and then identify the primary or first-listed diagnosis. Then report the code for the diagnosis.

11. Patient with a long history of shortness of breath and wheezing is diagnosed with moderate persistent asthma.

a. Primary diagnosis: ____

b. ICD-10-CM code: ____

12. 34-year-old female presents to the clinic complaining of severe upper right quadrant abdominal pain that is determined to be due to acute cholecystitis.

a. Primary diagnosis: ____

b. ICD-10-CM code: ____

13. Patient with sore throat and fever tests negative for streptococcal tonsillitis.

a. Primary diagnosis: ____

b. ICD-10-CM code: ____

14. 78-year-old female suffering from confusion presents to the office. Clinician suspects transient ischemic attack.

a. Primary diagnosis: ____

b. ICD-10-CM code: ____

Instructions: Report the ICD-10-CM diagnosis code(s) from the following diagnostic statements. Pay attention to sequencing conventions and instructions in the Tabular List to ensure that multiple codes are sequenced correctly.

15. Acute and chronic pancreatitis

ICD-10-CM code(s): ______________________, ______________________

16. Orthostatic headache

ICD-10-CM code(s): ______________________

17. Loefflerella mallei infection

ICD-10-CM code(s): ______________________

18. Laceration of the right index finger due to an accident in which patient was cut with a kitchen knife as he was preparing dinner in the kitchen of a single-family home while working as a personal chef, initial encounter

ICD-10-CM code(s) for laceration: ______________________

ICD-10-CM code(s) for the injury mechanism: ______________________

ICD-10-CM code(s) for the patient activity: ______________________

ICD-10-CM code(s) for the place of occurrence: ______________________

ICD-10-CM code(s) for the patient status: ______________________

19. Alligator skin disease

ICD-10-CM code(s): ______________________

20. Congenital aplastic anemia (Hint: This is an NEC code.)

ICD-10-CM code(s): ______________________

21. Black lung disease

ICD-10-CM code(s): ______________________

22. Sleep disorder due to sedative abuse

ICD-10-CM code(s): ______________________

23. Patient with primary malignant neoplasm of the prostate presents for treatment of neoplasm-related anemia

ICD-10-CM code(s): ______________________, ______________________

24. Patient with melanoma of the skin of the back is diagnosed with metastases to the left lung and brain

ICD-10-CM code(s) for the primary neoplasm: ______________________

ICD-10-CM code(s) for the secondary neoplasms: ______________________,

____

25. Head lice

ICD-10-CM code(s): ______________________

26. Meningitis due to Hemophilus influenza

ICD-10-CM code(s): ______________________

27. Patient presents to the clinic complaining of chest pain upon breathing after breathing in rubbing alcohol fumes, initial encounter. (Hint: Code for the manifestation of the toxic effect as well as the toxic effect code; look to the beginning of the section for sequencing instructions.)

ICD-10-CM code(s): ______________________, ______________________

28. Anaphylaxis due to adverse effect of nonsteroidal anti-inflammatory drug (NSAID)

ICD-10-CM code(s): ______________________, ______________________

29. Subsequent encounter for underdosing of antithrombotic drug

ICD-10-CM code(s): ______________________

30. Pain in right wrist

ICD-10-CM code(s): ______________________

31. Patient presents with intestinal obstruction in Crohn's disease of both small and large intestines

ICD-10-CM code(s): ______________________

32. Acute and chronic prostatitis

ICD-10-CM code(s): ______________________, ______________________

33. Hepatic ascites and chronic active hepatitis due to toxic liver disease

ICD-10-CM code(s): ______________________

34. Unstable angina co-occurrent and due to coronary arteriosclerosis

ICD-10-CM code(s): ______________________

35. Acute and chronic tonsillitis

ICD-10-CM code(s): ______________________, ______________________

36. Anemia in stage 4 chronic kidney disease

ICD-10-CM code(s): ______________________, ______________________

37. Postprocedural (postpancreatectomy) diabetes mellitus, uncomplicated. Patient is on long-term use of insulin.

ICD-10-CM code(s): ______________________, ______________________

38. Otitis externa due to impetigo, bilateral ears

ICD-10-CM code(s): ______________________, ______________________

39. Abscess of lung in *S. pneumoniae* pneumonia

ICD-10-CM code(s): ______________________, ______________________

40. Patient presents with classic hemophilia manifesting in hemophilic arthropathy

ICD-10-CM code(s): ______________________, ______________________

Instructions: In each of the following questions, compare the documentation and the code selected. Then identify the component of the diagnosis code missing from the documentation and rewrite the documentation to match the code description.

41. 15-year-old patient presents for a follow-up on her bronchitis. She is feeling better, is less short of breath, and the medications prescribed by the doctor have been helping.

Diagnosis code reported: **J41.0**

Rewrite the documentation to include the detail required in order to support the code reported.

____

____

____

42. Patient is seen for a fracture of the right humerus. Fracture was manipulated and immobilized.

Diagnosis code reported: **S42.331A**

Rewrite the documentation to include the detail required in order to support the code reported.

____

____

____

43. 62-year-old male presents with superficial foreign body in his finger.

Diagnosis code reported: **S60.451A**

Rewrite the documentation to include the detail required in order to support the code reported.

___

___

___

44. 2-year-old female presents for treatment for purulent otitis media.

Diagnosis code selected: **H66.004**

Rewrite the documentation to include the detail required in order to support the code reported.

___

___

___

Instructions: For each of the following questions, read through the diagnostic statement and then note that the ICD-10-CM code is missing one or more characters. Complete the ICD-10-CM code by identifying the missing character(s) and adding it/them in the correct location in the ICD-10-CM code, according to details given in the diagnostic statement.

45. Diagnostic statement: Atherosclerosis of bypass graft of coronary artery of transplanted heart with unstable angina.

Incomplete ICD-10-CM code: I25.7__0

Complete ICD-10-CM code: ___

46. Diagnostic statement: Pathological fracture in neoplastic disease of the right tibia, subsequent encounter for fracture with nonunion.

Incomplete ICD-10-CM code: M84.561____

Complete ICD-10-CM code: ___

47. Diagnostic statement: Laceration of the popliteal vein of the left leg, initial encounter.

Incomplete ICD-10-CM code: S____5.51____A

Complete ICD-10-CM code: ___

48. Diagnostic statement: Sequela of perforation due to foreign body accidentally left in body following removal of catheter.

Incomplete ICD-10-CM code: T81.53____ ____

Complete ICD-10-CM code: ________________________

49. Diagnostic statement: Mechanical ectropion of right upper eyelid.

Incomplete ICD-10-CM code: H02.___21

Complete ICD-10-CM code: ________________________

Case Studies Assigning ICD-10-CM Codes

Case Study 4.1

PATIENT: Pyotr Skopolov

DATE OF SERVICE: 05/01/20XX

REASON FOR VISIT: Wellness exam

HISTORY OF PRESENT ILLNESS:
Patient presents today for his wellness exam. He has been trying to eat better but has not been exercising regularly. He has a skin spot to look at. One bump on his foot and several small spots on his face.

Time up and go (TUG) test: normal (30 seconds or less)
Hearing test: right ear heard finger rub. Left ear heard finger rub.

Activities of daily living (ADLs): The patient does not need assistance with dressing, does not need assistance with feeding, does not need assistance with toileting, does not need assistance with personal hygiene, does not need assistance managing medications, does not need assistance managing money, and does not need assistance with transportation.

Documented and discussed: Patient provided with advanced care directive and medical directive power of attorney. Copy of advance care directive included in patient's electronic chart.

PHQ9: Over the past two weeks, how often have you been bothered by the following problems?

1. Little interest or pleasure in doing things? Not at all
2. Feeling down, depressed, or hopeless? Not at all

3. Trouble falling asleep or sleeping too much? Not at all
4. Feeling tired or having little energy? Not at all
5. Poor appetite or overeating? Not at all
6. Feeling bad about yourself, or that you are a failure, or have let your family down? Not at all
7. Trouble concentrating on things, such as reading a newspaper or watching television? Not at all
8. Moving or speaking so slowly that other people could have noticed, or the opposite, moving or speaking faster than usual? Not at all
9. Thoughts that you would be better off dead or hurting yourself in some way? Not at all

TOTAL SCORE: 0

There are no concerns regarding the patient's cognitive functions.

REVIEW OF SYSTEMS:
Complete review of systems, all within normal limits

PAST, FAMILY, SOCIAL HISTORY:
Allergies: No known drug allergies (NKDA)
History of: Cataract surgery, cornea transplant, bilateral eyes
Family history of COPD, severe: Father
Family history of Hypertension: Brother
Family history of Lymphoma: Mother
Patient is retired, married, enjoys volunteer work.

MEDICATION LIST:

1. Omeprazole 40 mg oral capsule delayed release; take one capsule by mouth every day.
2. Aspirin, 81 mg tabs. Take one tablet daily.
3. Atorvastatin Calcium 20 mg oral tablet. Take one tablet by mouth at bedtime.
4. Vitamin D 2000-unit oral capsule. Take one capsule daily.

PHYSICAL EXAMINATION:
Constitutional: in no acute distress, alert.
Skin: No rash, skin was normal—dry and warm, normal skin turgor. 3-mm papule that is rough on the left foot. The right temple has some vascular engorgement but no scaling. The left temple has reddened areas similar to actinic keratosis.

PROCEDURE:
Destruction of lesions by cryosurgery. Benefits and alternatives were discussed with the patient. Consent was obtained prior to the procedure.
Procedure note: Six actinic keratoses are treated with cryosurgery. One common wart is treated with cryosurgery. There were no complications. The patient tolerated the procedure well.

ASSESSMENT:

1. Encounter for preventive health examination. Discussed preventive care. He is up to date, but advanced directives were advised.
2. Abdominal aortic aneurysm (AAA) without rupture: 3.1 cm on US 01/20XX. Will monitor.
3. Benign essential hypertension. Improved with diet and exercise. Encourage more of the same. Monitor.
4. Mixed hyperlipidemia. Compensated with Atorvastatin. Continue same.
5. Patellofemoral syndrome of right knee. Illustrated knee exercises to increase range of motion (ROM) and decrease pain. If this does not help, I will refer to physical therapy.
6. Common wart, left foot. Treated with cryotherapy today. May return if a second application is needed.
7. Overweight (BMI 25.0–29.9). Goals are set, and he is advised weight loss will help his hypertension.
8. Actinic keratosis. Six lesions are treated with cryotherapy today. May return if a second application is needed.

PLAN:
Orders: 1. Colonoscopy, status—active

You have set the following goals: 1. Exercise 20 minutes per day; 2. Not eating after 6 p.m. Advised patient to create durable power of attorney and living will.

SIGNED: Dr. Ivan Foote, MD

Use the following steps to select the appropriate diagnosis codes for the case study. Note that the medical record provided is the same documentation from the case study presented in chapters 2 and 3 of this workbook. However, in this exercise you will need to identify and assign the ICD-10-CM diagnosis codes for the encounter:

1. Read through the case study in full. Use a medical dictionary or medical terminology textbook to define the following terms:
   a. *Actinic keratosis*:

   ____

   ____

   b. *Patellofemoral syndrome*:

   ____

   ____

2. Review the case study and answer the following question: *Why did the doctor do it?* Identify the patient's diagnoses and list them on the lines provided.

   Note: For this case study, you do not need to abstract the procedure (*what did the doctor do?*).

   ____

   ____

   ____

   ____

3. Now that the patient's diagnoses have been identified, use the following steps to locate the correct code(s) for each condition in the ICD-10-CM code book. Then list the ICD-10-CM codes on the lines provided.
   a. Search the Main Index for the name of the condition.
   b. Search through any applicable subterms and cross-references to locate the appropriate code for each diagnosis.
   c. Refer to the case study in chapter 4 of your textbook for steps to locate, assign, and sequence multiple diagnosis codes.

   ICD-10-CM code(s): ________, ________, ________,
   ________, ________, ________, ________,
   ____

Case Study 4.2

PATIENT: Skye McDougall

CHIEF COMPLAINT: Random vomiting × 5 days. Small amount of congestion but no other symptoms.

HISTORY OF PRESENT ILLNESS:
Here for an initial evaluation of vomiting for the last 5 days. Vomiting small amounts. Started Saturday on the way to a ski trip. Vomited first on the chair lift. Ate saltines and Gatorade on Tuesday and vomited. She was fine the next day but then threw up again this morning. Sister is at home with fever and cold. She is a picky eater but diet has been normal in the past few days.

REVIEW OF SYSTEMS:
No fever, sleeping well, no sore throat, no diarrhea, nasal congestion, decreased appetite

PAST, FAMILY, SOCIAL HISTORY:
Allergies: No known drug allergies (NKDA)

PHYSICAL EXAMINATION:
Constitutional: general appearance: active, alert, healthy appearing, in no acute distress, well developed, well nourished, and well hydrated.

Abdomen: normal bowel sounds, soft, nontender, no hepatosplenomegaly, and no abdominal mass palpated.
Pulmonary: no respiratory distress, normal respiratory rhythm and effort, and clear bilateral breath sounds.

ASSESSMENT:

1. Gastroesophageal reflux

PLAN:

1. Start Zantac 75 MG oral tablet. Take one every day.

SIGNED: Dr. Susan Alameda, DO

Use the following steps to select the appropriate diagnosis codes for the case study.

1. Read through the case study in full. Use a medical dictionary or medical terminology textbook to define the following terms:
   a. *Hepatosplenomegaly*:

   ____

   ____

   b. *Gastroesophageal reflux*:

   ____

   ____

2. Review the case study and answer the following question: *Why did the doctor do it?* Identify the patient's diagnoses and list them on the lines provided.

   Note: For this case study, you do not need to abstract the procedure (*what did the doctor do?*).

   ____

   ____

   ____

   ____

3. Now that the patient's diagnoses have been identified, use the following steps to locate the correct code(s) for each condition in the ICD-10-CM code book. Then list the ICD-10-CM codes on the lines provided.
   a. Search the Main Index for the name of the condition.
   b. Search through any applicable subterms and cross-references to locate the appropriate code for each diagnosis.
   c. Refer to the case study in chapter 4 of your textbook for steps to locate, assign, and sequence multiple diagnosis codes.

   ICD-10-CM code(s): ______________

Case Study 4.3

PATIENT: Dutch Johnson

CHIEF COMPLAINT: 60-year-old male presents today to establish new patient care and for medication review.

HISTORY OF PRESENT ILLNESS:
Patient is being seen for benign prostatic hyperplasia. No lower urinary tract symptoms other than nocturia. He reports drinking caffeine and large amounts of fluid in the evening time and before bed. Patient is being seen for an initial evaluation of preexisting diagnosis of hypertension with exacerbating factor of weight gain. He has not been on medication for the last two years. BPs are mostly in the 120s.
Patient is being seen for an initial evaluation of hyperlipidemia. He is not currently being treated for this problem. Past evaluation included total cholesterol and past treatment has included statins but is not currently on any medication for this condition.

REVIEW OF SYSTEMS:
Constitutional: not feeling poorly, no malaise
Genitourinary: no sensation of incomplete bladder emptying, no urinary frequency, no intermittency, no weak stream, no straining, no incontinence, no post-void dribbling, no suprapubic pain
Cardiovascular: no chest pain, no calf cramps with physical activity, no myalgias

PAST, FAMILY, SOCIAL HISTORY:
Allergies: Codeine

PHYSICAL EXAMINATION:
Constitutional: obese but is well developed, is healthy appearing, alert and in no acute distress.
Cardiovascular: peripheral edema, but heart rate and rhythm are normal, no murmurs heard, normal S1 and S2 and carotid pulses normal with no bruits. Trace nonpitting edema of the BLE with varicose veins.
Pulmonary: normal respiratory rhythm and effort, normal breath sounds, no accessory muscle use and auscultation clear with no wheezes, rhonchi, or rales.
Lymphatics: the lymph nodes were not tender, nonpalpable posterior cervical and nonpalpable anterior cervical nodes.
Skin: normal skin color and pigmentation, no ecchymosis, and no rash. Mid xerosis of the legs.

ASSESSMENT:

1. Hyperlipidemia
2. Hypertension
3. Benign prostatic hyperplasia with LUTS

PLAN:

1. Hyperlipidemia and hypertension uncontrolled, has been off medications greater than 1 year. Will restart ACE and BB and statin, respectively. EKG in office was normal. Ordered baseline labs today.

SIGNED: Dr. Susan Alameda, DO

Use the following steps to select the appropriate diagnosis codes for the case study.

1. Read through the case study in full. Use a medical dictionary or medical terminology textbook to define the following terms:

a. *Nocturia*:

____

____

b. *Peripheral edema*:

____

____

2. Review the case study and answer the following question: *Why did the doctor do it?* Identify the patient's diagnoses and list them on the lines provided.
Note: For this case study, you do not need to abstract the procedure (*what did the doctor do?*).

____

____

____

____

3. Now that the patient's diagnoses have been identified, use the following steps to locate the correct code(s) for each condition in the ICD-10-CM code book. Then list the ICD-10-CM codes on the lines provided.

a. Search the Main Index for the name of the condition.

b. Search through any applicable subterms and cross-references to locate the appropriate code for each diagnosis.

c. Refer to the case study in chapter 4 of your textbook for steps to locate, assign, and sequence multiple diagnosis codes.

ICD-10-CM code(s): ______________, ______________, ______________,
____

Case Study 4.4

PATIENT: Jackson Stewart

CHIEF COMPLAINT: Presents for removal of sutures

HISTORY OF PRESENT ILLNESS:
50-year-old male presents to have nine sutures removed from his right upper and mid-back. Sutures were placed after removal of seborrheic keratoses seven days ago. States that he feels like the sutures went really well. No pain or discomfort.

PROCEDURE:
Suture removal: the wound was located on the left back
Wound exam: well-healed with no signs of infection
Procedure note: nine sutures were removed
Complications: There were no complications

ASSESSMENT:

1. Seborrheic keratoses, left back

PLAN:

1. Patient was advised of pathology results.

SIGNED: Dr. Susan Alameda, DO

Use the following steps to select the appropriate diagnosis codes for the case study.

1. Read through the case study in full. Use a medical dictionary or medical terminology textbook to define the following term:

a. *Seborrheic keratosis*:

____

____

2. Review the case study and answer the following question: *Why did the doctor do it?* Identify the patient's diagnoses and list them on the lines provided.
Note: For this case study, you do not need to abstract the procedure (*what did the doctor do?*).

____

____

____

____

3. Now that the patient's diagnoses have been identified, use the following steps to locate the correct code(s) for each condition in the ICD-10-CM code book. Then list the ICD-10-CM codes on the lines provided.

a. Search the Main Index for the name of the condition.

b. Search through any applicable subterms and cross-references to locate the appropriate code for each diagnosis.

c. Refer to the case study in chapter 4 of your textbook for steps to locate, assign, and sequence multiple diagnosis codes.

ICD-10-CM code(s): ______________

Case Study 4.5

PATIENT: Evangeline Swenson

CHIEF COMPLAINT: 90-year-old female presents with adult daughter to discuss left wrist pain and swelling.

HISTORY OF PRESENT ILLNESS:
90-year-old widowed female, lives with her daughter. Here to follow up on multiple issues.
Wrist pain: saw an urgent care provider last week for this and x-ray was completed with no fracture found. Positive for soft-tissue swelling.
Edema: daughter states that she would like to discuss lower-leg swelling. Patient does have venous insufficiencies with some varicosities, mostly superficial.
Elevated blood pressure: elevated in clinic today. They do not check pressures at home. Daughter states that she is very dizzy most of the time.
Chronic kidney disease, stage 3 (CKD III): creatinine 0.93, eGFR 54 on 10/2018 labs. Avoids NSAIDS.

REVIEW OF SYSTEMS:
Cardiovascular: denies chest pain, SOB, or CVA symptoms

PHYSICAL EXAMINATION:
Constitutional: No fever, no chills, no malaise, and no fatigue
Cardiovascular: heart rate and rhythm were normal, normal S1 and S2, no gallops, no murmurs, no pericardial rub, and the apical impulse was normal. No peripheral edema, carotid pulses were normal with no bruits, the abdominal aorta was normal, and the pedal pulses were full. She has venous insufficiency with stasis changes around her ankles with hemosiderin deposit.
Pulmonary: normal respiratory distress, normal respiratory rhythm, and effort with clear bilateral breath sounds.
Musculoskeletal: Abnormal gait seen. Patient noted to have limitations in mobility including the use of a cane.

ASSESSMENT:

1. Wrist pain. Improved, discussed wrist x-ray with patient.
2. Elevated blood pressure. Labile, and with severe neck issue, do not want her to risk her blood pressure getting too low and causing possible falls. Patient's daughter agrees with this plan. Recommend getting a tape on seated exercises, three times a week.
3. Stage 3 CKD. Stable, see plan on elevated blood pressure, avoid NSAIDs. Will monitor with labs.
4. Venous stasis. Discussed with daughter. Bad veins and not edema. No real therapy needed at this stage. Will watch over time. I will see her back in 3 months.

PLAN:

1. Follow-up visit in three months
2. Do not take additional NSAIDs such as naproxen, ibuprofen, Aleve, or Motrin

SIGNED: Dr. Susan Alameda, DO

Use the following steps to select the appropriate diagnosis codes for the case study.

1. Read through the case study in full. Use a medical dictionary or medical terminology textbook to define the following terms:

a. *NSAID*:

____

____

b. *Varicosity*:

____

____

2. Review the case study and answer the following question: *Why did the doctor do it?* Identify the patient's diagnoses and list them on the lines provided.
Note: For this case study, you do not need to abstract the procedure (*what did the doctor do?*).

____

____

____

____

3. Now that the patient's diagnoses have been identified, use the following steps to locate the correct code(s) for each condition in the ICD-10-CM code book. Then list the ICD-10-CM codes on the lines provided.

a. Search the Main Index for the name of the condition.

b. Search through any applicable subterms and cross-references to locate the appropriate code for each diagnosis.

c. Refer to the case study in chapter 4 of your textbook for steps to locate, assign, and sequence multiple diagnosis codes

ICD-10-CM code(s): ____________, ____________, ____________, ____________

CHAPTER 5

Learning the CPT and HCPCS Code Books

Vocabulary

Instructions: Define each of the following key terms in the space provided.

1. Add-on code: ____________________

____

____

2. Anesthesia section: ____________________

____

____

3. Category I code: ____________________

____

____

4. Category II code: ____________________

____

____

5. Category III code: ____________________

____

____

6. Eponym: ____

____

____

7. Evaluation and Management Services section: ____

____

____

8. Indented code: ____

____

____

9. Medicine section: ____

____

____

10. Modifying term: ____

____

____

11. Parenthetical note: ____

____

____

12. Pathology and Laboratory section: ____

____

____

13. Radiology section: ____

____

____

14. Resequenced code: ____

____

____

15. Separate procedure: ______________________________

____

____

16. Special report: ______________________________

____

____

17. Standalone code: ______________________________

____

____

18. Surgery section: ______________________________

____

____

19. Synonym: ______________________________

____

____

20. Table of Drugs: ______________________________

____

____

21. Telemedicine service: ______________________________

____

____

22. Unlisted procedure codes: ______________________________

____

____

Fill in the Blank

Instructions: Complete the following statements.

1. Evaluation and management codes are found in the code range(s) ______________________.

2. Radiology codes are found in the code range(s) ______________________.

3. Medicine codes are found in the code range(s) ______________________.

4. Codes within the 33010 to 37799 range are found in the ______________________ subsection of the CPT code book.

5. Codes within the 50010 to 53899 range are found in the ______________________ subsection of the CPT code book.

6. Female genital subsection codes in the CPT manual begin with code ________________ and end with code ________________.

7. Nervous system subsection codes in the CPT manual begin with code ________________ and end with code ________________.

Complete the following figure by labeling the CPT headings.

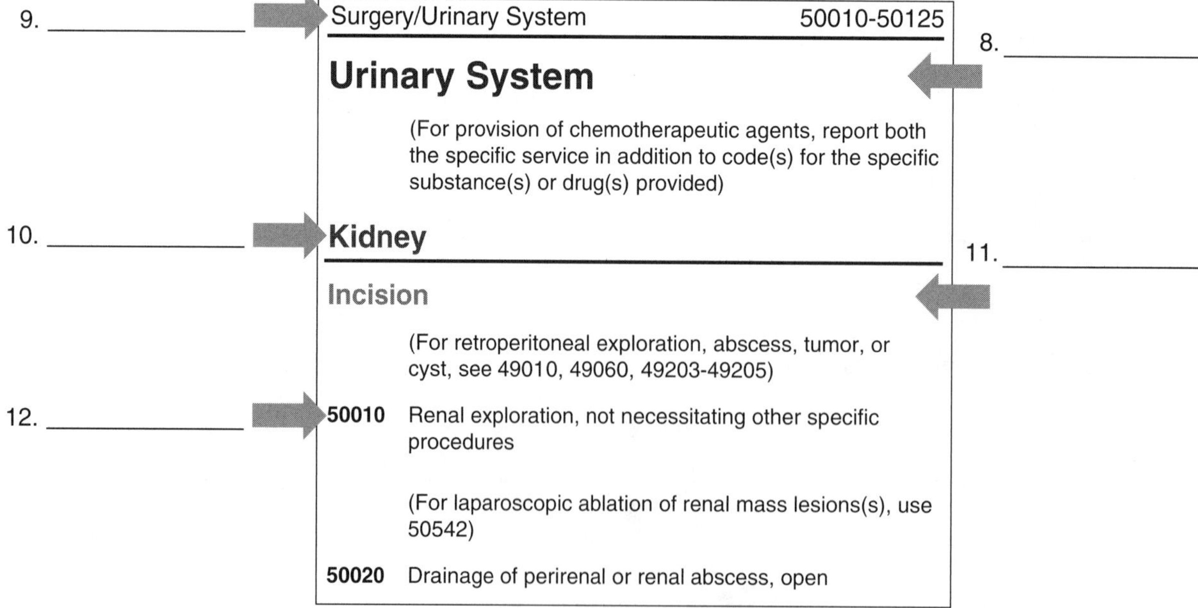

9. ____________
8. ____________
10. ____________
11. ____________
12. ____________
Surgery/Urinary System 50010-50125
Urinary System
(For provision of chemotherapeutic agents, report both the specific service in addition to code(s) for the specific substance(s) or drug(s) provided)
Kidney
Incision
(For retroperitoneal exploration, abscess, tumor, or cyst, see 49010, 49060, 49203-49205)
50010 Renal exploration, not necessitating other specific procedures
(For laparoscopic ablation of renal mass lesions(s), use 50542)
50020 Drainage of perirenal or renal abscess, open

Source: AMA 2019, 361.

Matching

Instructions: Match the terms with the appropriate descriptions.

1. ________ Category I codes	**A.** Reports a service in which the provider evaluates and then treats a patient's healthcare needs
2. ________ Category II codes	**B.** Two digits that alter the meaning of a code, appended to the end of a CPT/HCPCS code
3. ________ Category III codes	**C.** Set of temporary codes used to report new and emerging technologies
4. ________ Evaluation and Management codes	**D.** Make up the largest section of codes in the CPT book, describe invasive and noninvasive procedures
5. ________ Anesthesia codes	**E.** Identify procedures that use radiant energy to diagnose and treat medical conditions
6. ________ Surgery codes	**F.** Supplemental tracking codes that may be used for performance measurement
7. ________ Radiology codes	**G.** Identify services provided to reduce pain or alleviate sensation
8. ________ Pathology and Laboratory codes	**H.** Miscellaneous grouping of codes that represent a vast array of minimally and noninvasive services
9. ________ Medicine codes	**I.** Divided into subsections, organized by body area or organ system, and describe invasive procedures
10. ________ Modifiers	**J.** Represent diagnostic tests on human specimens

Instructions: Match the code type with the correct code.

11. _______ HCPCS **K.** 2060F

12. _______ ICD-10-CM **L.** 0NTV0ZZ

13. _______ ICD-10-PCS **M.** K0890

14. _______ CPT **N.** M86.479

15. _______ Category II CPT **O.** 59610

16. _______ Category III CPT **P.** 0209T

Multiple Choice

Instructions: Choose the best answer

1. Code 60520 is an example of which of the following?
a. CPT
b. ICD-10-CM
c. Category II
d. HCPCS

2. Code 60520 is an example of which of the following?
a. Category III
b. Category I
c. Category II
d. Performance measurement

3. Code 0085T is an example of which of the following?
a. Category II
b. Performance measurement
c. New technology
d. Category I

4. Code A4760 is an example of which of the following?
a. CPT
b. New technology
c. HCPCS
d. Category II

5. Code 00932 is an example of which of the following?
a. Category II
b. HCPCS
c. Evaluation and management
d. Anesthesia

6. Code 29750 is an example of which of the following?
a. Category II
b. Surgery
c. Evaluation and management
d. Medicine

7. Code 1066F is an example of which of the following?
a. Category II
b. New technology
c. Evaluation and management
d. HCPCS

8. Code E0130 is an example of which of the following?
a. Category III
b. Durable medical equipment
c. Radiology
d. Drugs administered in the medical setting

9. Code J9173 is an example of which of the following?
a. Durable medical equipment
b. CPT
c. Drugs administered in the medical setting
d. New technology

10. Code 99201 is an example of which of the following?
a. Performance measurement
b. New technology
c. Evaluation and management
d. Anesthesia

Coding

Instructions: Report the CPT or HCPCS code(s) from the following statements.

1. Evisceration of ocular contents of the left eye, without subsequent implantation of prosthetic eye

CPT code(s): ____________

2. Ventriculocisternostomy of the third ventricle

CPT code(s): ____________

3. Total thymectomy via transcervical approach

CPT code(s): ____________

4. Computed tomography of the brain without contrast

CPT code(s): ____________

5. Fluorescein angioscopy with interpretation and report
CPT code(s): ____________

6. Tobacco use assessed performed as part of preventive care performance measurement
CPT code(s): ____________

7. Automated speech audiometry threshold
CPT code(s): ____________

8. Needle biopsy of salivary gland
CPT code(s): ____________

9. Abrasion of 5 keratotic lesions
CPT code(s): ____________, ____________

10. Proetz therapy of the nose
CPT code(s): ____________

11. Level 3 molecular pathology procedure
CPT code(s): ____________

12. Unlisted procedure of urinary system
CPT code(s): ____________

13. Excision of bulbourethral gland
CPT code(s): ____________

14. Prophylactic pinning of clavicle
CPT code(s): ____________

15. Male to female intersex surgery
CPT code(s): ____________

16. 3 patch allergy tests
CPT code(s): ____________ × _____

17. SPECT brain imaging
CPT code(s): ____________

18. Floating kyphosis pad
HCPCS code(s): ____________

19. Alcohol misuse screening

HCPCS code(s): ____________

20. Tracheostomy tube collar

HCPCS code(s): ____________

21. 1 mg Clolar (Hint: This is a medication administered in the healthcare setting.)

HCPCS code(s): ____________

22. Amygdalin

HCPCS code(s): ____________

23. Injection of 20 units of taliglucerase alfa

HCPCS code(s): ____________ × _____

24. Wig

HCPCS code(s): ____________

25. Heat lamp with stand and infrared element

HCPCS code(s): ____________

26. Barium enema colorectal cancer screening

HCPCS code(s): ____________

27. 5 units of irradiated platelets

HCPCS code(s): ____________ × ____

Case Studies Procedures

Case Study 5.1

PATIENT: Phoenix Goldsmith

INDICATIONS: Nursemaid's elbow, right

PROCEDURE NOTE:
Patient suffered dislocation of right elbow on the playground today, approximately 2.5 hours ago. Presents with moderate pain and discomfort.
Reduction of nursemaid's elbow in this pediatric patient performed manually without incident. Patient tolerated the procedure well.

COMPLICATIONS: None, patient tolerated the procedure well

SIGNED: Dr. Susan Alameda, DO

Use the following steps to select the appropriate diagnosis and procedure codes for the case study.

1. Read through the case study in full. Use a medical dictionary or medical terminology textbook to define the following term:

   Nursemaid's elbow:

   ____

   ____

2. To identify the patient's diagnosis, answer the following question: *Why did the doctor do it?* List the diagnosis on the lines provided. Note that there may be multiple diagnoses.

   ____

   ____

3. Now that the patient's diagnosis has been identified, list the corresponding ICD-10-CM code(s):

   ICD-10-CM code(s): ________________

4. To identify the procedure(s), answer the following question: *What did the doctor do?* List the procedure(s) on the lines provided:

   ____

   ____

5. Now that you have the name of the procedure(s), locate the code(s) for each procedure in the CPT code book. List the CPT/HCPCS code(s) and any applicable modifiers:

   CPT code(s): ________________ - _____

6. List the procedure and diagnosis codes on the CMS-1500 form. Be sure to correctly link the procedure and diagnosis codes. Refer to figure 3.6 for an example.

21. DIAGNOSIS OR NATURE OF ILLNESS OR INJURY Relate A-L to service line below (24E) ICD Ind.

A.	B.	C.	D.
E.	F.	G.	H.
I.	J.	K.	L.

24. A. DATE(S) OF SERVICE From MM DD YY	To MM DD YY	B. PLACE OF SERVICE	C. EMG	D. PROCEDURES, SERVICES, OR SUPPLIES (Explain Unusual Circumstances) CPT/HCPCS	MODIFIER	E. DIAGNOSIS POINTER

Case Study 5.2

PATIENT: Elizabeth Negroni

PREOPERATIVE DIAGNOSIS: Foreign body (FB) right nostril

POSTOPERATIVE DIAGNOSIS: FB right nostril

ANESTHESIA: General inhalant

PROCEDURE NOTE:
3-year-old patient requiring general anesthesia was prepped and draped, and the right nostril was examined. FB appeared to be sponge of some sort, with noted degeneration indicating that FB had been in nasal passage for some time. FB was noted and was retrieved using forceps. Saline irrigation used to ensure all particles of the FB had been successfully removed. Patient tolerated the procedure well and was returned to the postanesthesia care unit in stable condition.

COMPLICATIONS: None, patient tolerated the procedure well

SIGNED: Dr. Susan Alameda, DO

Use the following steps to select the appropriate diagnosis and procedure codes for the case study.

1. To identify the patient's diagnosis, answer the following question: *Why did the doctor do it?* List the diagnosis on the lines provided. Note that there may be multiple diagnoses.

   ____

   ____

2. Now that the patient's diagnosis has been identified, list the corresponding ICD-10-CM code(s):
   ICD-10-CM code(s): ______________

3. To identify the procedure(s), answer the following question: *What did the doctor do?* List the procedure(s) on the lines provided:

   ____

   ____

4. Now that you have the name of the procedure(s), locate the code(s) for each procedure in the CPT code book. List the CPT/HCPCS code(s) and any applicable modifiers:
   CPT code(s): ______________ - _____

5. List the procedure and diagnosis codes on the CMS-1500 form. Be sure to correctly link the procedure and diagnosis codes. Refer to figure 3.6 for an example.

21. DIAGNOSIS OR NATURE OF ILLNESS OR INJURY Relate A-L to service line below (24E) ICD Ind.

A.	B.	C.	D.
E.	F.	G.	H.
I.	J.	K.	L.

24. A. DATE(S) OF SERVICE From MM DD YY	To MM DD YY	B. PLACE OF SERVICE	C. EMG	D. PROCEDURES, SERVICES, OR SUPPLIES (Explain Unusual Circumstances) CPT/HCPCS	MODIFIER	E. DIAGNOSIS POINTER

Case Study 5.3

PATIENT: Larry Moore

CHIEF COMPLAINT: Patient presents for mole biopsy.

HISTORY OF PRESENT ILLNESS: Patient with history of cytologic atypia presents for biopsy of a new mole located on the dorsal area of the right foot.

PROCEDURE NOTE:
Procedure: biopsy of lesion. Consent was obtained prior to procedure. The lesion was located on the right foot. The site was prepped with Betadine. The area was anesthetized with bupivacaine 0.5% with epinephrine.
Procedure note: a 3-mm punch biopsy of the lesion was taken. The cutaneous layer was closed with sutures of 4-0 vicryl. Horizontal mattress sutures were used for the skin closure.
Dressing: an antibiotic ointment was applied, and a sterile dressing was placed.
Patient status: the patient tolerated the procedure well.
Complications: there were no complications.

SIGNED: Dr. Susan Alameda, DO

Use the following steps to select the appropriate diagnosis and procedure codes for the case study.

1. Read through the case study in full. Use a medical dictionary or medical terminology textbook to define the following term:

   Cytologic atypia:

   ____

   ____

2. To identify the patient's diagnosis, answer the following question: *Why did the doctor do it?* List the diagnosis on the lines provided. Note that there may be multiple diagnoses.

   ____

   ____

3. Now that the patient's diagnosis has been identified, list the corresponding ICD-10-CM code(s):
ICD-10-CM code(s): ________________

4. To identify the procedure(s) answer the following question: *What did the doctor do?* List the procedure(s) on the lines provided:

____

____

5. Now that you have the name of the procedure(s), locate the code(s) for each procedure in the CPT code book. List the CPT/HCPCS code(s) and any applicable modifiers:
CPT code(s): ________________- _____

6. List the procedure and diagnosis codes on the CMS-1500 form. Be sure to correctly link the procedure and diagnosis codes. Refer to figure 3.6 for an example.

21. DIAGNOSIS OR NATURE OF ILLNESS OR INJURY Relate A-L to service line below (24E) ICD Ind.

A.	B.	C.	D.
E.	F.	G.	H.
I.	J.	K.	L.

24. A. DATE(S) OF SERVICE From MM DD YY	To MM DD YY	B. PLACE OF SERVICE	C. EMG	D. PROCEDURES, SERVICES, OR SUPPLIES (Explain Unusual Circumstances) CPT/HCPCS	MODIFIER	E. DIAGNOSIS POINTER

Case Study 5.4

PATIENT: Jamie Bencomo

INDICATIONS: The patient presents with symptomatic gallbladder disease and will undergo laparoscopic cholecystectomy.

PREOPERATIVE DIAGNOSIS: Biliary dyskinesia

POSTOPERATIVE DIAGNOSIS: Same

ANESTHESIA: General endotracheal

PROCEDURE NOTE:
The risks, benefits, complications, treatment options, and expected outcomes were discussed with the patient. The possibilities of reaction to medication, pulmonary aspiration, perforation of viscus, bleeding, recurrent infection, finding a normal gallbladder, the need for additional procedures, failure to diagnosis a condition, the possible need to convert to an open procedure, and creating a complication requiring a transfusion operation were discussed with the patient. The patient concurred with the proposed plan, giving informed consent. The patient was taken to the OR. A time-out was held and all information was verified.

Prior to the induction of general anesthesia, antibiotic prophylaxis was administered. General endotracheal anesthesia was then administered and tolerated well. After the induction, the abdomen was prepped in the usual sterile fashion. The patient was positioned in the supine position with some reverse Trendelenburg.

After injecting local anesthetic, a 5-mm incision was made in the right upper quadrant and, with the help of 5-mm Optiview trocar and a 5-mm camera, the peritoneal cavity was accessed without complications. Pneumoperitoneum was then created with CO_2 and tolerated well without any adverse changes in the patient's vital signs.

The gallbladder was identified, the fundus grasped and retracted cephalad. Adhesions were lysed bluntly and with the electrocautery where indicated, taking care not to injure any adjacent organs or viscus. The infundibulum was grasped and retracted laterally, exposing the peritoneum overlying the triangle of Calot. This was then divided and exposed in a blunt fashion. The cystic duct was clearly identified and bluntly dissected circumferentially. The junctions of the gallbladder, cystic duct, and common bile duct were clearly identified prior to the division of any linear structure.

The cystic duct was then doubly ligated with surgical clips on the patient side and singly clipped on the gallbladder side and divided. The cystic artery was identified, dissected free, ligated with clips, and divided as well.

The gallbladder was dissected from the liver bed in retrograde fashion with the electrocautery. The gallbladder was removed. The liver bed was inspected. Hemostasis was achieved with the electrocautery. No irrigation was performed.

Pneumoperitoneum was completely reduced after viewing removal of the trocars under direct supervision. The wound was thoroughly irrigated and the fascia was then closed with a figure-of-eight suture; the skin was then closed with a 4-0 Monocryl, and Dermabond was applied.

Instrument, sponge, and needle counts were correct at closure and at the conclusion of the case.

FINDINGS: Biliary dyskinesia

SPECIMENS: Gallbladder

COMPLICATIONS: None; the patient tolerated the procedure well

DISPOSITION: PACU—Hemodynamically stable

CONDITION: Stable

SIGNED: Dr. Steven Ray, DO

Use the following steps to select the appropriate diagnosis and procedure codes for the case study.

1. Read through the case study in full. Use a medical dictionary or medical terminology textbook to define the following term:

   Pneumoperitoneum:

   ____

   ____

2. To identify the patient's diagnosis, answer the following question: *Why did the doctor do it?* List the diagnosis on the lines provided. Note that there may be multiple diagnoses.

   ____

   ____

3. Now that the patient's diagnosis has been identified, list the corresponding ICD-10-CM code(s):

   ICD-10-CM code(s): ________________

4. To identify the procedure(s), answer the following question: *What did the doctor do?* List the procedure(s) on the lines provided:

   ____

   ____

5. Now that you have the name of the procedure(s), locate the code(s) for each procedure in the CPT code book. List the CPT/HCPCS code(s) and any applicable modifiers:

   CPT code(s): ________________- _____

6. List the procedure and diagnosis codes on the CMS-1500 form. Be sure to correctly link the procedure and diagnosis codes. Refer to figure 3.6 for an example.

21. DIAGNOSIS OR NATURE OF ILLNESS OR INJURY Relate A-L to service line below (24E) ICD Ind.

A.	B.	C.	D.
E.	F.	G.	H.
I.	J.	K.	L.

24. A. DATE(S) OF SERVICE From MM DD YY	To MM DD YY	B. PLACE OF SERVICE	C. EMG	D. PROCEDURES, SERVICES, OR SUPPLIES (Explain Unusual Circumstances) CPT/HCPCS | MODIFIER	E. DIAGNOSIS POINTER

Case Study 5.5

PATIENT: Faith Perkins

CHIEF COMPLAINT: Patient presents with recurrent epistaxis

HISTORY OF PRESENT ILLNESS: 58-year-old female presents complaining of several weeks of right-sided epistaxis. She states it happens with strenuous lifting and activity. She thinks it is posterior-based because it runs down the back of her throat. She denies any trauma, pain, or prior nasal surgery. No fevers, chills, or night sweats.

PROCEDURE NOTE:
Control anterior nasal hemorrhage, simple

INDICATION: Epistaxis

ANESTHESIA: Topical anesthesia with 4% lidocaine

DESCRIPTION OF PROCEDURE: After verbal consent was obtained and a surgical pause, Afrin and 4% lidocaine were atomized into the nose. Silver nitrate was used to cauterize an area of the nasal septum. Bactroban coating surgical was then applied over top of the cauterized area using a cotton top applicator. The patient tolerated the procedure well and there were no complications.

SIGNED: Dr. Susan Alameda, DO

Use the following steps to select the appropriate diagnosis and procedure codes for the case study.

1. Read through the case study in full. Use a medical dictionary or medical terminology textbook to define the following term:

Epistaxis:

____

____

2. To identify the patient's diagnosis, answer the following question: *Why did the doctor do it?* List the diagnosis on the lines provided. Note that there may be multiple diagnoses.

____

____

3. Now that the patient's diagnosis has been identified, list the corresponding ICD-10-CM code(s):

ICD-10-CM code(s): ________________

4. To identify the procedure(s), answer the following question: *What did the doctor do?* List the procedure(s) on the lines provided:

____

____

5. Now that you have the name of the procedure(s), locate the code(s) for each procedure in the CPT code book. List the CPT/HCPCS code(s) and any applicable modifiers:

CPT code(s): ________________- _____

6. List the procedure and diagnosis codes on the CMS-1500 form. Be sure to correctly link the procedure and diagnosis codes. Refer to figure 3.6 for an example.

21. DIAGNOSIS OR NATURE OF ILLNESS OR INJURY Relate A-L to service line below (24E)			ICD Ind.
A.	B.	C.	D.
E.	F.	G.	H.
I.	J.	K.	L.

24. A. DATE(S) OF SERVICE From MM DD YY	To MM DD YY	B. PLACE OF SERVICE	C. EMG	D. PROCEDURES, SERVICES, OR SUPPLIES (Explain Unusual Circumstances) CPT/HCPCS	MODIFIER	E. DIAGNOSIS POINTER

Reference

American Medical Association (AMA). 2021. *CPT 2022 Professional Edition*. Chicago: AMA.

Part II

Coding in the Real World

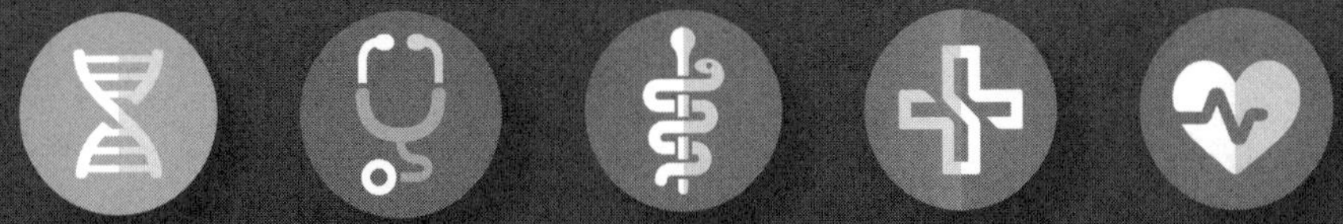

Supplies and Services

Vocabulary

Instructions: Define each of the following key terms in the space provided.

1. Advanced life support (ALS): ______________________________

____

____

2. Ambulance modifier: ______________________________

____

____

3. Ambulance supplier: ______________________________

____

____

4. Basic life support (BLS): ______________________________

____

____

5. Certificate of Medical Necessity (CMN): ______________________________

____

____

6. Destination: ______________________________

7. Durable medical equipment (DME): ______________________________

8. Durable medical equipment, prosthetics, orthotics, and supplies (DMEPOS): ___

9. Emergency transportation: ______________________________

10. Nonambulatory: ______________________________

11. Nonemergency transportation: ______________________________

12. Origin: ______________________________

13. Orthotics: ______________________________

14. Physician's Desk Reference (PDR): ______________________________

15. Prosthetics: ____

____

____

16. Route of administration: ____

____

____

17. Services: ____

____

____

18. Supplies: ____

____

____

19. Transportation indicator: ____

____

____

Matching

Instructions: Match the terms with the appropriate acronyms.

1. ________ IV	**A.** Intra-arterial
2. ________ VAR	**B.** Intravenous
3. ________ IA	**C.** Intramuscular
4. ________ ORAL	**D.** Intrathecal
5. ________ SC	**E.** Subcutaneous
6. ________ OTH	**F.** Inhaled
7. ________ INH	**G.** Various routes
8. ________ IT	**H.** Other routes
9. ________ IM	**I.** Oral

True/False

Instructions: Indicate whether the following statements are true or false (T or F). For false statements, rewrite the statement on the line below to make the statement true.

1. HCPCS Level II codes are used to report ambulance services.

____

____

2. The type of life support services provided during the ambulance services does not make a difference in code selection.

____

____

3. The type of vehicle used in ambulance transportation does not make a difference in code selection.

____

____

4. Transportation indicators are used to specify the type of supply provided for DME claims.

____

____

5. Medical necessity does not play a role in DMEPOS billing.

____

____

6. A certificate of medical necessity is used to indicate that a DME item is medically necessary.

____

____

7. When coding for drugs administered in the medical setting, the route of administration may impact code selection.

____

____

8. Drugs administered in the medical setting are identified with CPT level II codes.

____

____

9. If more than one HCPCS code exists for a specific drug, code selection will depend on the route of administration or unit per dose.

____

____

10. The majority of the codes used to identify drugs administered in the medical setting begin with the letter J.

____

____

Coding

Instructions: Answer the question with the appropriate HCPCS, ICD-10, modifier, or transportation indicator code.

1. Ambulance service ground mileage for 15 miles (include only the mileage code).

HCPCS code: ____________ × _____

2. Nonemergency taxi transportation.

HCPCS code: ____________

3. Fixed wing air transportation, 43 miles traveled.

HCPCS code: ____________

HCPCS code: ____________ × _____

4. Ambulance was dispatched to the scene of an accident, but no injuries were encountered on the scene. Code for the ambulance response with no transport provided.

HCPCS code: ____________

5. What transportation indicator would be used for an air transportation service that was provided due to a factory explosion?

Transportation indicator: _____

6. Ground ambulance dispatched to the scene of an accident. Woman at the scene had severe laceration of her upper right thigh area. She was transported via emergency ALS ambulance van to an acute-care hospital, 9 miles total.

HCPCS code: ____________ - _____

HCPCS code: ____________ × _____

ICD-10 code: ____________

7. Level 1 ALS ambulance transported a woman complaining of shortness of breath and chest pains to from her residence to an acute-care hospital, Level 1 emergency ALS transport, 12 miles total.

HCPCS code: ____________ - _____

HCPCS code: ____________ × _____

ICD-10 code: ____________, ____________

8. Pediatric patient with ESRD transferred via nonemergency ALS level 1 transport to location 236 miles away. Patient was transferred to another facility due to the nature of his medical needs, he requires specialized services not available in the local area.

HCPCS code: ____________

HCPCS code: ____________ × _____

Transportation indicator: _____

ICD-10 code: ____________

Enter these codes in the correct spaces on the following CMS-1500 claim form. Enter only the HCPCS codes (with units), transportation indicator (in box 19), and ICD-10 codes on the form.

19. ADDITIONAL CLAIM INFORMATION (Designated by NUCC)

20. OUTSIDE LAB? ☐ YES ☐ NO

21. DIAGNOSIS OR NATURE OF ILLNESS OR INJURY Relate A-L to service line below (24E) ICD Ind.

A. ______ B. ______ C. ______ D. ______

E. ______ F. ______ G. ______ H. ______

I. ______ J. ______ K. ______ L. ______

22. RESUBMISSION CODE

23. PRIOR AUTHORIZATION NU

	24. A. DATE(S) OF SERVICE From MM	DD	YY	To MM	DD	YY	B. PLACE OF SERVICE	C. EMG	D. PROCEDURES, SERVICES, OR SUPPLIES (Explain Unusual Circumstances) CPT/HCPCS	MODIFIER	E. DIAGNOSIS POINTER	F. $ CHARGES	G. DAYS OR UNITS
1													
2													
3													
4													
5													
6													

Source: CMS 2019.

9. Woman presents to the office of her OBGYN for the fitting of a diaphragm. Her provider counsels her on contraception and family planning and provides her with the diaphragm. (Code only for the HCPCS supply and ICD-10, not the CPT code for the service.)

HCPCS code: ____________

ICD-10 code: ____________

10. Custom fabricated plastic AFO provided to a patient with a healed complete traumatic right lower leg amputation. (Hint: Because the patient is not undergoing any active treatment at this time, use the seventh character extension for subsequent encounter.)

HCPCS code: ____________

ICD-10 code: ____________

11. Blood glucose monitor with integrated voice synthesizer for patient with uncomplicated diabetes mellitus type II.

HCPCS code: ____________

ICD-10 code: ____________

12. Pediatric size wheelchair with tilt-in-space, folding, adjustable, with seating system.

HCPCS code: ____________

13. CPAP device provided to 43-year-old male with obstructive sleep apnea. Additional length of CPAP tubing also provided.

HCPCS code: ____________

HCPCS code: ____________

ICD-10 code: ____________

14. Patient provided with nutritionally incomplete enteral formula (Propac), administered through feeding tube. 500 calories total.

HCPCS code: ____________ × _____

15. Rigid, wheeled, adjustable height walker provided to Medicare patient with ataxic gait.

HCPCS code: ____________

ICD-10 code: ____________

16. 10 mg IV Haldol.

HCPCS code: ____________ × _____

17. Patient provided with 200 mg of ciprofloxacin for intravenous infusion.

HCPCS code: ____________

18. 30 mCi therapeutic dose of IV 20 Zevalin.

HCPCS code: ____________

19. 20 units subcutaneous Vasopressin.

HCPCS code: ____________

20. 2 units incobotulinumtoxinA administered intramuscularly to 43-year-old female with glabellar lines.

HCPCS code: ____________ × _____

21. 5 sq. cm Integra Matrix provided to patient with diabetic (non-pressure) ulcer on left heel.

HCPCS code: ____________ × _____

ICD-10 code: ____________

22. Pentate Zinc Trisodium (25 mCi per study dose), intravenous form.

HCPCS code: ____________

23. 50 mg oral Etoposide.

HCPCS code: ____________

24. 25 mg Folex PFS.

HCPCS code: ____________ × _____

25. Blood glucose monitor with integrated voice synthesizer for legally blind patient with type 2 diabetes mellitus with hyperglycemia.

HCPCS code: ____________

ICD-10-CM codes: ____________, ____________

26. Foam collar orthoses provided to patient with cervical whiplash injury from a car accident. Patient was passenger in car that was rear-ended at a stop light in traffic by a pick-up truck.

HCPCS code: ____________

ICD-10-CM codes: ____________, ____________

27. Below-knee prosthesis with molded socket provided to patient with below-knee amputation (midcalf level) of the right leg.

HCPCS code: ______________

ICD-10-CM code: ______________

28. Inter-ear monaural hearing aid for patient with left-sided deafness.

HCPCS code: ______________

ICD-10-CM code: ______________

29. Urinary drainage latex leg bag, with extra pair of replacement latex leg straps, for patient with urinary incontinence.

HCPCS codes: ______________, ______________

ICD-10-CM code: ______________

30. Amputee wheelchair with detachable arms provided to patient with bilateral above-knee amputations.

HCPCS code: ______________

ICD-10-CM code: ______________

Case Studies Certificate of Medical Necessity (CMN)

Instructions: Complete the following Certificate of Medical Necessity forms using the information provided.

Case Study 6.1

A Medicare patient was provided with an electric, separate seat lift mechanism for use with her own furniture. Complete the CMS-849 Certificate of Medical Necessity form for this patient, using the information provided. Fill out the form as a supplier of the items/supplies, not as the medical provider.

Section A:

Initial Certification Date: 02/07/20XX

Place of Service: Home

Patient Information: Sally B. Good, 1234 Pleasant Road, Pleasantville, TX 12345. (555) 987-6543. DOB: 02/17/1965. Female. 5′1.5″ tall.

Supplier Name: National Medical Equipment and Supplies, 12345 Medical Lane, Pleasantville, TX 12345. (555) 576-8542. NPI # 123456789.

Name and address of facility: Not applicable.

Supply Item/Service Requested: HCPCS code: ______________

Physician Information: Dr. Susan Alameda, DO, 5678 Medical Parkway, Suite 1004, Pleasantville, TX 12345. (555) 987-6542. NPI # 987654321.

Section C: Provide a narrative description of the supply requested.

DEPARTMENT OF HEALTH AND HUMAN SERVICES
CENTERS FOR MEDICARE & MEDICAID SERVICES

Form Approved OMB
No. 0938-0679
Expires 02/2020

CERTIFICATE OF MEDICAL NECESSITY
CMS-849 — SEAT LIFT MECHANISMS

DME 07.03A

SECTION A: Certification Type/Date: INITIAL ___/___/___ REVISED ___/___/___ RECERTIFICATION___/___/___

PATIENT NAME, ADDRESS, TELEPHONE and MEDICARE ID (___ ___) ___ ___ - ___ ___ ___ Medicare ID ______________		SUPPLIER NAME, ADDRESS, TELEPHONE and NSC or NPI # (___ ___) ___ ___ - ___ ___ ___ NSC or NPI #__________
PLACE OF SERVICE ________	Supply Item/Service Procedure Code(s):	PT DOB ___/___/___ Sex ___ (M/F) Ht. ___(in) Wt ___
NAME and ADDRESS of FACILITY *if applicable (see reverse)*	__________ __________ __________ __________	PHYSICIAN NAME, ADDRESS, TELEPHONE and UPIN or NPI # (___ ___) ___ ___ - ___ ___ ___ UPIN or NPI #__________

SECTION B: Information in this Section May Not Be Completed by the Supplier of the Items/Supplies.

EST. LENGTH OF NEED (# OF MONTHS): _____ 1-99 *(99=LIFETIME)* | DIAGNOSIS CODES: _____ _____ _____ _____

ANSWERS	ANSWER QUESTIONS 1-5 FOR SEAT LIFT MECHANISM (Check Y for Yes, N for No, or D for Does Not Apply)
❑Y ❑N ❑D	1. Does the patient have severe arthritis of the hip or knee?
❑Y ❑N ❑D	2. Does the patient have a severe neuromuscular disease?
❑Y ❑N ❑D	3. Is the patient completely incapable of standing up from a regular armchair or any chair in his/her home?
❑Y ❑N ❑D	4. Once standing, does the patient have the ability to ambulate?
❑Y ❑N ❑D	5. Have all appropriate therapeutic modalities to enable the patient to transfer from a chair to a standing position (e.g., medication, physical therapy) been tried and failed? If YES, this is documented in the patient's medical records.

NAME OF PERSON ANSWERING SECTION B QUESTIONS, IF OTHER THAN PHYSICIAN (Please Print):
NAME: ______________________ TITLE: ______________ EMPLOYER:________________

SECTION C: Narrative Description of Equipment and Cost

(1) Narrative description of all items, accessories and options ordered; (2) Supplier's charge; and (3) Medicare Fee Schedule Allowance for each item, accessory, and option. (see instructions on back)

SECTION D: PHYSICIAN Attestation and Signature/Date

I certify that I am the treating physician identified in Section A of this form. I have received Sections A, B and C of the Certificate of Medical Necessity (including charges for items ordered). Any statement on my letterhead attached hereto, has been reviewed and signed by me. I certify that the medical necessity information in Section B is true, accurate and complete, to the best of my knowledge, and I understand that any falsification, omission, or concealment of material fact in that section may subject me to civil or criminal liability.

PHYSICIAN'S SIGNATURE______________________________ DATE ____/____/____

Signature and Date Stamps Are Not Acceptable.

Form CMS-849 (02/17)

Source: CMS 2017a.

Case Study 6.2

A Medicare patient was provided with a continuous positive airway pressure (CPAP) device for obstructive sleep apnea, for home use. Complete the CMS-10269 Certificate of Medical Necessity form for this patient, using the information provided. Fill out the form as a supplier of the items/supplies, not as the medical provider.

Section A:

Initial Certification Date: 05/08/20XX

Place of Service: Home

Patient Information: John Johnson, 5687 Main Street, Pleasantville, TX 12345. (555) 996-5874. DOB: 05/09/1965. Male. 5′11″ tall.

Supplier Name: National Medical Equipment and Supplies, 12345 Medical Lane, Pleasantville, TX 12345. (555) 576-8542. NPI # 123456789.

Name and address of facility: Not applicable.

Supply Item/Service Requested: HCPCS code: _______________

Physician Information: Dr. Susan Alameda, DO, 5678 Medical Parkway, Suite 1004, Pleasantville, TX 12345. (555) 987-6542. NPI# 987654321.

Section C: Provide a narrative description of the supply requested.

DEPARTMENT OF HEALTH AND HUMAN SERVICES
CENTERS FOR MEDICARE & MEDICAID SERVICES

Form Approved
OMB No. OMB 0938-0679

CERTIFICATE OF MEDICAL NECESSITY — DME 03.03

CMS-10269: POSITIVE AIRWAY PRESSURE (PAP) DEVICES FOR OBSTRUCTIVE SLEEP APNEA

SECTION A: **Certification Type/Date: INITIAL ___/___/___ RECERTIFICATION ___/___/___**

PATIENT NAME, ADDRESS, TELEPHONE and HICN	SUPPLIER NAME, ADDRESS, TELEPHONE and NSC or NPI #
(___) ___-____ HICN ________	(___) ___-____ NSC or NPI # ________

PLACE OF SERVICE ________	HCPCS CODE	PT DOB ___/___/___; Sex ___ (M/F); HT.___(in.); WT.___(lbs.)
NAME and ADDRESS of FACILITY if applicable (See Reverse)	________ ________ ________ ________	PHYSICIAN NAME, ADDRESS (Printed or Typed) PHYSICIAN'S NSC or NPI #: ________ PHYSICIAN'S TELEPHONE #: (___) ___-____

SECTION B: Information in this section may not be completed by the supplier of the items/supplies.

EST. LENGTH OF NEED (# OF MONTHS): ______ **1–99 (99=LIFETIME)** **DIAGNOSIS CODES (ICD-9):** ______ ______ ______ ______

ANSWERS	ANSWER QUESTIONS 1–7 FOR INITIAL EVALUATION ANSWER QUESTIONS 8–10 FOR FOLLOW-UP EVALUATION (RECERTIFICATION) (Check **Y** for Yes, **N** for No, **D** for Does Not Apply)
☐Y ☐N	1. Is the device being ordered for the treatment of obstructive sleep apnea (ICD-9 diagnosis code 327.23)? If YES, continue to Questions 2–5; If NO, Proceed to Section D
___/___/___	2. Enter date of initial face-to-face evaluation
___/___/___	3. Enter date of sleep test (If test spans multiple days, enter date of first day of test)
☐Y ☐N	4. Was the patient's sleep test conducted in a facility-based lab?
________	5. What is the patient's Apnea-Hypopnea Index (AHI) or Respiratory Disturbance Index (RDI)?
☐Y ☐N	6. Does the patient have documented evidence of at least one of the following? Excessive daytime sleepiness, impaired cognition, mood disorders, insomnia, hypertension, ischemic heart disease or history of stroke.
☐Y ☐N ☐D	7. If a bilevel device is ordered, has a CPAP device been tried and found ineffective?
___/___/___	8. Enter date of follow-up face-to-face evaluation.
☐Y ☐N	9. Is there a report documenting that the patient used PAP ≥ 4 hours per night on at least 70% of nights in a 30 consecutive day period?
☐Y ☐N	10. Did the patient demonstrate improvement in symptoms of obstructive sleep apnea with the use of PAP?

NAME OF PERSON ANSWERING SECTION B QUESTIONS, IF OTHER THAN PHYSICIAN (Please Print):

NAME: ________ TITLE: ________ EMPLOYER: ________

SECTION C: Narrative Description of Equipment and Cost

(1) Narrative description of all items, accessories and options ordered; **(2)** Supplier's charge; and **(3)** Medicare Fee Schedule Allowance for each item, accessory, and option. *(See instructions on back)*

SECTION D: Physician Attestation and Signature/Date

I certify that I am the physician identified in Section A of this form. I have received Sections A, B and C of the Certificate of Medical Necessity (including charges for items ordered). Any statement on my letterhead attached hereto, has been reviewed and signed by me. I certify that the medical necessity information in Section B is true, accurate and complete, to the best of my knowledge, and I understand that any falsification, omission, or concealment of material fact in that section may subject me to civil or criminal liability.

PHYSICIAN'S SIGNATURE ________ DATE ___/___/___ (SIGNATURE AND DATE STAMPS ARE NOT ACCEPTABLE)

Form CMS-10269 (12/09) 1

Source: CMS 2009.

Case Study 6.3

A Medicare patient purchased a portable oxygen system for continuous home use, including regulator, flowmeter, humidifier, cannula, and tubing. Complete the CMS-484 Certificate of Medical Necessity form for this patient, using the information provided. Fill out the form as a supplier of the items/supplies, not as the medical provider.

Section A:

Recertification Date: 11/30/20XX

Place of Service: Home

Patient Information: Javier Gomez, 9232 University Drive, Pleasantville, TX 12345. (555) 635-9847. DOB: 01/21/1953. Male. 5′9″ tall.

Supplier Name: National Medical Equipment and Supplies, 12345 Medical Lane, Pleasantville, TX 12345. (555) 576-8542. NPI # 123456789.

Name and address of facility: Not applicable.

Supply Item/Service Requested: HCPCS code: _______________

Physician Information: Dr. Susan Alameda, DO, 5678 Medical Parkway, Suite 1004, Pleasantville, TX 12345. (555) 987-6542. NPI # 987654321.

Section C: Provide a narrative description of the supply requested.

DEPARTMENT OF HEALTH AND HUMAN SERVICES
CENTERS FOR MEDICARE & MEDICAID SERVICES

Form Approved OMB
No. 0938-0679
Expires 02/2020

CERTIFICATE OF MEDICAL NECESSITY
CMS-484— OXYGEN

DME 484.5

SECTION A: Certification Type/Date: INITIAL ___/___/___ REVISED ___/___/___ RECERTIFICATION___/___/___

PATIENT NAME, ADDRESS, TELEPHONE and MEDICARE ID	SUPPLIER NAME, ADDRESS, TELEPHONE and NSC or NPI #
(___) ___-____ Medicare ID	(___) ___-____ NSC or NPI #_____

PLACE OF SERVICE _____	Supply Item/Service Procedure Code(s):	PT DOB ___/___/___ Sex ___ (M/F) Ht. ___(in) Wt ___
NAME and ADDRESS of FACILITY if applicable (see reverse)		PHYSICIAN NAME, ADDRESS, TELEPHONE and UPIN or NIP # (___) ___-____ UPIN or NPI # _____

SECTION B: Information in this Section May Not Be Completed by the Supplier of the Item Supplies.

EST. LENGTH OF NEED (# OF MONTHS): ___ 1–99 (99=LIFETIME) | DIAGNOSIS CODES: ___ ___ ___ ___

ANSWERS	ANSWER QUESTIONS 1–9. (Check Y for Yes, N for No, or D for Does Not Apply, unless otherwise noted.)
a)____mm Hg b)_____% c)___/___/___	1. Enter the result of recent test taken on or before the certification date listed in Section A. Enter (a) arterial blood gas PO2 and/or (b) oxygen saturation test; (c) date of test.
❑ 1 ❑ 2 ❑ 3	2. Was the test in Question 1 performed (1) with the patient in a chronic stable state as an outpatient, (2) within two days prior to discharge from an inpatient facility to home, or (3) under other circumstances?
❑ 1 ❑ 2 ❑ 3	3. Check the one number for the condition of the test in Question 1: (1) At Rest; (2) During Exercise; (3) During Sleep
❑ Y ❑ N ❑ D	4. If you are ordering portable oxygen, is the patient mobile within the home? If you are not ordering portable oxygen, check D.
_____LPM	5. Enter the highest oxygen flow rate ordered for this patient in liters per minute. If less than 1 LPM, enter an "X".
a)____mm Hg b)_____% c)___/___/___	6. If greater than 4 LPM is prescribed, enter results of recent test taken on 4 LPM. This may be an (a) arterial blood gas PO2 and/or (b) oxygen saturation test with patient in a chronic stable state. Enter date of test (c).

ANSWER QUESTIONS 7-9 ONLY IF PO2 = 56–59 OR OXYGEN SATURATION = 89 IN QUESTION 1

❑ Y ❑ N	7. Does the patient have dependent edema due to congestive heart failure?
❑ Y ❑ N	8. Does the patient have cor pulmonale or pulmonary hypertension documented by P pulmonale on an EKG or by an echocardiogram, gated blood pool scan or direct pulmonary artery pressure measurement.
❑ Y ❑ N	9. Does the patient have a hematocrit greater than 56%?

NAME OF PERSON ANSWERING SECTION B QUESTIONS, IF OTHER THAN PHYSICIAN (Please Print):
NAME__________ TITLE________ EMPLOYER________

SECTION C: Narrative Description of Equipment and Cost

(1) Narrative description of all items, accessories and option ordered; (2) Suppliers charge; and (3) Medicare Fee Schedule Allowance for each item, accessory, and option (see instructions on back)

SECTION D: PHYSICIAN Attestation and Signature/Date

I certify that I am the treating physician identified in Section A of this form. I have received Sections A, B and C of the Certificate of Medical Necessity (including charges for items ordered). Any statement on my letterhead attached hereto, has been reviewed and signed by me. I certify that the medical necessity information in Section B is true, accurate and complete, to the best of my knowledge, and I understand that any falsification, omission, or concealment of material fact in that section may subject me to civil or criminal liability.

PHYSICIAN'S SIGNATURE________________ DATE ___/___/___

Signature and Date Stamps Are Not Acceptable.

Form CMS–484 (12/18)

Source: CMS 2017b.

Case Study 6.4

A Medicare patient purchased a TENS device with four leads for stimulation of multiple spinal nerves. Complete the CMS-848 Certificate of Medical Necessity form for this patient, using the information provided. Fill out the form as a supplier of the items/supplies, not as the medical provider.

Section A:

Initial Certification Date: 09/09/20XX

Place of Service: Home

Patient Information: Steven Swanson, 66541 Union Blvd, Pleasantville, TX 12345. (555) 323-3347. DOB: 02/14/1979. Male. 6′0″ tall.

Supplier Name: National Medical Equipment and Supplies, 12345 Medical Lane, Pleasantville, TX 12345. (555) 576-8542. NPI # 123456789.

Name and address of facility: Not applicable.

Supply Item/Service Requested: HCPCS code: ______________

Physician Information: Dr. Susan Alameda, DO, 5678 Medical Parkway, Suite 1004, Pleasantville, TX 12345. (555) 987-6542. NPI# 987654321.

Section C: Provide a narrative description of the supply requested.

DEPARTMENT OF HEALTH AND HUMAN SERVICES
CENTERS FOR MEDICARE & MEDICAID SERVICES

Form Approved OMB
No. 0938-0679
Expires 02/2020

CERTIFICATE OF MEDICAL NECESSITY

DME 06.03B

CMS-848 — TRANSCUTANEOUS ELECTRICAL NERVE STIMULATOR (TENS)

SECTION A: Certification Type/Date: INITIAL ___/___/___ REVISED ___/___/___ RECERTIFICATION___/___/___

PATIENT NAME, ADDRESS, TELEPHONE and MEDICARE ID (__ __ __) __ __ __ - __ __ __ __ Medicare ID __________		SUPPLIER NAME, ADDRESS, TELEPHONE and NSC or NPI # (__ __ __) __ __ __ - __ __ __ __ NSC or NPI #__________
PLACE OF SERVICE ________	Supply Item/Service Procedure Code(s):	PT DOB ___/___/___ Sex ___ (M/F) Ht. ___(in) Wt ___(lbs
NAME and ADDRESS of FACILITY *if applicable (see reverse)*	________ ________ ________ ________	PHYSICIAN NAME, ADDRESS, TELEPHONE and UPIN or NPI # (__ __ __) __ __ __ - __ __ __ __ UPIN or NPI #__________

SECTION B: Information in this Section May Not Be Completed by the Supplier of the Items/Supplies.

EST. LENGTH OF NEED (# OF MONTHS): ____ 1–99 *(99=LIFETIME)* | DIAGNOSIS CODES: ____ ____ ____ ____

ANSWERS	ANSWER QUESTIONS 1–6 for purchase of TENS (Check Y for Yes, N for No,)
❑ Y ❑ N	1. Does the patient have chronic, intractable pain?
______ Months	2. How long has the patient had intractable pain? (Enter number of months, 1–99.)
❑ 1 ❑ 2 ❑ 3 ❑ 4 ❑ 5	3. Is the TENS unit being prescribed for any of the following conditions? (Check appropriate number) 1 - Headache 2 - Visceral abdominal pain 3 - Pelvic pain 4 - Temporomandibular joint (TMJ) pain 5 - None of the above
❑ Y ❑ N	4. Is there documentation in the medical record of multiple medications and/or other therapies that have been tried and failed?
❑ Y ❑ N	5. Has the patient received a TENS trial of at least 30 days?
___/___/___	6. What is the date that you reevaluated the patient at the end of the trial period?

NAME OF PERSON ANSWERING SECTION B QUESTIONS, IF OTHER THAN PHYSICIAN (Please Print):
NAME: ________________ TITLE: ____________ EMPLOYER: ____________

SECTION C: Narrative Description of Equipment and Cost

(1) Narrative description of all items, accessories and options ordered; (2) Supplier's charge; and (3) Medicare Fee Schedule Allowance for each item, accessory, and option. (see instructions on back)

SECTION D: PHYSICIAN Attestation and Signature/Date

I certify that I am the treating physician identified in Section A of this form. I have received Sections A, B and C of the Certificate of Medical Necessity (including charges for items ordered). Any statement on my letterhead attached hereto, has been reviewed and signed by me. I certify that the medical necessity information in Section B is true, accurate and complete, to the best of my knowledge, and I understand that any falsification, omission, or concealment of material fact in that section may subject me to civil or criminal liability.

PHYSICIAN'S SIGNATURE________________________ DATE ____/____/____

Signature and Date Stamps Are Not Acceptable.

Form CMS-848 (02/17)

Source: CMS 2017c.

Case Study 6.5

A Medicare patient with lymphedema was provided with a pneumatic compressor segmental home model with calibrated gradient pressure. This is a revision of her previous CMN, which was initially certified for a compressor system without calibrated gradient pressure. Complete the CMS-846 Certificate of Medical Necessity form for this patient, using the information provided. Fill out the form as a supplier of the items/supplies, not as the medical provider.

Section A:

Initial Certification Date: 04/16/20XX

Place of Service: Home

Patient Information: Edith Jackson, 1005 Parkway Drive, Pleasantville, TX 12345. (555) 635-4587. DOB: 10/02/1945. Female. 5′1″ tall.

Supplier Name: National Medical Equipment and Supplies, 12345 Medical Lane, Pleasantville, TX 12345. (555) 576-8542. NPI # 123456789.

Name and address of facility: Not applicable.

Supply Item/Service Requested: HCPCS code: ______________

Physician Information: Dr. Susan Alameda, DO, 5678 Medical Parkway, Suite 1004, Pleasantville, TX 12345. (555) 987-6542. NPI# 987654321.

Section C: Provide a narrative description of the supply requested.

Form Approved OMB
No. 0938-0679
Expires 02/2020

DEPARTMENT OF HEALTH AND HUMAN SERVICES
CENTERS FOR MEDICARE & MEDICAID SERVICES

CERTIFICATE OF MEDICAL NECESSITY
CMS-846 — PNEUMATIC COMPRESSION DEVICES

DME 04.04B

SECTION A: Certification Type/Date: INITIAL __/__/__ REVISED __/__/__ RECERTIFICATION__/__/__

PATIENT NAME, ADDRESS, TELEPHONE and MEDICARE ID (__ __ __) __ __ __ - __ __ __ __ Medicare ID ________		SUPPLIER NAME, ADDRESS, TELEPHONE and NSC or NPI # (__ __ __) __ __ __ - __ __ __ __ NSC or NPI #________
PLACE OF SERVICE ______	Supply Item/Service Procedure Code(s):	PT DOB __/__/__ Sex ___ (M/F) Ht. ___(in) Wt ___(lbs)
NAME and ADDRESS of FACILITY *if applicable (see reverse)*	______ ______ ______ ______	PHYSICIAN NAME, ADDRESS, TELEPHONE and UPIN or NPI # (__ __ __) __ __ __ - __ __ __ __ UPIN or NPI #________

SECTION B: Information in this Section May Not Be Completed by the Supplier of the Items/Supplies.

EST. LENGTH OF NEED (# OF MONTHS): ____ 1–99 *(99=LIFETIME)* | DIAGNOSIS CODE(S): ____ ____ ____ ____

ANSWERS	ANSWER QUESTIONS 1–5 FOR PNEUMATIC COMPRESSION DEVICES (Check Y for Yes, N for No, Unless Otherwise Noted)
❑ Y ❑ N	1. Does the patient have chronic venous insufficiency with venous stasis ulcers?
❑ Y ❑ N	2. If the patient has venous stasis ulcers, have you seen the patient regularly over the past six months and treated the ulcers with a compression bandage system or compression garment?
❑ Y ❑ N	3. Has the patient had radical cancer surgery or radiation for cancer that interrupted normal lymphatic drainage of the extremity?
❑ Y ❑ N	4. Does the patient have a malignant tumor with obstruction of the lymphatic drainage of an extremity?
❑ Y ❑ N	5. Has the patient had lymphedema since childhood or adolescence?

NAME OF PERSON ANSWERING SECTION B QUESTIONS, IF OTHER THAN PHYSICIAN (Please Print):
NAME: __________ TITLE: __________ EMPLOYER: __________

SECTION C: Narrative Description of Equipment and Cost

(1) Narrative description of all items, accessories and options ordered; (2) Supplier's charge; and (3) Medicare Fee Schedule Allowance for each item, accessory, and option. (see instructions on back)

SECTION D: PHYSICIAN Attestation and Signature/Date

I certify that I am the treating physician identified in Section A of this form. I have received Sections A, B and C of the Certificate of Medical Necessity (including charges for items ordered). Any statement on my letterhead attached hereto, has been reviewed and signed by me. I certify that the medical necessity information in Section B is true, accurate and complete, to the best of my knowledge, and I understand that any falsification, omission, or concealment of material fact in that section may subject me to civil or criminal liability.

PHYSICIAN'S SIGNATURE____________________ DATE ___/___/___

Signature and Date Stamps Are Not Acceptable.

Form CMS-846 (02/17)

Source: CMS 2017d.

References

Centers for Medicare and Medicaid Services (CMS). 2021. CMS 1500. https://www.cms.gov/Medicare/CMS-Forms/CMS-Forms/Downloads/CMS1500.pdf.

Centers for Medicare and Medicaid Services (CMS). 2021a. CMS 849. https://www.cms.gov/Medicare/CMS-Forms/CMS-Forms/CMS-Forms-Items/CMS006687.

Centers for Medicare and Medicaid Services (CMS). 2021b. CMS 484. https://www.cms.gov/Medicare/CMS-Forms/CMS-Forms/Downloads/CMS484.pdf.

Centers for Medicare and Medicaid Services (CMS). 2021c. CMS 848. https://www.cms.gov/Medicare/CMS-Forms/CMS-Forms/CMS-Forms-Items/CMS006684.

Centers for Medicare and Medicaid Services (CMS). 2021d. CMS 846. https://www.cms.gov/Medicare/CMS-Forms/CMS-Forms/CMS-Forms-Items/CMS006674.

Centers for Medicare and Medicaid Services (CMS). 2009. CMS 10269. https://www.cms.gov/Medicare/CMS-Forms/CMS-Forms/CMS-Forms-Items/CMS1220725.

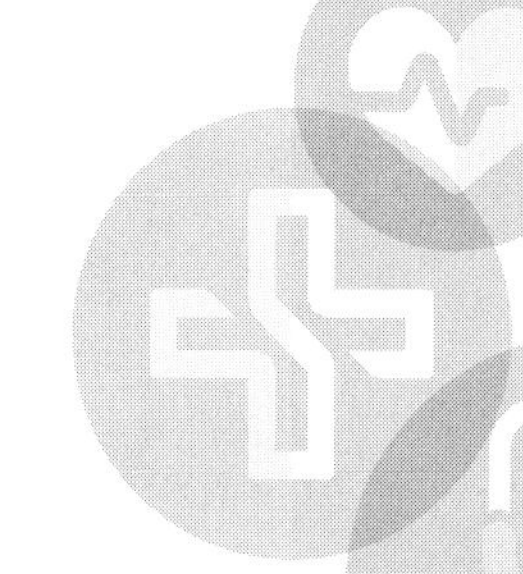

Behavioral Health Services

Vocabulary

Instructions: Define each of the following key terms in the space provided.

1. Anxiety disorders: ______________________________

____

____

2. Attention-deficit hyperactivity disorder (ADHD): ______________________________

____

____

3. Behavioral health services: ______________________________

____

____

4. Bipolar disorder: ______________________________

____

____

5. Contributory factors: ______________________________

____

____

6. Coordination of care: ______

7. Counseling: ______

8. Depression: ______

9. Diagnostic and Statistical Manual of Mental Disorders (DSM-5): ______

10. Eating disorders: ______

11. Electroconvulsive therapy (ECT): ______

12. Established patient: ______

13. Examination: ______

14. History: ______

15. Inpatient: ____

____

____

16. Interactive complexity: ____

____

____

17. Medical decision-making (MDM): ____

____

____

18. Mental health: ____

____

____

19. Mental illness: ____

____

____

20. Narcosynthesis for psychiatric purposes: ____

____

____

21. Nature of the presenting problem: ____

____

____

22. New patient: ____

____

____

23. Outpatient: ____

____

____

24. Partial hospitalization: ______________________________

25. Place of service (POS): ______________________________

26. Psychiatrist: ______________________________

27. Psychologist: ______________________________

28. Psychotherapy: ______________________________

29. Remission: ______________________________

30. Schizophrenia: ______________________________

31. Screening, Brief Intervention and Referral to Treatment (SBIRT): ______________________________

32. SOAP note: ______________________________

33. Social determinants of health (SDoH): ______________________________

____

____

34. Spectrum concept: ______________________________

____

____

35. Substance abuse: ______________________________

____

____

36. Total time: ______________________________

____

____

37. Transcranial magnetic stimulation (TMS): ______________________________

____

____

Multiple Choice

Instructions: Choose the best answer.

1. Which of the following specialties focuses specifically on the misuse of alcohol or drugs?
   a. Substance abuse
   b. Mental health
   c. Behavioral health
   d. Psychology

2. Which of the following is a type of mid-level provider that may provide behavioral health services?
   a. Medical Doctor (MD)
   b. Doctor of Osteopathy (DO)
   c. Medical Assistant (MA)
   d. Clinical Psychologist (CP)

3. What is the term for the two-digit code that identifies the setting in which the service was provided?
   a. Modifier
   b. Place of service code
   c. Transportation indicator
   d. HCPCS modifier

4. A new patient is a patient who has not received any professional services from the same provider or another provider of the same specialty and subspecialty in the same group practice in how many years?
   a. Two
   b. Three
   c. Four
   d. Five

5. An established patient is one who has received professional services from the same provider or another provider of the same specialty and subspecialty in the same group practice in how many years?
   a. Two
   b. Three
   c. Four
   d. Five

6. Which of the following types of patients has been formally admitted to a healthcare facility?
   a. Inpatient
   b. Outpatient
   c. Observation
   d. Established

7. Which of the following key components is the subjective information (given by the patient)?
   a. History
   b. Examination
   c. Counseling
   d. Coordination of care

8. Which of the following key components is the objective information (as determined by the healthcare provider)?
   a. Examination
   b. Time
   c. Medical decision-making
   d. Nature of the presenting problem

9. Which of the following key components involves the provider's determination of the patient's diagnoses and a course of treatment?
a. Examination
b. Medical decision-making
c. Coordination of care
d. History

10. Which of the following contributory factors identifies the type of condition for which the patient is receiving treatment?
a. Coordination of care
b. Counseling
c. Nature of presenting problem
d. Time

11. In order to select time as the determining factor in the level of an E/M code, what percentage of time must be spent on counseling or coordination of care?
a. 30%
b. 45%
c. 100%
d. 50%

12. Which of the following are the most commonly used behavioral health procedure codes (besides E/M service codes)?
a. Narcosynthesis
b. Transcranial magnetic stimulation (TMS)
c. Psychotherapy
d. Vagus nerve stimulation

13. When a medical E/M and psychotherapy are provided at the same encounter, how is the psychotherapy coded?
a. It is not coded; it is bundled into the code for the E/M service.
b. It is reported only with the medical E/M code.
c. It is reported with the psychotherapy add-on code.
d. It is reported with the psychotherapy standalone code.

14. When a behavioral health service is provided via a telemedicine platform, what modifier should be used?
a. -95
b. -59
c. -51
d. -25

15. If abuse and dependence are both documented for a single substance, what should the coder do?
a. Assign the diagnosis codes for both.
b. Assign the diagnosis code for the abuse only.
c. Assign the diagnosis code for the dependence only.
d. Assign the diagnosis code that combines the two conditions.

Fill in the Blank

Instructions: Complete each figure with the levels of each of the key components, in order from lowest to highest.

1. Levels of key component: History

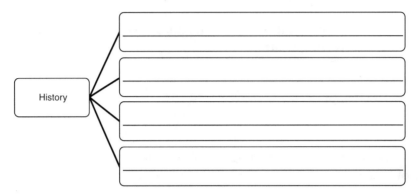

2. Levels of key component: Examination

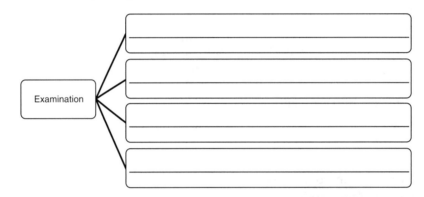

3. Levels of key component: Medical Decision-Making

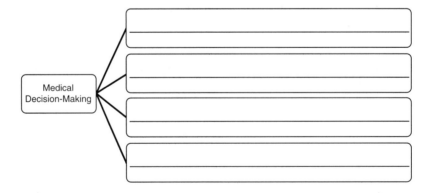

4. Anatomy of an E/M code

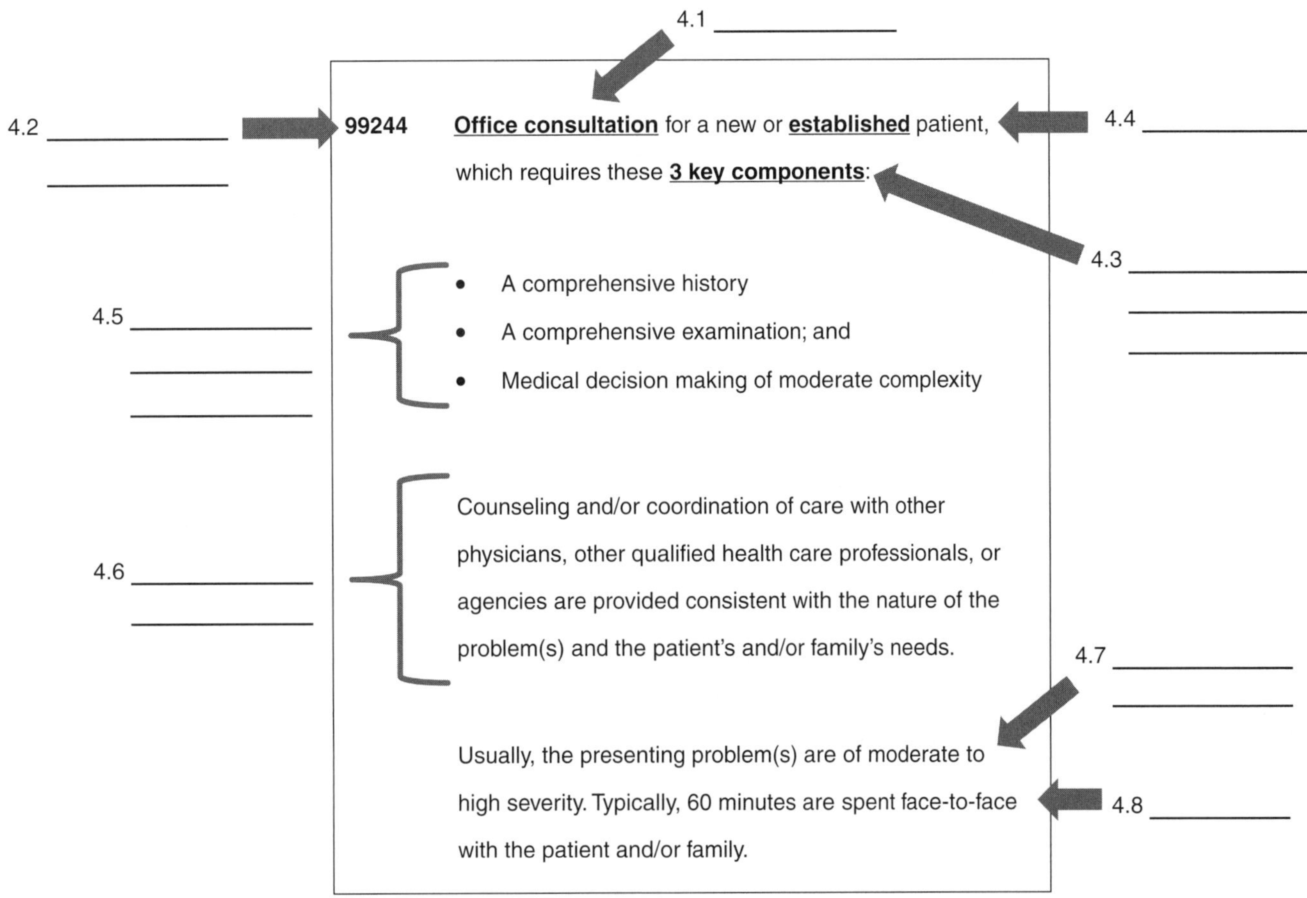

4.1 ____________
4.2 ____________
____
99244
Office consultation for a new or established patient,
which requires these 3 key components:
4.4 ____________
4.3 ____________
____
____
4.5 ____________
____
____
A comprehensive history
A comprehensive examination; and
Medical decision making of moderate complexity
4.6 ____________
____
Counseling and/or coordination of care with other physicians, other qualified health care professionals, or agencies are provided consistent with the nature of the problem(s) and the patient's and/or family's needs.
4.7 ____________
____
Usually, the presenting problem(s) are of moderate to high severity. Typically, 60 minutes are spent face-to-face with the patient and/or family.
4.8 ____________

Source: AMA 2019, 13.

Coding

Instructions: Answer the question with the appropriate CPT and ICD-10-CM code(s).

1. Factitious disorder with predominantly physical signs.
ICD-10-CM code(s): ____________

2. Patient with Down syndrome (trisomy 21 translocation) and severe intellectual disabilities (patient has a measured IQ of 40).
ICD-10-CM code(s): ____________, ____________

3. Sexual sadism.
ICD-10-CM code(s): ____________

4. ADHD in 32-year-old male.
ICD-10-CM code(s): ____________

5. Post-concussion encephalopathy with intractable post-traumatic headache.

ICD-10-CM code(s): ____________, ____________

6. 50 minutes of family psychotherapy without patient present, delivered via interactive telemedicine portal.

CPT code(s): ____________ - _____

7. Two hours (120 minutes) of psychotherapy for crisis.

CPT code(s): ____________, ____________ × _____

8. Unlisted psychiatric service.

CPT code(s): ____________

9. Diagnostic psychiatry evaluation with interactive complexity.

CPT code(s): ____________, ____________

10. E/M of an established 7-year-old patient in the outpatient office with selective mutism, which involved a detailed history, problem-focused examination, and MDM of moderate complexity.

CPT code(s): ____________

ICD-10-CM code(s): ____________

11. E/M for a new patient in the outpatient office with phobic issues. Male is 45 years old and is scared to leave the house, open the blinds, and generally fearful of other people and answering the door. After a comprehensive history, a detailed examination and MDM of moderate complexity, patient was diagnosed with agoraphobia without panic disorder.

CPT code(s): ____________

ICD-10-CM code(s): ____________

12. Consultation for an inpatient with suicidal ideation. E/M involved a detailed history, a detailed examination, and MDM of low complexity.

CPT code(s): ____________

ICD-10-CM code(s): ____________

13. Psychiatric diagnostic evaluation for a patient with patient with heroin (opioid) dependence, with heroin-induced psychotic disorder. Patient has been experiencing auditory and visual hallucinations.

CPT code(s): ____________

ICD-10-CM code(s): ____________

14. Code for the evaluation and management of an established patient with unspecified depression. Detailed history, expanded problem-focused examination, and moderate-complexity MDM.

CPT code(s): ____________

ICD-10-CM code(s): ____________

15. On-call psychiatrist was called in to emergency department to treat a 23-year-old female with severe panic attack. Patient also has a history of bipolar disorder. E/M service (which included a detailed history, a detailed examination, and moderate-complexity MDM) led to a clinical diagnosis of: bipolar disorder with current moderate manic episode; panic attack.

CPT code(s): ____________

ICD-10-CM code(s): ____________, ____________

16. Medical E/M of established patient with paranoid schizophrenia (expanded problem-focused history and examination, low-complexity MDM), along with 30 minutes of psychotherapy.

CPT code(s): ____________, ____________

ICD-10-CM code(s): ____________

17. 8 minutes of tobacco cessation counseling for a 37-year-old male current cigarette smoker (dependent on approximately 1.5 packs per day).

CPT code(s): ____________

ICD-10-CM code(s): ____________

18. Electroconvulsive therapy (ECT) for severe recurrent major depressive disorder with psychotic features.

CPT code(s): ____________

ICD-10-CM code(s): ____________

19. Psychoanalysis of patient with oppositional defiant disorder.

CPT code(s): ____________

ICD-10-CM code(s): ____________

20. Sedative withdrawal delirium.

ICD-10-CM code(s): ____________

21. Cannabis withdrawal with severe use disorder.

ICD-10-CM code(s): ____________

22. Factitious disorder imposed on another person.

ICD-10-CM code(s): ____________

23. Psychogenic dysphonia.

ICD-10-CM code(s): ____________

24. Patient with multiple phobias, including claustrophobia, agoraphobia, and generalized social phobia, as well as generalized anxiety disorder with panic attacks.

ICD-10-CM code(s): ____________, ____________, ____________, ____________

25. Office visit for an established patient with detailed history, detailed examination, and moderate MDM.

CPT code(s): ____________

26. Office visit for a new patient with detailed history, detailed examination, and moderate MDM.

CPT code(s): ____________

27. Office visit for a new patient with comprehensive history and examination and moderate MDM.

CPT code(s): ____________

28. Office visit for an established patient with expanded problem focused history, detailed examination, and moderate MDM.

CPT code(s): ____________

29. Office visit for an established patient with comprehensive history and examination with high MDM.

CPT code(s): ____________

30. Subsequent visit for a psychiatric patient in partial hospitalization setting, expanded history, problem-focused examination, and moderate MDM.

CPT code(s): ____________

Case Studies Behavioral Health Services

Case Study 7.1

PATIENT: Glenn Kim

SUBJECTIVE: (Detailed History)
Chief Complaint: Patient c/o headache, sleeping problems

History of Present Illness: This established patient has had a recurrent headache and difficulty sleeping for the last four days. He has not taken any medications and has not seen any other doctors for this problem. He has suffered from insomnia in the past but is not currently on medication. Recurrent migraines since teenage years. Mild depression for the last year, not currently being treated.

Review of Systems:
Constitutional: negative general constitutional systems review
Neurological: reports headache, no additional neurological symptoms
Musculoskeletal: neck pain, head pain
Psychiatric: insomnia for the past four days, reports feeling depressed/sad/apathetic/worried

Past, Family, Social History:
Current medications reviewed. No known drug allergies (NKDA).

OBJECTIVE: (Problem-focused Examination)
Physical Examination:
Constitutional: alert and in no acute distress. Well-nourished and healthy appearing. Thin but appears healthy.
Eyes: pupils were equal in size, round, reactive to light, with normal accommodation. No strabismus was seen.
ENMT: ears and nose were normal in appearance, both tympanic membranes were normal, and the nasal mucosa and septum were normal. The oropharynx was normal.
Musculoskeletal: neck examination normal, ROM normal, no abnormalities noted.

ASSESSMENT and PLAN: (Moderate Complexity MDM)

1. Headache. OTC NSAIDS for pain relief. Return to clinic in one week if pain does not subside.
2. Depression, mild, recurrent. Currently not being treated. Patient does not want treatment for this condition. Return to clinic in three months for re-evaluation.
3. Insomnia. Currently uncontrolled.

SIGNED: Dr. Susan Alameda, DO

Use the following these steps to select the appropriate diagnosis and procedure codes for the case study.

1. To identify the patient's diagnosis, answer the following question: *Why did the doctor do it?* List the diagnosis on the lines provided. Note that there may be multiple diagnoses.

____

____

2. Now that the patient's diagnosis has been identified, list the corresponding ICD-10-CM code(s):

ICD-10-CM code(s): ____________, ____________, ____________

3. To identify the procedure(s), answer the following question: *What did the doctor do?* List the procedure(s) on the lines provided:

____

____

4. Now that you have the name of the procedure(s), locate the code(s) for each procedure in the CPT code book. List the CPT/HCPCS code(s) and any applicable modifiers:

CPT code(s): ____________

5. List the procedure and diagnosis codes on the CMS-1500 form. Be sure to correctly link the procedure and diagnosis codes.

21. DIAGNOSIS OR NATURE OF ILLNESS OR INJURY Relate A-L to service line below (24E) ICD Ind.

A.	B.	C.	D.
E.	F.	G.	H.
I.	J.	K.	L.

24. A. DATE(S) OF SERVICE From MM DD YY	To MM DD YY	B. PLACE OF SERVICE	C. EMG	D. PROCEDURES, SERVICES, OR SUPPLIES (Explain Unusual Circumstances) CPT/HCPCS	MODIFIER	E. DIAGNOSIS POINTER

Case Study 7.2

PATIENT: Richard Abraham

SUBJECTIVE:
Chief Complaint: Patient c/o drinking problems and liver disease

History of Present Illness: 45-year-old established patient has significant history of alcoholism. Currently drinks approx. 24 beers per day but has cut out all hard alcohol for the last three months. Being seen by GI for alcoholic cirrhosis. Presents today to discuss referral to psych for depression and anxiety.

Review of Systems:
Constitutional: no fever, not feeling poorly, has been anxious lately
Gastrointestinal: No symptoms or significant changes since last visit

Past, Family, Social History:
Current medications reviewed. No known drug allergies (NKDA).

OBJECTIVE:
Physical Examination:
Constitutional: alert and in no acute distress. Well-nourished and healthy appearing. Overweight.

ASSESSMENT and PLAN:

1. Alcohol dependence with related anxiety disorder. Refer to psych.
2. Alcoholic liver cirrhosis. Continue with GI. Next appointment in 1 month.
3. Depression. Uncontrolled, refer to psych.
4. Overweight.

Spent over 40 minutes counseling patient on alcohol-related behavioral issues and referral to psychiatrist for counseling and medication options. Over 50% of this encounter was spent on counseling and/or coordination of care.

SIGNED: Dr. Susan Alameda, DO

Use the following these steps to select the appropriate diagnosis and procedure codes for the case study:

1. To identify the patient's diagnosis, answer the following question: *Why did the doctor do it?* List the diagnosis on the lines provided. Note that there may be multiple diagnoses.

   ____

   ____

2. Now that the patient's diagnosis has been identified, list the corresponding ICD-10-CM code(s):

   ICD-10-CM code(s): ____________, ____________, ____________, ____________

3. To identify the procedure(s), answer the following question: *What did the doctor do?* List the procedure(s) on the lines provided:

   ____

   ____

4. Now that you have the name of the procedure(s), locate the code(s) for each procedure in the CPT code book. List the CPT/HCPCS code(s) and any applicable modifiers:

   CPT code(s): ____________

5. List the procedure and diagnosis codes on the CMS-1500 form. Be sure to correctly link the procedure and diagnosis codes.

21. DIAGNOSIS OR NATURE OF ILLNESS OR INJURY Relate A-L to service line below (24E)			ICD Ind.
A.	B.	C.	D.
E.	F.	G.	H.
I.	J.	K.	L.

24. A. DATE(S) OF SERVICE From MM DD YY	To MM DD YY	B. PLACE OF SERVICE	C. EMG	D. PROCEDURES, SERVICES, OR SUPPLIES (Explain Unusual Circumstances) CPT/HCPCS	MODIFIER	E. DIAGNOSIS POINTER

Case Study 7.3

PATIENT: Gordon Brickell

SUBJECTIVE:
Chief Complaint: Follow-up on agoraphobia and social anxiety

History of Present Illness: This established patient has had agoraphobia and social anxiety since his teenage years and is now being treated via a telemedicine platform to reduce social anxiety and stressors related to presenting face-to-face in the clinic.

PSYCHOTHERAPY SERVICE:
Approximately 30 minutes spent with patient over telemedicine platform (patient not in office) discussing social-related stressors and behavioral interventions on how to cope with anxiety in a social setting.

ASSESSMENT and PLAN: (Moderate-Complexity MDM)

1. Agoraphobia. Currently uncontrolled. Patient self-restricted to the home setting. He does have family that assists with groceries and other needs. Lives with mother.
2. Social anxiety. Stable, improved. Patient is feeling less anxious about meeting new people in his home or talking with people over the phone. Does not engage in social media.

SIGNED: Dr. Susan Alameda, DO

Use the following these steps to select the appropriate diagnosis and procedure codes for the case study:

1. To identify the patient's diagnosis, answer the following question: *Why did the doctor do it?* List the diagnosis on the lines provide. Note that there may be multiple diagnoses.

____

____

2. Now that the patient's diagnosis has been identified, list the corresponding ICD-10-CM code(s):
ICD-10-CM code(s): ________________, ________________

3. To identify the procedure(s), answer the following question: *What did the doctor do?* List the procedure(s) on the lines provided:

____

____

4. Now that you have the name of the procedure(s), locate the code(s) for each procedure in the CPT code book. List the CPT/HCPCS code(s) and any applicable modifiers:
CPT code(s): ________________ - _____

5. List the procedure and diagnosis codes on the CMS-1500 form. Be sure to correctly link the procedure and diagnosis codes.

21. DIAGNOSIS OR NATURE OF ILLNESS OR INJURY Relate A-L to service line below (24E) ICD Ind.

A.	B.	C.	D.
E.	F.	G.	H.
I.	J.	K.	L.

24. A. DATE(S) OF SERVICE From MM DD YY	To MM DD YY	B. PLACE OF SERVICE	C. EMG	D. PROCEDURES, SERVICES, OR SUPPLIES (Explain Unusual Circumstances) CPT/HCPCS	MODIFIER	E. DIAGNOSIS POINTER

Case Study 7.4

PATIENT: Roberta Staff

REASON FOR VISIT:
Patient presents for psychiatric diagnostic evaluation for bipolar disorder

PSYCHIATRIC DIAGNOSTIC EVALUATION:
History: Patient has been suffering from manic episodes and severe depressed episodes for the last 6 months. Manic episodes typically last around 3–5 days, during which she sleeps only 3–5 hours per night. Depressed episodes are lasting from 7 to 9 days, during which she sleeps approximately 10–15 hours per day. No suicidal ideation. She is having trouble maintaining a work-life balance. She currently lives alone, children are out of the house, divorced. Maternal family history of bipolar disorder.

Mental Status: She seems depressed at visit today, a bit distracted. Cognition does not seem to be impaired.

Recommendations: Bipolar disorder, start lithium 900 mg; take one tablet daily. Return to clinic in two months.

SIGNED: Dr. Avinash Singh, MD

Use the following steps to select the appropriate diagnosis and procedure codes for the case study.

1. To identify the patient's diagnosis, answer the following question: *Why did the doctor do it?* List the diagnosis on the lines provided. Note that there may be multiple diagnoses.

____

____

2. Now that the patient's diagnosis has been identified, list the corresponding ICD-10-CM code(s):

   ICD-10-CM code(s): _______________

3. To identify the procedure(s), answer the following question: *What did the doctor do?* List the procedure(s) on the lines provided:

____

____

4. Now that you have the name of the procedure(s), locate the code(s) for each procedure in the CPT code book. List the CPT/HCPCS code(s) and any applicable modifiers:

   CPT code(s): _______________

5. List the procedure and diagnosis codes on the CMS-1500 form. Be sure to correctly link the procedure and diagnosis codes.

21. DIAGNOSIS OR NATURE OF ILLNESS OR INJURY Relate A-L to service line below (24E) ICD Ind.

A.	B.	C.	D.
E.	F.	G.	H.
I.	J.	K.	L.

24. A. DATE(S) OF SERVICE From MM DD YY	To MM DD YY	B. PLACE OF SERVICE	C. EMG	D. PROCEDURES, SERVICES, OR SUPPLIES (Explain Unusual Circumstances) CPT/HCPCS	MODIFIER	E. DIAGNOSIS POINTER

Reference

American Medical Association (AMA). 2021. *CPT 2022 Professional Edition*. Chicago: AMA.

Primary Care Services

Vocabulary

Instructions: Define each of the following key terms in the space provided.

1. Annual wellness visit (AWV): ______________________________

____

____

2. Body area: ______________________________

____

____

3. Care plan oversight (CPO): ______________________________

____

____

4. Chief complaint (C/C): ______________________________

____

____

5. Chronic care management (CCM): ______________________________

____

____

6. Chronic obstructive pulmonary disease (COPD): ____________________

____

____

7. CLIA-waived: ____________________

____

____

8. Congenital condition: ____________________

____

____

9. Diabetes mellitus: ____________________

____

____

10. Electrocardiogram (ECG/EKG): ____________________

____

____

11. Foreign body: ____________________

____

____

12. Heart failure: ____________________

____

____

13. History of present illness (HPI): ____________________

____

____

14. Hypercholesterolemia: ____________________

____

____

15. Hyperlipidemia: ____

____

____

16. Hypertension: ____

____

____

17. Immune globulin: ____

____

____

18. Incision and drainage (I&D): ____

____

____

19. Initial Preventive Physical Examination (IPPE): ____

____

____

20. Minor surgical procedure: ____

____

____

21. Organ system: ____

____

____

22. Otitis: ____

____

____

23. Overcoding: ____

____

____

24. Past, family, social history (PFSH): ______

25. Perinatal condition: ______

26. Preventive medicine services: ______

27. Primary care: ______

28. Primary care provider (PCP): ______

29. Prolonged services: ______

30. Review of systems (ROS): ______

31. Status asthmaticus: ______

32. Transient hypertension: ______

33. Transitional Care Management (TCM): ______________________________

____

____

34. Undercoding: ____

____

____

35. Underdose: ____

____

____

36. Vaccine administration: ______________________________________

____

____

37. Vaccine toxoid: ____

____

____

Multiple Choice

Instructions: Choose the best answer.

1. Which of the following types of codes are the most commonly reported procedures in primary care?
a. Evaluation and management
b. Medicine procedures
c. Vaccinations
d. In-office procedures

2. How many key components are there to E/M codes?
a. Two
b. Three
c. Four
d. Five

3. Which of the following is not an element of the key component of history?
a. Chief complaint
b. Risk of complications or morbidity or mortality
c. History of present illness
d. Review of systems

4. Which of the following elements of history is the patient's description of his or her reason for encounter?
a. Chief complaint
b. History of present illness
c. Review of systems
d. Past, family, social history

5. In the history of present illness, the characteristics of the sign(s) or symptom(s) are which of the following?
a. Location
b. Severity
c. Context
d. Quality

6. Which of the following elements of the key component history is aimed at obtaining more information regarding the patient's signs or symptoms?
a. Examination
b. History of present illness
c. Review of systems
d. Associated signs and symptoms

7. Which of the following elements of MDM considers the relative danger that a medical condition can pose to the patient if left untreated?
a. Risk of complications, morbidity, or mortality
b. Number of diagnoses and management options
c. Amount and/or complexity of data
d. Review of present illness

8. Which of the following modifiers may not be used with an E/M service?
a. Modifier -25
b. Modifier -32
c. Modifier -59
d. Modifier -57

9. There are two components to vaccine coding, the administration of the vaccine and which of the following?
a. Vaccine order
b. Immunoglobulin
c. Toxic substance
d. Toxoid or serum

10. Which of the following is a chronic lung disease characterized by chronically poor airflow?
a. Asthma
b. COPD
c. DM
d. Hypertension

Completion

Instructions: Define each of the following elements of history of present illness (HPI) and give an example of each.

1. Location: ______________________________

Example: ______________________________

2. Quality: ______________________________

Example: ______________________________

3. Severity: ______________________________

Example: ______________________________

4. Duration: ______________________________

Example: ______________________________

5. Timing: ______________________________

Example: ______________________________

6. Context: ______________________________

Example: ______________________________

7. Modifying factors: ______________________________

Example: ______________________________

8. Associated signs and symptoms: ______________________________

Example: ______________________________

Instructions: List and define the 14 elements (body systems) included in the review of systems.

9. ______________________________

10. ______________________________

11. ______________________________

12. ______________________________

13. ______________________________

14. ______________________________

15. ______

16. ______

17. ______

18. ______

19. ______

20. ______

21. ______

22. ______

Coding

Instructions: Read the documentation of the following E/M service and determine the levels of each of the elements.

C/C: Swollen tonsils, congestion, fever, and nausea

HPI: Patient began experiencing swollen tonsils, congestion, and fever two days ago. Also experiencing dizziness, hot flashes, and vomiting for two weeks. Hot flashes seem to happen when she goes to bed at night and when she wakes up in the morning. Nausea only happens after meals. She's been taking aspirin for the fever.

ROS: Constitutional: reports having fever for the last two days
Eyes: negative findings
Respiratory: negative
Cardiovascular: patient reports no problems
Gastrointestinal: patient reports nausea and vomiting
Neurological: patient reports dizziness and vertigo
Integumentary: negative finding
HENT: reports symptoms of throat problems congestion
Endocrine: negative findings
Musculoskeletal: negative findings
Psychiatric: negative findings
Genitourinary: reports having scanty and/or late menses

PFSH: Allergic to hydrocodone, no family history of early menopause

1. What is the level of HPI for this encounter?

____

____

2. What is the level of ROS for this encounter?

____

____

3. What is the level of PFSH for this encounter?

____

____

4. Using the following table, determine the level of history for this encounter (remember that all three of the three elements must meet or exceed the same level).

____

____

Level of History	HPI	ROS	PFSH
Problem focused	Brief	N/A	N/A
Expanded problem focused	Brief	Problem pertinent	N/A
Detailed	Extended	Extended	Pertinent
Comprehensive	Extended	Complete	Complete

Source: Table 8.1, p. 268.

EXAMINATION:
BMI 25.4 BP: 98/64 H: 59.00 in P: 90/min RR: 20/min T: 99.1 F W: 125lbs 6oz
Gen: general appearance fine, seems tired
HEENT: oropharynx red/erythematous, NOSE: positive erythema
NECK: n/a
LUNGS: Respiration within normal limits (wnl)
CHEST/BREASTS: n/a
HEART: wnl
ABD: wnl
GENT: wnl, pelvic examination deferred
MUSC: wnl
NEURO: wnl
SKIN: wnl
STUDIES: none

5. Using the 1997 guidelines and the following table, determine the level of examination for this encounter.

____

____

Level of Exam	Exam Components	Number of Body Areas/Organ Systems: 1995 Guidelines	Number of Body Areas/Organ Systems: 1997 Guidelines
Problem focused	Limited exam of affected body area/organ system	1 body area or organ system	1 to 5 body areas or organ systems
Expanded problem focused	Limited exam of affected area and other related/ symptomatic organ systems	2 to 7 body areas or organ systems	6 to 11 body areas or organ systems
Detailed	Extended exam of affected area and other related/ symptomatic organ systems	Extended exam of 2 to 7 body areas or organ systems	2 areas of examination from 6 organ systems
Comprehensive	General multisystem exam or complete exam of single organ system	8 or more organ systems	2 areas of examination from 9 organ systems

Source: Table 8.4, p. 271.

ASSESSMENT: Irregular menses (ICD-10 N92.6)
Dizziness (ICD-10 R42)
Acute Upper Respiratory Infection (J06.9)
Acute Pharyngitis (J02.9)
Vomiting (R11.10)

PLAN: Strep swab in office (negative)
Continue with aspirin to treat fever
Return if symptoms worsen
HCG pregnancy two weeks ago at home was negative

6. Using the following table, determine the number of diagnoses or treatment options for this encounter.

____

____

Number of Diagnoses and Management Options	Points
Minor problem (self-resolving)	1 each for a maximum of 2
Established (stable or improving)	1 each
Established (worsening)	2 each
New problem (no additional workup)	3
New problem (with additional workup)	4
Total	

Source: Table 8.5, p. 275.

7. Using the following table, determine the amount and/or complexity of data to be reviewed.

____

____

Amount and/or Complexity of Data	Points
Lab ordered or reviewed	1 maximum
Radiology exam ordered or reviewed	1 maximum
Medicine section test ordered or reviewed	1 each
Discussion of results with performing provider	1
Decision to obtain old records or history	1
Reviewing and summarizing old records, history, or discussion with other health provider	2
Independent interpretation of test results	2
Total	

Source: Table 8.6, p. 276.

8. Determine the risk of complications and/or morbidity or mortality for this encounter.

____

____

9. Using the following table, determine the level of MDM for this encounter.

____

____

Level of MDM	Number of Diagnosis or Management Options	Amount and/or Complexity of Data	Risk Involved
Straightforward	Minimal	Minimal or none	Minimal
Low	Limited	Limited	Low
Moderate	Multiple	Moderate	Moderate
High	Extensive	Extensive	High

Source: Table 8.7, p. 278.

10. Using the levels of history, examination, and medical decision-making determined previously, report the code for this emergency department encounter.

CPT code(s): ________________

Instructions: Assign the correct CPT and ICD-10-CM codes for the following.

11. Type 1 patient with diabetes mellitus presents for evaluation of her long-term insulin regimen.

ICD-10-CM code(s): ________________

12. Underdosing of insulin in patient with type 1 DM due to mechanical breakdown of pump. Patient has been experiencing hyperglycemia.

ICD-10-CM code(s): ________________, ________________

13. Patient with poorly controlled type 2 DM and long-term use of insulin presents for treatment of diabetic ulcer of left heel (limited to breakdown of skin).

ICD-10-CM code(s): ________________, ________________

14. Administration of MMR vaccine to 4-year-old patient, with counseling.

CPT code(s): ________________, ________________, ________________, ________________

ICD-10-CM code(s): ________________

15. 48-year-old established male patient with COPD and moderate persistent asthma presents for exacerbation of both chronic conditions. Detailed history and examination with moderate complexity MDM.

CPT code(s): ________________, ________________, ________________

ICD-10-CM code(s): ________________

16. An outpatient office visit for an established 15-year-old male with moderate persistent asthma with status asthmaticus required a detailed history and examination, with MDM of moderate complexity. Patient was also provided with a pressurized breathing treatment in the office and an additional 35 minutes of time was spent monitoring the patient before he was sent home. Total time spent during this prolonged encounter was 55 minutes.

CPT code(s): ________________, ________________, ________________

ICD-10-CM code(s): ________________

17. 63-year-old male established patient presented to the office of his PCP for routine examination; no abnormal findings.

CPT code(s): ________________

ICD-10-CM code(s): ________________

18. 31-year-old pregnant female received IM annual flu vaccine (trivalent IIV3 0.5 mL dosage) as well as Tdap booster shots.

CPT code(s): ________________, ________________, ________________, ________________

ICD-10-CM code(s): ________________

19. HCG urinalysis performed on 25-year-old female patient complaining of amenorrhea.

CPT code(s): ________________

ICD-10-CM code(s): ________________

20. Routine physical examination performed on a 50-year-old new male patient with uncontrolled type 2 DM and essential hypertension. Patient has a family history of cardiovascular disease and his current BMI is 32.3. Intranasal flu vaccine administered upon request.

CPT code(s): ________________, ________________, ________________

ICD-10-CM code(s): ________________, ________________, ________________, ________________, ________________, ________________

21. Outpatient office visit for established 54-year-old male with a history of smoking and COPD. Currently experiencing acute bronchitis and exacerbation of COPD. Comprehensive examination and high-complexity MDM.

CPT code(s): ________________

ICD-10-CM code(s): ________________, ________________, ________________, ________________

22. Routine newborn care provided to 39-week-old single liveborn infant in the inpatient setting. (Subsequent daily hospital care, vaginal birth.)

CPT code(s): ________________

ICD-10-CM code(s): ________________

23. Admission to skilled nursing facility including comprehensive examination and history and moderate MDM for 92-year-old patient with emphysema and continuous oxygen dependence.

CPT code(s): ________________

ICD-10-CM code(s): ________________

24. 62-year-old female patient with suspected pneumonia discharged from observation care. Patient was evaluated for productive cough and fever, but imaging studies were negative for pneumonia.

CPT code(s): ________________

ICD-10-CM code(s): ________________

25. 67-year-old male Medicare patient given seasonal influenza (trivalent [IIV3], spit virus, 0.5 mL, intramuscular) vaccination (Hint: Search for Medicare vaccine administration code.)

CPT code(s): ________________, ________________

ICD-10-CM code(s): ________________

26. Care plan oversight services provided to a patient receiving home health services. Patient has commercial insurance. Provider personally spent 35 minutes providing care plan oversight services during the reporting month.

CPT code(s): ________________

27. Transitional care management service provided to a patient with acute DVT of the left lower leg and multiple pulmonary emboli. Patient seen on day 8 since discharge. High MDM.

CPT code(s): ________________

ICD-10-CM code(s): ________________

28. Pediatric well-child exam provided to 5-year-old female new patient. Patient was also given varicella booster at this encounter with counseling from the physician.

CPT code(s): ________________, ________________, ________________

ICD-10-CM code(s): ________________, ________________

29. Office visit for a pediatric established patient with detailed history, problem-focused examination, and moderate MDM. Patient was evaluated for ADHD, and provider also went over one Vanderbilt behavioral assessment with patient's parent at the encounter. Patient diagnosed with ADHD, combined presentation. ADHD medication started at this visit and patient will return to the clinic in three months.

CPT code(s): ________________, ________________

ICD-10-CM code(s): ________________

30. 4-day-old newborn (new patient) seen in the office for a routine newborn wellness examination. During examination, patient was also diagnosed with neonatal jaundice and referred to home health to set up bili blanket treatment. Additional evaluation and management service documented an expanded problem-focused history, detailed examination, and low MDM.

CPT code(s): ________________, ________________ - _____

ICD-10-CM code(s): ________________, ________________

Case Studies Primary Care Services

Case Study 8.1

PATIENT: Jayce Singer

CHIEF COMPLAINT: Follow-up from urgent care, fever, and strep throat. Fingernail pain.

HISTORY OF PRESENT ILLNESS: Established patient was seen in the urgent care three days ago due to fever and strep throat. Patient also reports fingernail pain in bilateral hands for the last three days. Also reports that there are itchy blisters in her pelvic area.

REVIEW OF SYSTEMS:
Constitutional: no fever since started on strep meds three days ago
Integumentary: rash on torso, otherwise normal
Musculoskeletal: pain in fingernails on both hands, no recent trauma, no joint pain

PAST, FAMILY, SOCIAL HISTORY:
Allergies: No known drug allergies (NKDA)
Medications: Amoxicillin PO daily

EXAMINATION:
General: alert, healthy appearing, in no acute distress.
Musculoskeletal: fingernails, digits were normal. No lumps palpated, no erythema, no edema.
Integumentary: skin/subcutaneous exam positive for rash around midsection and groin area.

ASSESSMENT/PLAN:

1. Rash and nonspecific skin eruption. Likely related to current infectious process and antibiotic use. Return to clinic if worse or does not resolve within five days, or if swelling, hives, or trouble breathing.
2. Pain in bilateral fingertips.

SIGNED: Dr. Susan Alameda, DO

Select the appropriate codes for the case study.

1. ICD-10-CM code(s): ________________
2. CPT code(s): ________________
3. List the procedure and diagnosis codes on the CMS-1500 form. Be sure to correctly link the procedure and diagnosis codes.

21. DIAGNOSIS OR NATURE OF ILLNESS OR INJURY Relate A-L to service line below (24E) ICD Ind.

A. ______	B. ______	C. ______	D. ______
E. ______	F. ______	G. ______	H. ______
I. ______	J. ______	K. ______	L. ______

24. A. DATE(S) OF SERVICE From MM	DD	YY	To MM	DD	YY	B. PLACE OF SERVICE	C. EMG	D. PROCEDURES, SERVICES, OR SUPPLIES (Explain Unusual Circumstances) CPT/HCPCS	MODIFIER	E. DIAGNOSIS POINTER

Case Study 8.2

PATIENT: Dani Carson

CHIEF COMPLAINT: 15-year-old established patient well-child exam

HISTORY OF PRESENT ILLNESS: Doing well. Mom declines HPV. Otherwise UTD on vaccines. General health since last visit has been good. Dental care includes good dental hygiene and regular dental visits. Immunizations are up to date. No sensory or developmental concerns are expressed. Current diet includes a normal healthy diet. The patient does not use dietary supplements. No nutritional concerns are expressed. He sleeps alone in a bed. He is in basketball and track. Currently in the 9th grade. Depression screening negative.

CURRENT MEDS:
None

ALLERGIES:
No known drug allergies (NKDA)

EXAMINATION:
General: active, alert, healthy appearing, in no acute distress, well developed, well nourished, and well hydrated.
Eyes: sclera and conjunctiva normal, pupils were equal in size, round, reactive to light, with normal accommodation, extraocular movements were intact, and no strabismus was seen.
ENT: the external ears and nose were normal in appearance, both tympanic membranes were normal, the external auditory canals were normal, the nasal mucosa and septum were normal, and the lips and gums were normal.
Neck: the appearance of the neck was normal, and the neck was supple.
Chest: chest was normal in appearance.
Pulmonary: no respiratory distress, normal respiratory rhythm and effort, and clear bilateral breath sounds.
Cardiac: heart rate and rhythm were normal and normal S1 and S2. Soft 2/6 systolic murmur heard at LLSB and increases minimally when supine.
Abdomen: normal bowel sounds, soft, nontender, no hepatosplenomegaly, and no abdominal mass.
Genitourinary: the penis was normal. Tanner stage 4.
Musculoskeletal: normal gait, no clubbing or cyanosis of the fingernails, normal movements of all extremities, and the muscle tone was normal. Inspection of the back showed normal curvature and no scoliosis.
Neurological: cranial nerves 2–12 were intact, deep tendon reflexes were 2+ and symmetric and the motor exam was normal.
Skin: normal skin color and pigmentation, normal capillary refill, no rash, and no skin lesions.

ASSESSMENT/PLAN:

1. Well-child exam with abnormal findings. Anticipatory guidance for age, and handouts given as appropriate for age. Reviewed growth charts, developmental assessments, and vaccination records available. Recommend flu vaccine in the fall.
2. Heart murmur. New diagnosis. Will have cardiology eval. since this is a new murmur. Discussed with parent and completed referral to cardiology. Follow-up pending evaluation from cardio.

SIGNED: Dr. Jean Obregon, MD

Select the appropriate codes for the case study.

1. ICD-10-CM code(s): ________________

2. CPT code(s): ________________, ________________- _____

3. List the procedure and diagnosis codes on the CMS-1500 form. Be sure to correctly link the procedure and diagnosis codes.

21. DIAGNOSIS OR NATURE OF ILLNESS OR INJURY Relate A-L to service line below (24E) ICD Ind.

A. ________ B. ________ C. ________ D. ________

E. ________ F. ________ G. ________ H. ________

I. ________ J. ________ K. ________ L. ________

	24. A. DATE(S) OF SERVICE From MM	DD	YY	To MM	DD	YY	B. PLACE OF SERVICE	C. EMG	D. PROCEDURES, SERVICES, OR SUPPLIES (Explain Unusual Circumstances) CPT/HCPCS	MODIFIER	E. DIAGNOSIS POINTER
1											
2											
3											

Case Study 8.3

PATIENT: Doyle Neifert

CHIEF COMPLAINT: Hypertension follow-up

HISTORY OF PRESENT ILLNESS: Established patient presents for follow-up on primary hypertension. The patient states that her blood pressure has been stable since her last visit three months ago. The only high blood pressures she had was after eating Chinese takeout.

Home monitoring: the patient checks her blood pressure regularly. Typical morning BPs are 120–139 systolic and 80–89 diastolic. Blood pressure control has been good.

Medications: the patient has been compliant with her medication regimen. She denies medication side effects. She is compensated with losartan. She is doing Resperate.

REVIEW OF SYSTEMS:

Eyes: no impaired vision

Respiratory: no dyspnea

Cardiovascular: no chest pains, no leg claudication, no lower-extremity edema

Neurological: no headache

PAST, FAMILY, SOCIAL HISTORY:

Allergies: No known drug allergies (NKDA).

Medications: Losartan potassium 25 mg oral tablet. Take one tablet daily.

EXAMINATION:

Constitutional: well nourished and healthy appearing.

Pulmonary: no respiratory distress, normal respiratory rhythm and effort, no accessory muscle use, and clear bilateral breath sounds heard on auscultation.

Cardiovascular: Heart rate and rhythm normal. No murmurs heard.
Musculoskeletal: Normal gait.
Skin: Normal skin color and pigmentation and normal skin turgor.

ASSESSMENT/PLAN:

1. Benign essential hypertension. Stable on losartan and Resperate. Continue same and follow up in six months. Medications were reviewed and reconciled. Allergies were reviewed and reconciled.

SIGNED: Dr. Jean Obregon, MD

Select the appropriate codes for the case study.

1. ICD-10-CM code(s): ________________
2. CPT code(s): ________________ - ____
3. List the procedure and diagnosis codes on the CMS-1500 form. Be sure to correctly link the procedure and diagnosis codes.

21. DIAGNOSIS OR NATURE OF ILLNESS OR INJURY Relate A-L to service line below (24E) ICD Ind.

A.	B.	C.	D.
E.	F.	G.	H.
I.	J.	K.	L.

24. A. DATE(S) OF SERVICE From MM DD YY	To MM DD YY	B. PLACE OF SERVICE	C. EMG	D. PROCEDURES, SERVICES, OR SUPPLIES (Explain Unusual Circumstances) CPT/HCPCS	MODIFIER	E. DIAGNOSIS POINTER

Case Study 8.4

PATIENT: Wilma Fredrickson

CHIEF COMPLAINT: Family discussion of health issues, patient not present

HISTORY OF PRESENT ILLNESS: Patient's daughter here to talk about patient's general decline and her recent normal mammogram. Mammogram was ordered due to lump found in her breast, and mammogram results were normal. Patient has dementia and has become even more confused since getting this news. Patient worse in general. Family is starting to interview for home care. Patient's daughter is having her own health issues and cannot escalate care needs for her mother. Family also strongly considering a memory care facility. Patient does have a neurologist but daughter states that she has not begun medication as neuro thinks she will be unlikely to respond. Patient has a demonstrated unwillingness to take her medications for dementia and refuses to take her anxiety medications. Daughter states that she and her brother are watching the patient's finances and the bank has notice to check with brother on any transactions. Daughter is filling patient's medications and is looking into getting a timed-opening medication box to assist with taking Coumadin for secondary hypercoagulable state.

PAST, FAMILY, SOCIAL HISTORY:
Allergies: No known drug allergies (NKDA)
Medications: Amoxicillin PO daily

MEDICAL DECISION-MAKING:
Counseling/coordination of care total time spent was 25 minutes. Greater than 50% of the encounter time was spent on counseling and/or coordination of care for discussion with daughter regarding patient's healthcare needs.

ASSESSMENT/PLAN:

1. Person consulting on behalf of another person. Recent encounters have been detrimental to the patient's mental well-being. Decision made with daughter to minimize medical interventions and forego any further treatment or testing for breast lump.
2. Dementia without behavioral disturbance.
3. Noncompliance with medication regimen due to mental disturbance.
4. Secondary hypercoagulable state.
5. Long-term use of Coumadin.

SIGNED: Dr. Jean Obregon, MD

Selecting the appropriate codes for the case study.

1. ICD-10-CM code(s): ________________, ________________, ________________, ________________, ________________
2. CPT code(s): ________________ - ____
3. List the procedure and diagnosis codes on the CMS-1500 form. Be sure to correctly link the procedure and diagnosis codes.

21. DIAGNOSIS OR NATURE OF ILLNESS OR INJURY Relate A-L to service line below (24E) ICD Ind.

A.	B.	C.	D.
E.	F.	G.	H.
I.	J.	K.	L.

24. A. DATE(S) OF SERVICE From MM DD YY	To MM DD YY	B. PLACE OF SERVICE	C. EMG	D. PROCEDURES, SERVICES, OR SUPPLIES (Explain Unusual Circumstances) CPT/HCPCS	MODIFIER	E. DIAGNOSIS POINTER

Case Study 8.5

PATIENT: Eduardo Rodriguez

CHIEF COMPLAINT: Established patient is here for his 68-year annual physical examination. Patient is a current smoker.

HISTORY OF PRESENT ILLNESS: He is being seen for a health maintenance evaluation. General health since last visit described as good. Colorectal cancer screening includes fecal occult blood testing last year. Metabolic screening includes lipid profile within the past five years, glucose screening last year, and thyroid function test last year. Dental care includes a dental visit more than a year ago and dentures. Vision care includes an eye examination with the last year. Immunization status: flu immunization is needed. Current diet includes well-balanced meals. The patient is a current cigarette smoker.

REVIEW OF SYSTEMS:
Constitutional: not feeling poorly (malaise) and not feeling tired (fatigue)
ENT: no epistaxis
Gastrointestinal: no melena
The review of systems was otherwise negative

PAST, FAMILY, SOCIAL HISTORY:
Allergies: sulfa drugs
Medications: levothyroxine sodium 100 mcg oral tablet. Take one tablet by mouth daily.

EXAMINATION:
General: well developed; vital signs reviewed.
Eyes: sclera and conjunctiva were clear and lids symmetrical, pupils equal, round, and reactive to light.
ENT: external ears and nose are without deformity or lesions, no obvious dental caries, and the lips and gums appear healthy. Hearing was normal. Examination of the teeth revealed lower dentures and upper dentures.
Neck: no neck mass. The thyroid gland was not enlarged.
Cardiovascular: heart rate and rhythm were normal. No peripheral edema.
Pulmonary: auscultation clear with no wheezes, rhonchi, or rales, respiratory effort normal.
Abdomen: Soft, nontender, and without masses. No obvious hernias. Right fourth finger partial amputation, well-healed.
Skin: No rash, normal skin turgor.
Psychiatric: Oriented to person, place, and time, and insight and judgment were intact.

ASSESSMENT/PLAN:

1. Encounter for adult preventive health examination. Counseled on preventive care schedule. Encourage routine vision and dental care. Encourage healthy diet and regular exercises. Labs reviewed. Flu immunization in office today (inactivated [IIV], subunit, adjuvanted, intramuscular).
2. Hypothyroidism. Stable, continue current medications.
3. Anemia. Controlled since last visit. Repeat labs.
4. Elevated fasting blood sugar. Moderate, repeat labs.

SIGNED: Dr. Jean Obregon, MD

Select the appropriate codes for the case study.

1. ICD-10-CM code(s): ________________, ________________, ________________, ________________, ________________

2. CPT code(s): ________________, ________________, ________________

3. List the procedure and diagnosis codes on the CMS-1500 form. Be sure to correctly link the procedure and diagnosis codes.

21. DIAGNOSIS OR NATURE OF ILLNESS OR INJURY Relate A-L to service line below (24E)			ICD Ind.
A.	B.	C.	D.
E.	F.	G.	H.
I.	J.	K.	L.

	24. A. DATE(S) OF SERVICE From MM DD YY	To MM DD YY	B. PLACE OF SERVICE	C. EMG	D. PROCEDURES, SERVICES, OR SUPPLIES (Explain Unusual Circumstances) CPT/HCPCS	MODIFIER	E. DIAGNOSIS POINTER
1							
2							
3							

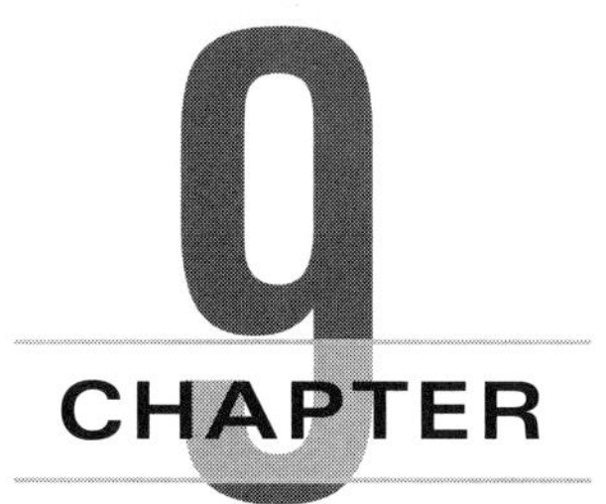

CHAPTER 9

Eye and Vision Services

Vocabulary

Instructions: Define each of the following key terms in the space provided.

1. Acquired condition: ______________________________

____

____

2. Comprehensive ophthalmological services: ______________________________

____

____

3. Cortical cataract: ______________________________

____

____

4. Enucleation: ______________________________

____

____

5. Evisceration: ______________________________

____

____

6. Exenteration: ____

____

____

7. Extracapsular cataract extraction (ECCE): ____

____

____

8. Glaucoma: ____

____

____

9. Gonio lens: ____

____

____

10. Intermediate ophthalmological services: ____

____

____

11. Intracapsular cataract extraction (ICCE): ____

____

____

12. Intraocular pressure: ____

____

____

13. Keratoplasty: ____

____

____

14. Lifestyle impairments: ____

____

____

15. Macular degeneration: ____

____

____

16. Nuclear cataract: ____

____

____

17. Ocular adnexa: ____

____

____

18. Ophthalmologist: ____

____

____

19. Ophthalmology: ____

____

____

20. Optometrist: ____

____

____

21. Optometry: ____

____

____

22. Paired organs: ____

____

____

23. Phacoemulsification: ____

____

____

24. Pseudophakia: ______________________________

____

____

25. Refraction: ______________________________

____

____

26. Refractive surgery: ______________________________

____

____

27. Retinal detachment: ______________________________

____

____

28. Slit lamp: ______________________________

____

____

29. Strabismus: ______________________________

____

____

30. Subcapsular cataract: ______________________________

____

____

31. Trabeculectomy: ______________________________

____

____

32. Vision insurance: ______________________________

____

____

Multiple Choice

Instructions: Choose the best answer.

1. Which of the following types of insurance covers routine eye wellness exams, contact lens fitting, and hardware and corrective lenses?
a. Behavioral health insurance
b. Health insurance
c. Vision insurance
d. Dental insurance

2. Which of the following services would be covered by health insurance rather than vision insurance?
a. Diagnostic screenings
b. Refraction
c. Injuries of the eye
d. Contact lens fitting

3. Which of the following includes the accessory structure of the eye, including the extraocular muscles, eyelids, and lacrimal system?
a. Ocular adnexa
b. Anterior segment
c. Extrinsic eye muscles
d. Posterior segment

4. Which of the following codes would be used to report an intermediate ophthalmological service provided to a new patient?
a. 92004
b. 92012
c. 92014
d. 92002

5. Which of the following codes would be used to report a comprehensive ophthalmological service provided to an established patient?
a. 92002
b. 92004
c. 92012
d. 92014

6. Which of the following types of codes would be used to report the supply provided to patients for corrective lenses?
a. HCPCS
b. CPT
c. ICD-10-CM
d. None, these items are not reported separately

7. Which of the following types of surgeries are performed to reshape the cornea and improve eye sight?
a. Trabeculectomy
b. Refractive surgeries
c. Gonioscopy
d. Goniotomy

8. Which of the following types of glaucoma is due to a narrow angle between the iris and cornea?
a. Open-angle
b. Angle-closure
c. Congenital
d. Secondary

9. If a patient is admitted for glaucoma, and the stage of the glaucoma evolves during admission, what should the coder do?
a. Assign the code for the highest stage of glaucoma documented.
b. Assign the code for the stage of glaucoma documented at admission.
c. Assign the code for the state of glaucoma documented at discharge.
d. Assign the one code for each stage of glaucoma documented.

10. Which of the following modifiers would be used to identify a procedure performed on the lower left eyelid?
a. E1
b. E2
c. E3
d. E4

Labeling

Instructions: Complete the following anatomical diagrams with the correct labels to identify the anatomy of the eye, eye muscles, and lacrimal apparatus.

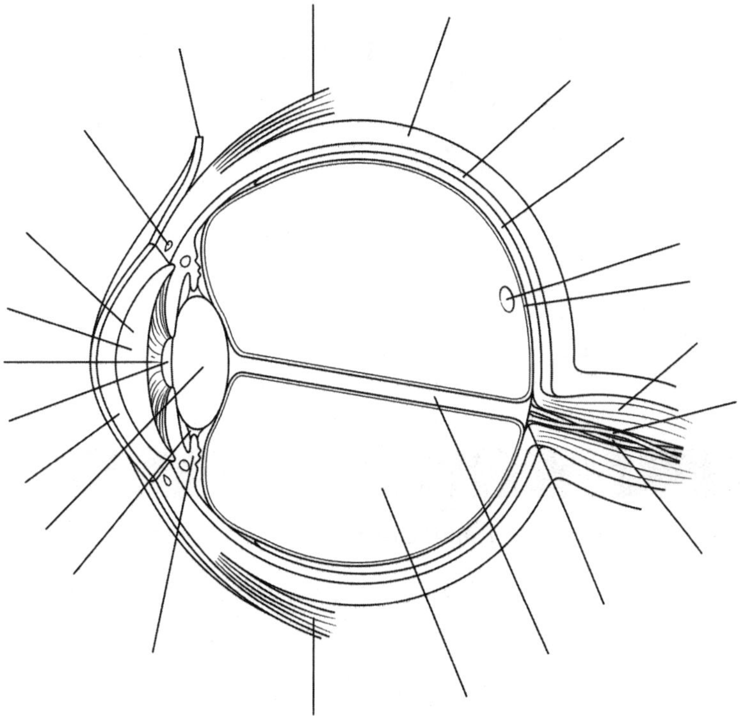

Source: ©AHIMA.

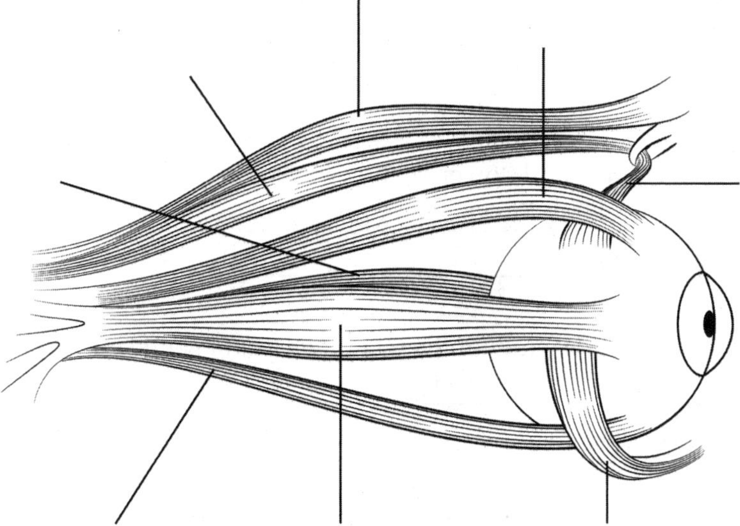

Source: ©AHIMA.

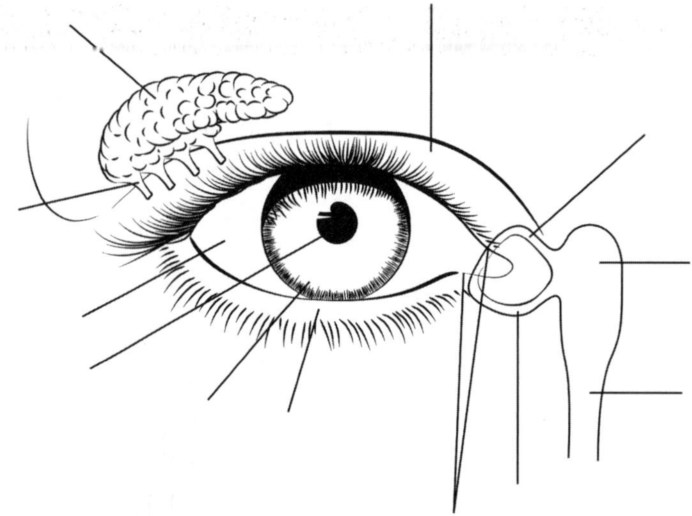

Source: ©AHIMA.

Coding

Instructions: Assign the correct CPT and ICD-10-CM codes for the following.

1. Code for the evisceration of ocular contents without subsequent implant due to chronic vitreous abscess of the right eye

CPT code(s): ____________-_____

ICD-10-CM code(s): ____________

2. Anterior removal of retained metallic foreign body of the posterior wall of the globe of the left eye via magnetic extraction

CPT code(s): ____________-_____

ICD-10-CM code(s): ____________, ____________

3. Bilateral correction of both lower eyelids via electrosurgery epilation

CPT code(s): ____________-_____, ____________-_____

ICD-10-CM code(s): ____________, ____________

4. Single-stage ICCE procedure of the bilateral eyes for senile nuclear cataracts

CPT code(s): ____________-_____

ICD-10-CM code(s): ____________

5. Repair of retinal detachment with single break of the right eye via photocoagulation

CPT code(s): ____________-_____

ICD-10-CM code(s): ____________

6. Bilateral fluorescein angiography with interpretation and report, performed on 56-year-old male with type 2 DM and stable prolific diabetic retinopathy of the bilateral eyes

CPT code(s): ____________

ICD-10-CM code(s): ____________

7. Ophthalmological services for new patient, intermediate; patient has presbyopia

CPT code(s): ____________

ICD-10-CM code(s): ____________

8. Fitting of contact lens for patient with stable keratoconus of the bilateral eyes; patient provided with two spherical gas-permeable contact lenses

CPT code(s): ____________

HCPCS code(s): ____________ × _____

ICD-10-CM code(s): ____________

9. Patient supplied with one pair of spectacle frames fitted with two lenses: trifocal sphere plano to 4.00d (right lens) and triphocal sphere plan to 6.50 (left lens) in patient with presbyopia

HCPCS code(s): ____________, ____________-_____, ____________-_____

ICD-10-CM code(s): ____________

10. Prescription of corneal lens for congenital aphakia of the right eye, with fitting provided by independent technician

CPT code(s): ____________-_____

ICD-10-CM code(s): ____________

11. Type II diabetes with mild nonproliferative retinopathy without macular edema of bilateral eyes with diabetic cataract of the left eye. On long-term use of insulin. Patient also has lupus erythematosus.

ICD-10-CM code(s): ____________, ____________, ____________, ____________

12. An 80-year-old female patient presents for evaluation of senile nuclear cataracts of the bilateral eyes and macular degeneration of the right eye.

ICD-10-CM code(s): ____________, ____________

13. Established patient presents to the office for evaluation of pseudomembranous conjunctivitis of the bilateral eyes. EPF history and examination with low-complexity MDM.

CPT code(s): ____________

ICD-10-CM code(s): ____________

14. A 42-year-old male patient presents for evaluation of his acute angle-closure glaucoma and transient myopia, which was caused by topiramate (Topamax) taken for epilepsy and migraines.

ICD-10-CM code(s): ____________, ____________, ____________, ____________, ____________

15. Patient with benign essential hypertension and long-term simvastatin use is being evaluated for diplopia.

ICD-10-CM code(s): ____________, ____________, ____________

Case Studies Eye and Vision Services

Case Study 9.1

PATIENT: Roger Roberts

CHIEF COMPLAINT: Six-month glaucoma evaluation

HISTORY OF PRESENT ILLNESS: Established patient presents today for an evaluation of glaucoma OU. Patient reports stable visual assessments since his last visit. Denies any pain, pressure, or irritation. Patient compliant with medication and testing. Need refill on Brimonidine Tartrate. Denies any other physical ocular symptoms.

REVIEW OF SYSTEMS:
Constitutional: no problems
Eyes: eyesight problems

CURRENT MEDS:

1. Brimonidien Tartrate 0.2% ophthalmic solution
2. Dozolamide HCl/Timolol Mal 22.3-6.8 mg/ml ophthalmic solution. One drop into both eyes daily.
3. Latanoprost 0.005% ophthalmic solution; I gtt OU qhs

ALLERGIES:

1. Oxycodone–Acetaminophen tabs
2. Vicodin tabs

EXAMINATION:
General: alert and in no acute distress
Neurological: the patient was oriented to person, place, and time. Mood and affect were appropriate.

SCANNING COMPUTERIZED OPHTHALMIC IMAGING (POSTERIOR SEGMENT):

	OD (right eye)	OS (left eye)
Visual field	Full	Full
Pupils	Normal. No afferent pupil defect. Pupil reacts to light.	Normal. No afferent pupil defect. Pupil reacts to light.
Lids	Eyelid normal	Eyelid normal
Conjunctiva	Clear	Clear
Cornea	Clear	Clear
Lens	NS 2+	NS 2+
Ocular Motility	Extraocular movements intact. Primary gaze orthotropic. Motility full.	Extraocular movements intact. Primary gaze orthotropic. Motility full.
Anterior chamber	Clear	Clear
Intraocular pressure	17 mmHg	17 mmHg
Iris	Normal	Normal
Retina	No holes, breaks, or tears	No holes, breaks, or tears
Optic nerve	Optic disc normal. Cupping 1+.	Optic disc normal. Cupping 2+. Sloping OS
Macula	Normal. No macular edema. No macular hemorrhage.	Normal. No macular edema. No macular hemorrhage.
Vitreous	Intact	Intact

ASSESSMENT/PLAN:

1. Primary open-angle glaucoma of both eyes, severe stage. Progressing. Additional treatment options discussed in detail today. After being able to ask questions and have them answered to his satisfaction, patient denies surgical treatment at this time. Patient to return to clinic in three months for intraocular pressure (IOP) check.
2. Diabetes mellitus with glaucoma. Patient was instructed on optimizing diabetes control in order to minimize the development of diabetic retinopathy.
3. Nuclear sclerotic cataract of both eyes. Not visually significant. Discussion and education about cataract. Will recheck in six months or as desired.

SIGNED: Dr. Hugh C. Mee, MD

Select the appropriate codes for the case study.

1. List the ICD-10-CM code(s):

   ICD-10-CM code(s): ________________, ________________, ________________
2. List the CPT/HCPCS code(s) and any applicable modifiers:

   CPT code(s): ________________ - _____, ________________

3. List the procedure and diagnosis codes on the CMS 1500 form. Be sure to correctly link the procedure and diagnosis codes.

21. DIAGNOSIS OR NATURE OF ILLNESS OR INJURY Relate A-L to service line below (24E) ICD Ind.

A.	B.	C.	D.
E.	F.	G.	H.
I.	J.	K.	L.

	24. A. DATE(S) OF SERVICE From MM	DD	YY	To MM	DD	YY	B. PLACE OF SERVICE	C. EMG	D. PROCEDURES, SERVICES, OR SUPPLIES (Explain Unusual Circumstances) CPT/HCPCS	MODIFIER	E. DIAGNOSIS POINTER
1											
2											
3											

Case Study 9.2

PATIENT: Roger Roberts

DATE OF PROCEDURE: 09/19/20XX

TIME: 1550

INDICATIONS: Primary open-angle glaucoma of both eyes, severe stage. Left eye more severe. Treatment today aimed at left eye only.

PROCEDURE: SELECTIVE LASER TRABECULOPLASTY
Eye treated: left eye
Power: 0.9–1.0
Bursts: 100
Lens Used: 360°
Comments: patient tolerated the procedure well. No complications.

Laser postprocedure orders:

1. Rinse eye if Goniosol is used
2. Take postoperative vitals
3. Meds: none
4. There should not be much, if any, pain
5. If there is intense pain, or for other concerns, please call the eye clinic during the day. In emergencies or after hours, please call the after-hours provider line.
6. Follow-up appointment on 11/06/20XX

SIGNED: Dr. Hugh C. Mee, MD

Select the appropriate codes for the case study.

1. List the ICD-10-CM code(s):

ICD-10-CM code(s): ________________

2. List the CPT/HCPCS code(s) and any applicable modifiers:

CPT code(s): ________________

3. List the procedure and diagnosis codes on the CMS-1500 form. Be sure to correctly link the procedure and diagnosis codes.

21. DIAGNOSIS OR NATURE OF ILLNESS OR INJURY Relate A-L to service line below (24E) ICD Ind.

A.	B.	C.	D.
E.	F.	G.	H.
I.	J.	K.	L.

	24. A. DATE(S) OF SERVICE From MM	DD	YY	To MM	DD	YY	B. PLACE OF SERVICE	C. EMG	D. PROCEDURES, SERVICES, OR SUPPLIES (Explain Unusual Circumstances) CPT/HCPCS	MODIFIER	E. DIAGNOSIS POINTER
1											
2											
3											

Case Study 9.3

PATIENT: Roger Roberts

REASON FOR VISIT: Follow-up visual field examination.

INDICATIONS: Primary open-angle glaucoma of both eyes, severe stage.

PROCEDURE: Visual field examination; extended (documentation in chart).

DISCUSSION/SUMMARY: Patient is here for HFV 24-2 Sita fast follow-up. Trial lens used today was OD: +1.75 and OS: +2.75. Patient had no problems with fixation light. Very unusual and concerning change in visual field. The right eye has a few interior depressed points that have appeared previously. The left eye has very dense diffuse loss that has progressed from 2015 and from earlier in the year. Because of the asymmetry, I am considering the possibility of imaging. Intraocular pressure is 11 in both eyes, and this is following selective laser trabeculoplasty. I have some concerns about adherence to medical treatment. Again, this is concerning and will require follow-up and discussion with patient.

SIGNED: Dr. Hugh C. Mee, MD

Select the appropriate codes for the case study.

1. List the ICD-10-CM code(s):

   ICD-10-CM code(s): ________________

2. List the CPT/HCPCS code(s) and any applicable modifiers:

   CPT code(s): ________________

3. List the procedure and diagnosis codes on the CMS-1500 form. Be sure to correctly link the procedure and diagnosis codes.

21. DIAGNOSIS OR NATURE OF ILLNESS OR INJURY Relate A-L to service line below (24E) ICD Ind.

A. ______	B. ______	C. ______	D. ______
E. ______	F. ______	G. ______	H. ______
I. ______	J. ______	K. ______	L. ______

	24. A. DATE(S) OF SERVICE From MM	DD	YY	To MM	DD	YY	B. PLACE OF SERVICE	C. EMG	D. PROCEDURES, SERVICES, OR SUPPLIES (Explain Unusual Circumstances) CPT/HCPCS	MODIFIER	E. DIAGNOSIS POINTER
1											
2											
3											

Case Study 9.4

PATIENT: Roger Roberts

DATE OF PROCEDURE: 02/05/20XX

PREOPERATIVE DIAGNOSIS: Primary open-angle glaucoma, severe stage, left eye

POSTOPERATIVE DIAGNOSIS: same

PROCEDURE: XEN GEL STENT IMPLANTATION: Insertion of aqueous drainage device, without extraocular reservoir, internal approach, into the subconjunctival space; initial device.

ANESTHESIA: Peribulbar block

COMPLICATIONS: none

PROCEDURE DESCRIPTION:
A time-out was performed, and the correct patient, correct site, and correct procedure was confirmed. The eye was prepped with betadine solution and draped in a sterile fashion. A subconjunctival injection of MMC mixed with lidocaine was injected superotemporally and moved to the superonasal quadrant with cotton tip applicators and pushed away from the limbus. Calipers were used to make superotemporal target area. A paracentesis was made nasally, and the anterior chamber was filled

with preservative free lidocaine. The anterior chamber was then filled with viscoelastic. A main wound was then made 1 mm into clear cornea, temporally angled toward the target quadrant. The Xen implant was confirmed in the injector under the microscope and placed into the eye. A gonioprism was placed on the eye and the needle seated anterior to the scleral spur. The needle was passed through the sclera underneath the conjunctiva in the quadrant area. The Xen implant was deployed with 1 mm remaining in the anterior chamber. The implant was mobile underneath the conjunctiva. The viscoelastic was irrigated from the anterior chamber using BSS on a cannula. There was a forming blen around the Xen implant. Wounds were checked and found to be watertight. Anterior chamber was deep and at physiologic pressure. The eye was then patched and covered with a fox shield. The patient tolerated the procedure well.

SIGNED: Dr. Hugh C. Mee, MD

Select the appropriate codes for the case study.

1. List the ICD-10-CM code(s):

   ICD-10-CM code(s): ________________

2. List the CPT/HCPCS code(s) and any applicable modifiers:

   CPT code(s): ________________ - _____

3. List the procedure and diagnosis codes on the CMS-1500 form. Be sure to correctly link the procedure and diagnosis codes.

21. DIAGNOSIS OR NATURE OF ILLNESS OR INJURY Relate A-L to service line below (24E) ICD Ind.

A.	B.	C.	D.
E.	F.	G.	H.
I.	J.	K.	L.

	24. A. DATE(S) OF SERVICE From MM	DD	YY	To MM	DD	YY	B. PLACE OF SERVICE	C. EMG	D. PROCEDURES, SERVICES, OR SUPPLIES (Explain Unusual Circumstances) CPT/HCPCS	MODIFIER	E. DIAGNOSIS POINTER
1											
2											
3											

Case Study 9.5

PATIENT: Roger Roberts

CHIEF COMPLAINT: One-day follow up from gel stent implant

HISTORY OF PRESENT ILLNESS: One-day post-op Xen gel implantation, doing well. Good stent filter and acceptable intraocular pressure. Topical steroid and antibiotic.

EXAMINATION:
Distance uncorrected: OS20/-; OD 20/200
Conjunctiva: good bleb.
Lens: OS lens pseudophakia
Anterior chamber: OS cell grade tr+
Intraocular pressure: OS intraocular pressure 14 mmHg

ASSESSMENT/PLAN:

1. Primary open-angle glaucoma, severe stage, left eye. One-day post-op, doing well. Follow-up next week for medication adjustments.

SIGNED: Dr. Hugh C. Mee, MD

Select the appropriate codes for the case study.

1. List the ICD-10-CM code(s):
   ICD-10-CM code(s): ________________
2. List the CPT/HCPCS code(s) and any applicable modifiers:
   CPT code(s): ________________
3. List the procedure and diagnosis codes on the CMS-1500 form. Be sure to correctly link the procedure and diagnosis codes.

21. DIAGNOSIS OR NATURE OF ILLNESS OR INJURY Relate A-L to service line below (24E) ICD Ind.

A.	B.	C.	D.
E.	F.	G.	H.
I.	J.	K.	L.

	24. A. DATE(S) OF SERVICE From MM DD YY	To MM DD YY	B. PLACE OF SERVICE	C. EMG	D. PROCEDURES, SERVICES, OR SUPPLIES (Explain Unusual Circumstances) CPT/HCPCS	MODIFIER	E. DIAGNOSIS POINTER
1							
2							
3							

Chapter 10

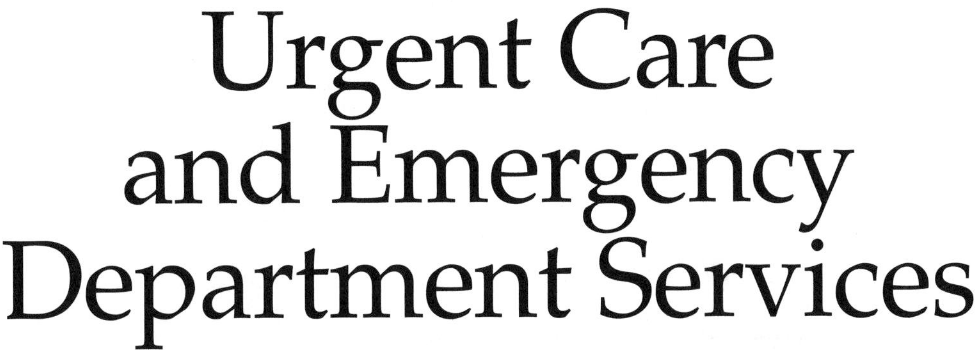

Urgent Care and Emergency Department Services

Vocabulary

Instructions: Define each of the following key terms in the space provided.

1. Appendicitis: ______________________________

____

____

2. Burn codes: ______________________________

____

____

3. Cardiopulmonary resuscitation (CPR): ______________________________

____

____

4. Closed procedure: ______________________________

____

____

5. Corrosion: ______________________________

____

____

6. Dislocation reduction: ______________________________

____

____

7. Emergency services: ______________________________

____

____

8. Emergent: ______________________________

____

____

9. Endotracheal intubation: ______________________________

____

____

10. Foreign body (FB): ______________________________

____

____

11. Hemothorax: ______________________________

____

____

12. Incision and drainage (I&D): ______________________________

____

____

13. Lumbar puncture: ______________________________

____

____

14. Lund-Browder classification: ______________________________

____

____

15. Moderate (conscious) sedation: ______________________________

____

____

16. Motor vehicle accident (MVA): ______________________________

____

____

17. Myocardial infarction: ______________________________

____

____

18. Nasal packing: ______________________________

____

____

19. Open procedure: ______________________________

____

____

20. Oximetry: ______________________________

____

____

21. Penetrating wound: ______________________________

____

____

22. Pleural effusion: ______________________________

____

____

23. Pneumothorax: ______________________________

____

____

24. Professional component: ____

____

____

25. Rule of nines: ____

____

____

26. Sepsis: ____

____

____

27. Septic shock: ____

____

____

28. Systemic inflammatory response syndrome (SIRS): ______________________

____

____

29. Technical component: ____

____

____

30. Thoracostomy: ____

____

____

31. Tracheostomy: ____

____

____

32. Tracheotomy: ____

____

____

33. Urgent care: ______________________________

____

____

Multiple Choice

Instructions: Choose the best answer.

1. If an emergency service is not indicated as "Y" for emergency in box 24.C of the CMS-1500 claim form, which of the following things might happen?
   a. The service will require a prior authorization before it can be performed.
   b. The patient will have to wait until the next business day to receive the procedure.
   c. The insurance company may not pay for the service.
   d. The insurance will pay for the service; this box is for informational purposes only.

2. If an urgent care center does not have the resources to treat a patient's medical condition, what might the urgent care center do?
   a. Call an ambulance to transport the patient to the emergency department.
   b. Call the patient's family to come and take the patient home.
   c. Call the patient's primary care provider to make an appointment.
   d. Provide as much care as possible and then discharge the patient.

3. Which of the following types of urgent care procedures involves the use of diagnostic procedures to test patient specimens?
   a. X-rays and imaging procedures
   b. Laboratory tests
   c. Wound repair
   d. Oximetry

4. Which of the following ECG procedures describes only the technical component of the procedure?
   a. 93000
   b. 93005
   c. 93010
   d. No ECG codes describe only the technical components of the procedure

5. Which of the following types of wound repair includes layered closure of one or more deeper layers of subcutaneous tissue?
   a. Simple
   b. Complex
   c. Complete
   d. Intermediate

6. Which of the following are the three components of wound repair procedure codes?
a. Site, depth, and extent
b. Complexity, site, and length
c. Length, site, and area
d. Depth, width, and complexity

7. Which of the following procedure codes identifies an emergency procedure in which a tube is inserted through the mouth and into the trachea?
a. 31500
b. 31603
c. 31605
d. 31600

8. Which of the following external causes of injury codes identifies what the patient was doing when the injury occurred?
a. External cause status
b. Injury mechanism
c. Place of occurrence
d. Patient activity

9. Sepsis is considered severe sepsis when it presents with which of the following?
a. Acute organ failure
b. Septicemia
c. Systemic inflammatory response syndrome (SIRS)
d. Septic shock

10. Which of the following divides the body's surface into differing percentage based on the age of the patient?
a. Rule of nines
b. Extent of the burn
c. Lund-Browder classification
d. Corrosive classification system

Completion

Instructions: Complete the following flowchart with the decision process for when to code signs and symptoms versus a definitive diagnosis.

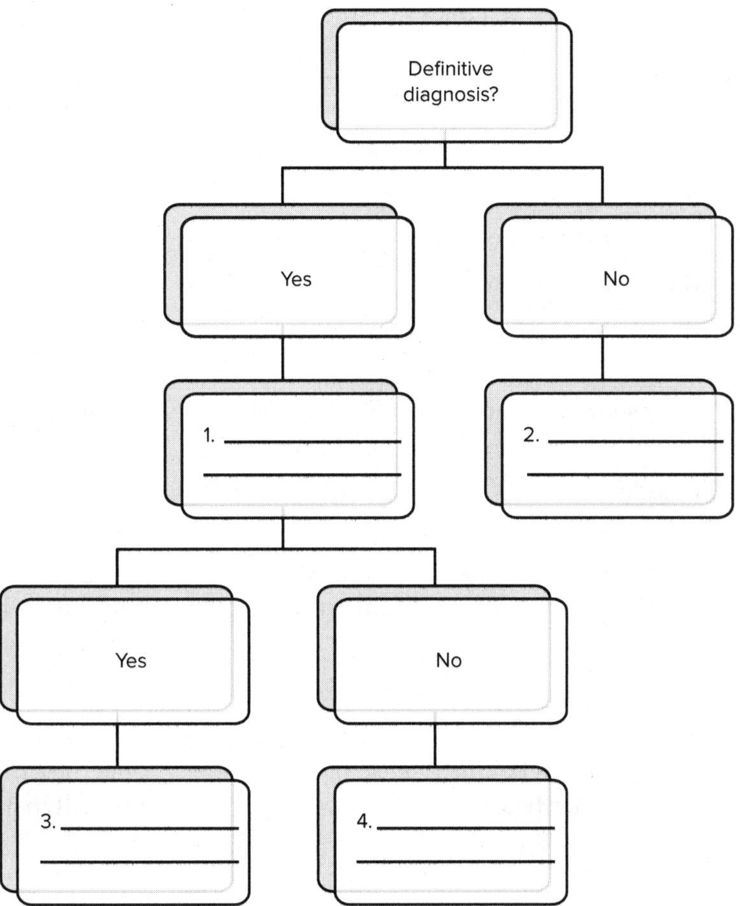

Coding

Instructions: Assign the correct CPT and ICD-10-CM codes for the following.

1. 43-year-old patient presents to the emergency department with sepsis of unknown infectious origin, experiencing acute respiratory failure without septic shock. Provider completes a detailed history, comprehensive examination, and high-complexity MDM.

CPT code(s): ________________

ICD-10-CM code(s): ________________, ________________, ________________

2. A 14-year-old male patient presents to the ED after having suffered burns to both hands, arms, and chest. Burns are as follows: second-degree burns of bilateral hands, 6 percent TBSA; second-degree burns of the bilateral forearms, 6 percent TBSA; second-degree burn of upper chest, 10 percent TBSA; also has a small area of third-degree burn on the left cheek, approximately 1 percent TBSA. ED provider performed a detailed history and examination with moderate complexity MDM.

   CPT code(s): _______________

   ICD-10-CM code(s) for burns of hands: _______________, _______________

   ICD-10-CM code(s) for burns of forearms: _______________, _______________

   ICD-10-CM code for burn of chest: _______________

   ICD-10-CM code for burn of face: _______________

   ICD-10-CM code for total body surface area: _______________

3. Patient XYZ presents with acute non-ST anterior wall MI. Patient also has atrial fibrillation.

   ICD-10-CM code(s): _______________

4. Patient XYZ returns two weeks later with acute anterior wall STEMI. Still under care for her initial MI that occurred two weeks ago and continues to have A Fib.

   ICD-10-CM code(s): _______________

5. Patient XYZ returns to the ED three months after her last heart attack, this time complaining of an overwhelming sense of dread. She is concerned that she is experiencing another heart attack. All tests are negative for MI; patient is diagnosed with panic attack.

   ICD-10-CM code(s): _______________, _______________

6. 18-year-old female presents to ED complaining of severe RLQ pain. Computed tomography of abdomen without contrast reveals enlarged appendix. Clinical impression: acute appendicitis. Expanded problem-focused history and examination, MDM of low complexity.

   CPT code(s): _______________, _______________

   ICD-10-CM code(s): _______________

7. Patient presents with multiple open wounds, which were closed as follows: intermediate repair of 4 cm laceration of right chest wall (no penetration into thoracic cavity); complex 2 cm repair of puncture wound of right abdomen (left upper quadrant, no puncture of peritoneal cavity); intermediate repair of two 3 cm lacerations of the left forearm, and simple repair of 1 cm laceration of the left hand. (Tip: When sequencing, remember to sequence the most complex repairs first, and to use a modifier to identify that additional repairs were distinct procedural services.)

   CPT code(s): _______________, _______________-______,
   _______________-______

ICD-10-CM code(s): ______________, ______________, ______________,
____

8. 18-year-old male patient presents to the urgent care clinic in the evening hours on a weekday complaining of trouble breathing after a soccer match. He has a history of exercise-induced asthma, which is mostly controllable with a rescue inhaler, but he is currently experiencing shortness of breath, wheezing, and faintness. Pulse oximetry performed in the office reveals oxygen level of 89, and patient states that he has used his rescue inhaler three times in the last two hours with no relief. Inhaled pressurized nebulizer treatment administered in clinic. Physician documented a comprehensive history, comprehensive examination, and high-complexity MDM for this new patient encounter. Clinical impression: exercise-induced bronchospasm. (Tip: Use additional codes to identify that the service was performed during regularly scheduled evening hours as well as the HCPCS code to identify that the service was performed in an urgent care center.)

CPT code(s): ______________-______, ______________, ______________,
______________, ______________

ICD-10-CM code(s): ______________

9. 27-year-old established female presents to the urgent care clinic during normal working hours complaining of nausea, vomiting, and lethargy. After a detailed history, expanded problem-focused examination, and MDM of low complexity, the provider diagnoses the patient with acute gastroenteritis. Patient also elects to get the flu mist nasal vaccine (LAIV3) while in the office, which is administered at the time of the encounter.

CPT code(s): ______________-______
______________, ______________, ______________

ICD-10-CM code(s): ______________

10. Transtracheal tracheostomy performed emergently in the ED for patient with laryngeal fracture.

CPT code(s): ______________

ICD-10-CM code(s): ______________

11. Simple repair of a two-inch laceration on the right forearm.

CPT code(s): ______________

ICD-10-CM code(s): ______________

12. 45-year-old female suffered second-degree burns to her face and shoulder when she was splashed with flaming liquid from a flambé dessert. While at a business dinner, the waiter accidentally poured too much alcohol in the pan, and it splashed her shoulder and hair as it caught flames at the tableside. She has second-degree burns over 8 percent of her body surface, mostly on the left side of her face and neck and on her left shoulder.

ICD-10-CM code(s): ______________, ______________, ______________,
______________, ______________, ______________, ______________

13. 42-year-old male presents to the ED complaining of burns on both of his feet. On his day off from work, he was using a pressure washer to clean his driveway in front of his house in bare feet when he noticed that his feet had gotten dirty, so he sprayed the tops of both of his feet with the pressure washer, causing immediate second-degree burns on the tops of both of his feet (approximately 2 percent of total body surface).

ICD-10-CM code(s): ________________, ________________, ________________, ________________, ________________, ________________, ________________

14. Provider performed a comprehensive history and physical examination on an established 70-year-old male patient encounter with high MDM. During the visit, IV access was started, and the patient was given three separate pushes of morphine (10 mg each) and one push of Zofran (1 mg). Patient was also given a Tdap vaccine in clinic. (List out all procedures separately.)

CPT code(s): ________________, ________________, ________________, ________________, ________________, ________________, ________________, ________________

HCPCS codes(s): ________________, ________________, ________________, ________________

15. 35-year-old male presents to the urgent care clinic complaining of fever, headache, and nausea. Provider performs an evaluation and management encounter with moderate MDM and a rapid COVID-screening (Infectious agent detection by nucleic acid (DNA or RNA); COVID-19, amplified probe technique), which is negative.

CPT code(s): ________________, ________________

ICD-10-CM code(s): ________________, ________________, ________________, ________________

16. A 64-year-old female presented to the urgent care clinic complaining of severe headache, body aches, and fever. She was recently at a party at which she suspects that she was exposed to COVID-19. The nurse practitioner performed a rapid COVID swab in the office (Infectious agent detection by nucleic acid (DNA or RNA); COVID-19, amplified probe technique), which revealed that the patient was positive for COVID-19. NP documented that 32 minutes of total time were spent on this encounter on the date of service.

CPT code(s): ________________, ________________

ICD-10-CM code(s): ________________

Case Studies Urgent Care and Emergency Department Encounters

Case Study 10.1

Emergency Department Treatment Log

PATIENT: Douglas Kaiser

DATE OF SERVICE: 11/16/20XX

SUBJECTIVE:
F/u cellulitis RLE.
All resolved with residual knot in the medial aspect of the right knee where all problems seem to have emanated. No other pains, fever, sweats, or chills. No edema reported. Continues to take erythromycin (last two days).

OBJECTIVE:
Zero erythema. 3-cm hard area on the right proximal medial tibia. Zero edema. No additional skin abnormalities. Not directly tender. Full range of motion (ROM) at right knee.

ASSESSMENT and PLAN:

1. RLE cellulitis (resolving). Unknown etiology. Continue medication regimen and return if pain, redness, swelling, or symptoms return.
2. Allergy to penicillin.

SIGNED: Dr. Alejandro Jaramillo, MD

Select the appropriate codes for the case study.

1. List the ICD-10-CM code(s):
   ICD-10-CM code(s): __________, __________
2. List the CPT/HCPCS code(s) and any applicable modifiers:
   CPT code(s): __________
3. List the procedure and diagnosis codes on the CMS-1500 form. Be sure to correctly link the procedure and diagnosis codes.

21. DIAGNOSIS OR NATURE OF ILLNESS OR INJURY Relate A-L to service line below (24E) ICD Ind.

A.	B.	C.	D.
E.	F.	G.	H.
I.	J.	K.	L.

	24. A. DATE(S) OF SERVICE From MM	DD	YY	To MM	DD	YY	B. PLACE OF SERVICE	C. EMG	D. PROCEDURES, SERVICES, OR SUPPLIES (Explain Unusual Circumstances) CPT/HCPCS	MODIFIER	E. DIAGNOSIS POINTER
1											
2											
3											

Case Study 10.2

Emergency Department Treatment Log

PATIENT: Holland Young

DATE OF SERVICE: 04/26/20XX

SUBJECTIVE:
25-year-old male presents complaining to "flash burn" to left arm and forehead, which occurred approximately 20 minutes ago while he was at work. He states that he was lighting a tar kettle and it "coughed back" onto his forehead and outstretched arms. Patient was burned with flames as no tar landed on his bare skin. Pain is currently at 5/10.

OBJECTIVE:
Approximately 7% total body surface burn. 4% second-degree burns to bilateral forearms. 2% first-degree burns along forehead and bridge of nose. Also 1% first-degree burn to left forearm. Lung examination normal—no carbonaceous particles noted in airway.

ASSESSMENT and PLAN:

1. First- and second-degree burns to face and forearms, not exceeding 7% TBS. Apply wet-to-dry dressing for approximately 30 minutes, then light dressing. Refer to MD for narcotic therapy. Tylenol #3 PO now. Follow up in ER in one day.

SIGNED: Dr. Alejandro Jaramillo, MD

Select the appropriate codes for the case study.

1. List the ICD-10-CM code(s):
   ICD-10-CM code(s): ________, ________, ________,
   ________, ________, ________, ________
2. List the CPT/HCPCS code(s) and any applicable modifiers:
   CPT code(s): ________
3. List the procedure and diagnosis codes on the CMS-1500 form. Be sure to correctly link the procedure and diagnosis codes.

21. DIAGNOSIS OR NATURE OF ILLNESS OR INJURY Relate A-L to service line below (24E) ICD Ind.

A.	B.	C.	D.
E.	F.	G.	H.
I.	J.	K.	L.

	24. A. DATE(S) OF SERVICE From MM	DD	YY	To MM	DD	YY	B. PLACE OF SERVICE	C. EMG	D. PROCEDURES, SERVICES, OR SUPPLIES (Explain Unusual Circumstances) CPT/HCPCS	MODIFIER	E. DIAGNOSIS POINTER
1											
2											
3											

Case Study 10.3

Emergency Department Treatment Log

PATIENT: Douglas Kaiser

DATE OF SERVICE: 04/27/20XX

SUBJECTIVE:
25-year-old male presents for follow-up. Flash burns suffered yesterday to forearms and face. Patient states the areas are tender and throb mildly. No shortness of breath or coughing. Tetanus is up to date. Patient burned while at work lighting tar kettle and flames coughed back up into his face.

OBJECTIVE:
Burned areas are still tender to the touch. All skin is viable. 4% shallow second-degree burn to left forearm. Not circumferential. Small first-degree burn to bridge of nose.

ASSESSMENT and PLAN:

1. 4% second-degree burn on bilateral forearms. Continue Silvadene applications. Erythromycin 250 QID × 4 days prophylaxis. Continue Tylenol #3 as needed. Dry gauze dressing. Limit work duty for 3–5 days.

SIGNED: Dr. Alejandro Jaramillo, MD

Select the appropriate codes for the case study.

1. List the ICD-10-CM code(s):
   ICD-10-CM code(s): ________________, ________________, ________________,
   ________________, ________________, ________________
2. List the CPT/HCPCS code(s) and any applicable modifiers:
   CPT code(s): ________________
3. List the procedure and diagnosis codes on the CMS-1500 form. Be sure to correctly link the procedure and diagnosis codes.

21. DIAGNOSIS OR NATURE OF ILLNESS OR INJURY Relate A-L to service line below (24E) ICD Ind.

A.	B.	C.	D.
E.	F.	G.	H.
I.	J.	K.	L.

	24. A. DATE(S) OF SERVICE From MM	DD	YY	To MM	DD	YY	B. PLACE OF SERVICE	C. EMG	D. PROCEDURES, SERVICES, OR SUPPLIES (Explain Unusual Circumstances) CPT/HCPCS	MODIFIER	E. DIAGNOSIS POINTER
1											
2											
3											

Case Study 10.1

Urgent Care Office Visit Summary

PATIENT: Jorge Canales

DATE OF SERVICE: 02/17/20XX

SUBJECTIVE:
23-year-old male was working in a crane and attempted to throw an empty glass bottle out of the cab. Bottle hit the door frame and shattered. A piece of glass cut his right thumb. Tetanus UTD.

OBJECTIVE:
Distal phalanx (R thumb) volar surface with deep avulsion-type laceration. No pulsatile bleeding.

WOUND REPAIR:
Wound exploration: Administered anesthesia with total 8 cc 1% lidocaine/0.25% Marcaine. Wound explored to subcutaneous fat layer.
Wound repair: Additional anesthesia of 3 cc used. Irrigated with 1000 cc of sterile saline. Sutured with eight 5.0 nylon sutures on one layer. No complications. Bacitracin with tube gauze applied. Approx. 2.5 wound repaired.

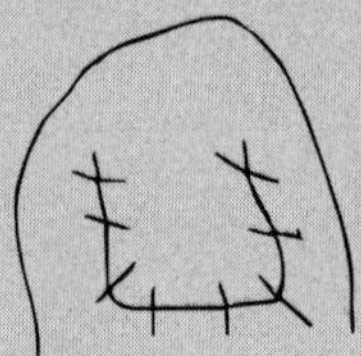

X-RAY:
Right thumb (two views), no foreign body particles seen.

ASSESSMENT and PLAN:

1. Laceration right thumb. Return in one week for suture removal. If otherwise sick, call clinic. Gave patient wound instruction sheet.

SIGNED: Dr. Alejandro Jaramillo, MD

Select the appropriate codes for the case study:

1. List the ICD-10-CM code(s):
   ICD-10-CM code(s): ________________, ________________, ________________
2. List the CPT/HCPCS code(s) and any applicable modifiers:
   CPT code(s): ________________, ________________

3. List the procedure and diagnosis codes on the CMS-1500 form. Be sure to correctly link the procedure and diagnosis codes.

21. DIAGNOSIS OR NATURE OF ILLNESS OR INJURY Relate A-L to service line below (24E) ICD Ind.

A.	B.	C.	D.
E.	F.	G.	H.
I.	J.	K.	L.

	24. A. DATE(S) OF SERVICE From MM	DD	YY	To MM	DD	YY	B. PLACE OF SERVICE	C. EMG	D. PROCEDURES, SERVICES, OR SUPPLIES (Explain Unusual Circumstances) CPT/HCPCS	MODIFIER	E. DIAGNOSIS POINTER
1											
2											
3											

Case Study 10.5

Urgent Care Office Visit Summary

PATIENT: Jorge Canales

DATE OF SERVICE: 02/29/20XX

SUBJECTIVE:
RTC to clinic today for removal of stitches. Patient was seen 12 days ago for wound repair. He suffered laceration from shattered glass bottle while at work. No pain, no additional symptoms. No other concerns.

OBJECTIVE:
Distal phalanx (R thumb) volar surface horseshoe-shaped wound with eight stitches intact. Appears well healed. Removed all eight sutures without complication.

ASSESSMENT and PLAN:

1. Laceration right thumb; well healed.

SIGNED: Dr. Alejandro Jaramillo, MD

Select the appropriate codes for the case study.

1. List the ICD-10-CM code(s):

ICD-10-CM code(s): ________________, ________________

2. List the CPT/HCPCS code(s) and any applicable modifiers:

CPT code(s): ________________

3. List the procedure and diagnosis codes on the CMS-1500 form. Be sure to correctly link the procedure and diagnosis codes.

21. DIAGNOSIS OR NATURE OF ILLNESS OR INJURY Relate A-L to service line below (24E) ICD Ind.

A.	B.	C.	D.
E.	F.	G.	H.
I.	J.	K.	L.

	24. A. DATE(S) OF SERVICE From MM	DD	YY	To MM	DD	YY	B. PLACE OF SERVICE	C. EMG	D. PROCEDURES, SERVICES, OR SUPPLIES (Explain Unusual Circumstances) CPT/HCPCS	MODIFIER	E. DIAGNOSIS POINTER
1											
2											
3											

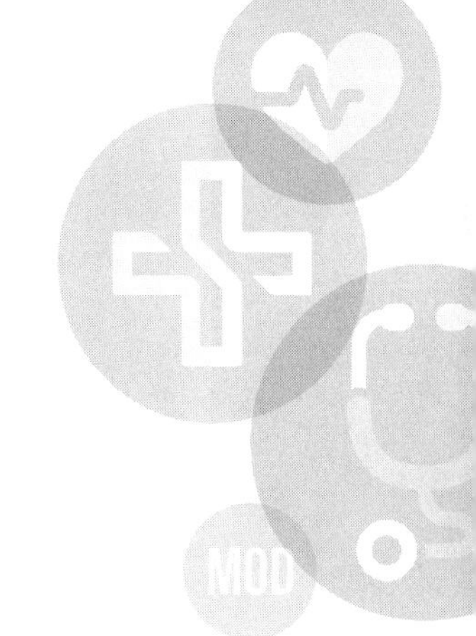

11 CHAPTER

Surgical Services

Vocabulary

Instructions: Define each of the following key terms in the space provided.

1. Ablation: ______

2. Admitting provider: ______

3. Allograft: ______

4. Ambulatory surgical center (ASC): ______

5. Appendectomy: ______

6. Appendicitis: ______________________________

____

____

7. Autograft: ______________________________

____

____

8. Block: ______________________________

____

____

9. Cadaver donor: ______________________________

____

____

10. Cholangiography: ______________________________

____

____

11. Cholangitis: ______________________________

____

____

12. Cholecystectomy: ______________________________

____

____

13. Cholecystitis: ______________________________

____

____

14. Choledocholithiasis: ______________________________

____

____

15. Cholelithiasis: ______________________________

____

____

16. Code edit: ______________________________

____

____

17. Comorbid condition: ______________________________

____

____

18. Complication of care: ______________________________

____

____

19. Debridement: ______________________________

____

____

20. Destruction: ______________________________

____

____

21. Diagnostic procedure: ______________________________

____

____

22. Diaphragm: ______________________________

____

____

23. Endoscopy: ______________________________

____

____

24. Excised diameter: ______________________________

25. Excision: ______________________________

26. Global period: ______________________________

27. Global surgical package: ______________________________

28. Homograft: ______________________________

29. Incidental appendectomy: ______________________________

30. Incision: ______________________________

31. Introduction: ______________________________

32. Laparoscopy: ______________________________

33. Living donor: ____

____

____

34. Manipulation: ____

____

____

35. Margin: ____

____

____

36. Mediastinum: ____

____

____

37. Mohs micrographic surgery: ____

____

____

38. National Correct Coding Initiative (NCCI): ____

____

____

39. Never events: ____

____

____

40. Nonpressure ulcer: ____

____

____

41. Outpatient: ____

____

____

42. Outpatient hospital: ______________________________

____

____

43. Paring: ______________________________

____

____

44. Performing provider: ______________________________

____

____

45. Peritonitis: ______________________________

____

____

46. Postoperative diagnosis: ______________________________

____

____

47. Preoperative diagnosis: ______________________________

____

____

48. Pressure ulcer: ______________________________

____

____

49. Removal: ______________________________

____

____

50. Repair: ______________________________

____

____

51. Resection: ______________________________

____

____

52. Rhinoplasty: ______________________________

____

____

53. Robot-assisted surgery: ______________________________

____

____

54. Separate procedure: ______________________________

____

____

55. Shaving: ______________________________

____

____

56. Skin lesion: ______________________________

____

____

57. Skin ulcer: ______________________________

____

____

58. Stage: ______________________________

____

____

59. Surgical procedure: ______________________________

____

____

60. Therapeutic procedure: ____

____

____

61. Transplantation: ____

____

____

62. Unbundling: ____

____

____

63. Xenograft: ____

____

____

Word Bank

Instructions: Using the procedures listed, complete the following table to describe the components of surgical packages. You do not need to assign codes for these procedures.

Complex wound repair
Diagnostic endoscopy
Pacemaker insertion
Major surgical procedure
Simple procedure
Minor surgical procedure

	Zero Day Global Period	10-Day Global Period	90-Day Global Period
Procedure type			
Example of procedure			

Matching

Instructions: Match the Surgery subsection with the code range for that section.

1. _______	Integumentary	**A.** 54000 to 55899
2. _______	Musculoskeletal	**B.** 69000 to 69979
3. _______	Respiratory	**C.** 30000 to 32999
4. _______	Cardiovascular	**D.** 60000 to 60699
5. _______	Hemic and Lymphatic	**E.** 39000 to 39599
6. _______	Mediastinum and Diaphragm	**F.** 10030 to 19499
7. _______	Digestive	**G.** 56405 to 58999
8. _______	Urinary	**H.** 33010 to 37799
9. _______	Male Genital	**I.** 20005 to 29999
10. _______	Female Genital	**J.** 40490 to 49999
11. _______	Maternity Care and Delivery	**K.** 38100 to 38999
12. _______	Endocrine System	**L.** 59000 to 59899
13. _______	Nervous System	**M.** 61000 to 64999
14. _______	Eye and Ocular Adnexa	**N.** 65091 to 68899
15. _______	Auditory System	**O.** 50010 to 53899

Completion

Instructions: There are three components to endoscopy coding. Name and describe each of the three components and give one example of how each of these components may impact code selection.

1. ____

____

2. ______________________________

____

3. ______________________________

____

Coding

Instructions: Identify only the modifier for the following procedural descriptions.

1. General anesthesia provided by the surgeon for a child undergoing a foreign body removal procedure

Modifier: ______________

2. Procedure performed on the bilateral arms

Modifier: ______________

3. Surgical team of four physicians completed a complex surgery of the skull base

Modifier: ______________

4. Patient undergoing an endoscopic examination of the bronchus began experiencing respiratory difficulties, so the endoscope was removed, and the procedure was discontinued

Modifier: ______________

5. Ophthalmological surgeon performed the intraoperative services only for a procedure involving the removal and insertion of a cataract prosthesis

Modifier: ______________

6. Open heart procedure performed on a two-month-old infant weighing 7 lbs (3.5 kg)

Modifier: ______________

7. A normally bilateral procedure (CPT code for procedure identifies a bilateral service) is completed unilaterally

Modifier: ______________

8. Anterior cervical discectomy with arthrodesis required additional work to dissect through unusually thick tissue and ligaments (extra work was substantially greater than what is typically required for the service)

Modifier: ______________

9. Patient with Alzheimer's dementia with behavioral disturbances suffered chest lacerations after falling in his kitchen; due to extreme aggression, the patient was placed under general anesthesia in order to repair the chest wounds

Modifier: _______________

10. Ten days after pacemaker insertion, the patient was returned to the operating room (in the global period) because the patient was experiencing electrical shocks from the device; the entire pacemaker and all leads were removed and replaced with new functioning parts

Modifier: _______________

11. Plastic surgeon assisted in wound repair surgery for patient with multiple open wounds

Modifier: _______________

12. Team of surgeons consisting of one cardiologist and one pulmonologist performed a thoracic repair procedure

Modifier: _______________

13. General surgeon minimally assisted in transplantation surgery

Modifier: _______________

14. Colorectal surgeon completed only the postoperative and follow-up care for a patient who underwent a colectomy

Modifier: _______________

15. Orthopedic specialist performed only the preoperative evaluation and consultation services to a patient undergoing a bilateral total knee arthroplasty

Modifier: _______________

Instructions: Identify only the procedure(s) and diagnosis code(s) for the following.

16. Excision of tumor of carotid body with sparing of carotid artery

CPT code(s): _______________

ICD-10-CM code(s): _______________

17. Surgical treatment of papillary thyroid carcinoma with total unilateral thyroid lobectomy of the left thyroid, with contralateral subtotal lobectomy of the right lobe, including isthmusectomy; functional activity of the neoplasm includes corticoadrenal insufficiency and hypopituitarism

CPT code(s): _______________

ICD-10-CM code(s): _______________, _______________, _______________

18. Excision of stage 4 coccygeal pressure ulcer with removal of portion of coccyx bone and flap closure

    CPT code(s): ________________

    ICD-10-CM code(s): ________________

19. Biopsy of uvula (palate) for neoplasm of uncertain behavior of the uvula

    CPT code(s): ________________

    ICD-10-CM code(s): ________________

20. Open drainage of renal abscess

    CPT code(s): ________________

    ICD-10-CM code(s): ________________

21. Laparoscopic unilateral orchiectomy of the right descended testicle for testicular cancer

    CPT code(s): ________________ - _____

    ICD-10-CM code(s): ________________

22. Destruction (chemodenervation) of axillary eccrine sweat glands for primary focal hyperhidrosis of the axilla

    CPT code(s): ________________

    ICD-10-CM code(s): ________________

23. Unlisted procedure of the accessory sinuses

    CPT code(s): ________________

24. Bronchoscopy with revision of previously placed bronchial stent and bronchial dilation for congenital stenosis of bilateral bronchus

    CPT code(s): ________________

    ICD-10-CM code(s): ________________

25. Bronchoscopy with bronchial alveolar lavage and endobronchial biopsy for patient with alveolar pneumopathy

    CPT code(s): ________________, ________________ - _____

    ICD-10-CM code(s): ________________

26. Robotic-assisted cholecystectomy in patient with calculus of gallbladder with chronic cholecystitis with obstruction. (Hint: Check for an HCPCS code to indicate that the surgery was performed with robotic assistance.)

    CPT code(s): ________________, ________________

    ICD-10-CM code(s): ________________

27. An open appendectomy was started for a patient when it was discovered (after anesthesia and primary incision) that the wrong patient had been incised. The procedure was quickly discontinued and the patient was returned to the PACU in stable condition.

CPT code(s): ________________ - _____ - _____

28. Removal of bilateral permanent TM ventilation tubes for patient with recurrent suppurative bilateral otitis media. Due to patient's young age, general anesthesia was required.

CPT code(s): ________________ - _____

ICD-10-CM code(s): ________________

29. Initial left-sided tympanoplasty with ossicular chain reconstruction was performed on a patient with traumatic tympanic membrane perforation of the left side.

CPT code(s): ________________ - _____

ICD-10-CM code(s): ________________

Case Studies Surgery

Case Study 11.1

PATIENT: Catherine Speedman

DATE OF PROCEDURE: 02/12/20XX

INDICATIONS:

1. Chest lesion with irregular border
2. Anterior left abdomen lesion, raised regular brown speckled lesion
3. Left upper back/shoulder area, raised regular dark brown lesion
4. Low right lumbar pedunculated flesh-toned lesion

PROCEDURE:

1. Chest lesion with irregular border
   Risks, benefits, and alternatives were discussed with the patient. Informed consent obtained prior to the procedure. The site was prepped with Betadine.
   Anesthesia: The area around the lesion was anesthetized with 0.5 ml of lidocaine 1% with epinephrine.
   An 8-mm punch biopsy of the lesion was taken. The cutaneous layer was closed with three sutures of 5-0 Ethilon. Simple sutures were used for the skin closure. The lesion was place in buffered formalin and sent for histopathology.
   Dressing: An antibiotic ointment was applied, and a sterile dressing was placed.
   Patient status: Wound care instructions and OTC analgesics advised. The patient tolerated the procedure well.
   Complications: There were no complications.

2. Anterior left abdomen lesion, raised regular brown speckled lesion
   Risks, benefits, and alternatives were discussed with the patient. Informed consent obtained prior to the procedure. The site was prepped with Betadine.
   Anesthesia: The area around the lesion was anesthetized with 0.5 ml of lidocaine 1% with epinephrine.
   An 8-mm punch biopsy of the lesion was taken. The cutaneous layer was closed with three sutures of 5-0 Ethilon. Simple sutures were used for the skin closure. The lesion was placed in buffered formalin and sent for histopathology.
   Dressing: An antibiotic ointment was applied, and a sterile dressing was placed.
   Patient status: Wound care instructions and OTC analgesics advised. The patient tolerated the procedure well.
   Complications: There were no complications.
3. Left upper back/shoulder area, raised regular dark brown lesion
   Risks, benefits, and alternatives were discussed with the patient. Informed consent obtained prior to the procedure. The site was prepped with Betadine.
   Anesthesia: The area around the lesion was anesthetized with 0.5 ml of lidocaine 1% with epinephrine.
   An 8-mm punch biopsy of the lesion was taken. The cutaneous layer was closed with three sutures of 5-0 Ethilon. Simple sutures were used for the skin closure. The lesion was placed in buffered formalin and sent for histopathology.
   Dressing: An antibiotic ointment was applied, and a sterile dressing was placed.
   Patient status: Wound care instructions and OTC analgesics advised. The patient tolerated the procedure well.
   Complications: There were no complications.
4. Low right lumbar, pedunculated flesh-toned lesion
   Risks, benefits, and alternatives were discussed with the patient. Informed consent obtained prior to the procedure. The site was prepped with Betadine.
   Anesthesia: The area around the lesion was anesthetized with 0.5 ml of lidocaine 1% with epinephrine.
   Sharp excisional biopsy with silver nitrate for hemostasis. The subcutaneous layer was closed with silver nitrate hemostasis. The excised lesion was place in buffered formalin and sent for histopathology.
   Dressing: An antibiotic ointment was applied and a sterile dressing was placed.
   Patient status: Wound care instructions and OTC analgesics advised. The patient tolerated the procedure well.
   Complications: There were no complications.
   All lesions sent for pathology.

IMPRESSION: Multiple benign nevi, as follows:

1. Chest lesion with irregular border
2. Anterior left abdomen lesion, raised regular brown speckled lesion
3. Left upper back/shoulder area, raised regular dark brown lesion
4. Low right lumbar, pedunculated flesh-toned lesion

SIGNED: Dr. Allan Daniel, MD

Select the appropriate codes for the case study.

1. List the ICD-10-CM code(s):

ICD-10-CM code(s): ________________, ________________

2. List the CPT/HCPCS code(s) and any applicable modifiers:

CPT code(s): ________________, ________________ × _____

3. List the procedure and diagnosis codes on the CMS-1500 form. Be sure to correctly link the procedure and diagnosis codes.

21. DIAGNOSIS OR NATURE OF ILLNESS OR INJURY Relate A-L to service line below (24E)			ICD Ind.	22. RESUBMISSION CODE
A.	B.	C.	D.	
E.	F.	G.	H.	23. PRIOR AUTHORIZATION NU
I.	J.	K.	L.	

	24. A. DATE(S) OF SERVICE From MM	DD	YY	To MM	DD	YY	B. PLACE OF SERVICE	C. EMG	D. PROCEDURES, SERVICES, OR SUPPLIES (Explain Unusual Circumstances) CPT/HCPCS	MODIFIER	E. DIAGNOSIS POINTER	F. $ CHARGES	G. DAYS OR UNITS
1													
2													
3													
4													

Case Study 11.2

PATIENT: Michael James

DATE OF PROCEDURE: 04/06/20XX

PREOPERATIVE DIAGNOSES:

1. Basal cell carcinoma, right shoulder
2. Basal cell carcinoma, left side of back
3. Basal cell carcinoma, left lateral canthal area of the left lower eyelid
4. Basal cell carcinoma of nose
5. Basal cell carcinoma of right eyebrow

POSTOPERATIVE DIAGNOSES:

1. Basal cell carcinoma, right shoulder
2. Basal cell carcinoma, left side of back
3. Basal cell carcinoma, left lateral canthal area of the left lower eyelid
4. Basal cell carcinoma of nose
5. Basal cell carcinoma of right eyebrow

OPERATION PERFORMED:

1. Excision and complex layered closure
2. Excision and complex layered closure

3. Excision and reconstruction with adjacent tissue transfer
4. Excision and reconstruction with adjacent tissue transfer
5. Excision and layered primary closure

DESCRIPTION OF PROCEDURE:
The patient was initially placed in the lateral decubitus position. Then, 1% Xylocaine and 1:100,000 epinephrine buffered with sodium bicarbonate was infiltrated. Appropriate prepping and draping was accomplished. The lesion to the shoulder was excised first. It was excised as a surgical ellipse oriented from anterior to posterior. It was tagged with a suture to orient the pathologist and sent for frozen section examination. This showed basal cell carcinoma with clear margins. The adjacent wound margins were undermined. Hemostasis was obtained with the bipolar cautery. Layered closure was accomplished with interrupted 3-0 PDS in the dermis and running 4-0 Prolene. Excised diameter was 9 cm.

Next, a lesion of the back was excised with an adequate-appearing margin on uninvolved-appearing surrounding skin and subcutaneous tissue. It was tagged with a suture to orient the pathologist and sent for frozen section examination. After 3 frozen sections, clear margins were obtained. The wound margins were undermined. Hemostasis obtained with the bipolar cautery. Layered closure was accomplished with interrupted 3-0 PDS in the dermis and running 4-0 Prolene. Excised diameter was 8 cm. Bacitracin and sterile gauze dressings were applied.

The patient was placed in the supine position. Then, 1% Xylocaine and 1:100,000 epinephrine buffered with sodium bicarbonate was infiltrated. Appropriate prepping and draping was accomplished. The lesion of the left lateral canthus was excised as a rhomboid. It was tagged with a suture to orient the pathologist and sent for frozen section examination. This showed a basal cell carcinoma with clear margins. Reconstruction was carried out by means of a Limberg type of adjacent tissue transfer. The appropriate markings were made. The incisions were made. The flaps were elevated, mobilized, and transposed. Hemostasis was obtained with the bipolar cautery. Closure was accomplished with interrupted 5-0 and interrupted 6-0 Prolene. Total repair size was 1.5 sq. cm.

Next, the nose was operated upon. The lesion was situated on the left side of the nose, just above the nostril rim. It was excised with an adequate-appearing margin of uninvolved-appearing surrounding skin and subcutaneous tissue. It was tagged with a suture to orient the pathologist and sent for frozen section examination. This showed a basal cell carcinoma with positive margin. Additional tissue was excised, and this now showed clear margins. Reconstruction was carried out with a transposition-type flap. The appropriate markings were made. The incisions were made. The flaps were elevated, mobilized, and transposed. Hemostasis was obtained with the bipolar cautery. Closure was accomplished with interrupted horizontal half-buried mattress sutures of 5-0 Prolene. Total repair size was 1 sq. cm.

Next, the right eyebrow was operated upon. This was excised as a surgical ellipse. It was tagged with a suture to orient the pathologist and sent for frozen section examination. This showed a basal cell carcinoma with involvement of the deep margin. Additional tissue was excised and this time showed clear margins. Hemostasis was obtained with the bipolar cautery. Layered closure was accomplished with interrupted 5-0 PDS and running 5-0 Prolene. Excised diameter was 3 cm. Bacitracin and sterile gauze dressing were applied. Estimated blood loss was negligible. The patient tolerated the procedure well and was removed from the operating room in satisfactory condition.

SIGNED: Dr. Allan Daniel, MD

Select the appropriate codes for the case study.

1. List the ICD-10-CM code(s):

ICD-10-CM code(s): ________________, ________________, ________________,
________________, ________________

2. List the CPT/HCPCS code(s) and any applicable modifiers:

CPT code(s): ________________, ________________ - _____, ________________ - _____- _____,
________________ - _____, ________________ - _____, ________________ - _____

3. List the procedure and diagnosis codes on the CMS-1500 form. Be sure to correctly link the procedure and diagnosis codes.
Note: Because the reconstruction procedure is the most complicated procedure, it should be listed as the primary procedure.

21. DIAGNOSIS OR NATURE OF ILLNESS OR INJURY Relate A-L to service line below (24E) ICD Ind.

A. ______ B. ______ C. ______ D. ______
E. ______ F. ______ G. ______ H. ______
I. ______ J. ______ K. ______ L. ______

22. RESUBMISSION CODE

23. PRIOR AUTHORIZATION NU

	24. A. DATE(S) OF SERVICE From MM	DD	YY	To MM	DD	YY	B. PLACE OF SERVICE	C. EMG	D. PROCEDURES, SERVICES, OR SUPPLIES (Explain Unusual Circumstances) CPT/HCPCS	MODIFIER	E. DIAGNOSIS POINTER	F. $ CHARGES	G. DAYS OR UNITS
1													
2													
3													
4													
5													
6													

Case Study 11.3

PATIENT: Tania Lopez

PREOPERATIVE DIAGNOSIS: Cystic lesion of right mandibular body

POSTOPERATIVE DIAGNOSIS: Traumatic bone cyst of right mandibular body

PRODECURES PERFORMED: Removal/treatment/curettage of traumatic bone cyst

ANESTHESIA: General nasoendotracheal

ESTIMATED BLOOD LOSS: 5 ml

COMPLICATIONS: None

SPECIMENS REMOVED: Wall and curettage of lesion

INDICATIONS FOR SURGERY:
The patient is a 13-year-old white female who was found to have a 1 × 1 radiolucency associated with the right body of the mandible on routine dental examination. Cone-beam CT scan of this lesion showed slight expansion of the lateral surface of the mandible and significant thinning of the cortical bone in the area between the roots of teeth #28 and #29 and extending to the lingual cortex. Due to the relatively small size of the lesion and its proximity to the mental nerve at the mental foramen, she was scheduled for outpatient excision and appropriate management.

PROCEDURE IN DETAIL:
The patient was taken to the operating room and placed in the supine position. After induction of anesthesia, nasoendotracheal intubation, she was prepped and draped in a routine fashion for intraoral surgery. A throat pack was placed, and a total of 5 ml of Xylocaine with 1:100,000 epinephrine, along with 2 ml of 0.5% Marcaine with 1:200,000 epinephrine was given to anesthetize the right side of the mandible.

An incision was made crestal from the mesial of tooth #30 forward to the distal of tooth #27, and then an angled vertical incision from this point was made down to the depth of the vestibule. A full-thickness subperiosteal dissection was carried out, and it could be seen that the bone overlying the lesion was extremely thin and had some slight expansion evident as well. An 18-gauge needle on a 5-ml syringe was placed within the lesion and some blood and air were able to be suctioned from the lesion. This was not, however, evident of a potential vascular lesion. The needle was withdrawn and hand instruments were used to create a bony osteotomy through the thin outer wall of the lesion, which was placed in the specimen jar. It could soon be seen that there was no true cystic lining and that the lesion was indeed a traumatic bone cyst. The osteotomy was enlarged to gain access both visually and with all instruments to all areas of the lesion. No evidence of cystic lining or tumor was seen. Curettage of some of the inner portions of the cystic was accomplished and, after thorough irrigation, the lesion was filled with Gelfoam to control oozing, and the incision was closed with 3-0 and 4-0 chromic suture.

The patient tolerated the procedure well.

It should be mentioned that the lesion had thinned the superior wall of the mental foramen to the point where this bone could easily be removed with a small mosquito hemostat. There was no overt injury to the mental nerve.

SIGNED: Dr. Bob Welkins, DO

Select the appropriate codes for the case study.

1. List the ICD-10-CM code(s):

ICD-10-CM code(s): _______________

2. List the CPT/HCPCS code(s) and any applicable modifiers:

CPT code(s): _______________

3. Link the procedure and diagnosis codes on the CMS-1500 form. Be sure to correctly link the procedure and diagnosis codes.

21. DIAGNOSIS OR NATURE OF ILLNESS OR INJURY Relate A-L to service line below (24E) ICD Ind.

A. B. C. D.
E. F. G. H.
I. J. K. L.

22. RESUBMISSION CODE

23. PRIOR AUTHORIZATION NU

	24. A. DATE(S) OF SERVICE From MM DD YY	To MM DD YY	B. PLACE OF SERVICE	C. EMG	D. PROCEDURES, SERVICES, OR SUPPLIES (Explain Unusual Circumstances) CPT/HCPCS	MODIFIER	E. DIAGNOSIS POINTER	F. $ CHARGES	G. DAYS OR UNITS
1									
2									
3									
4									

Case Study 11.4

PATIENT: Jacob Marks

DATE OF PROCEDURE: 09/15/20XX

INDICATIONS:

1. Congenital cleft lip

PROCEDURES PERFORMED:

1. Cleft lip rhinoplasty, secondary to congenital deformity

2. Conchal cartilage graft harvest for nasal reconstruction

DESCRIPTION OF PROCEDURE:

In the operating room, the patient was induced under general anesthesia, following which he was prepped and draped in a sterile fashion. Lidocaine 1% with 1:100,000 parts epinephrine was used for local infiltration and infraorbital foramen block.

An external right rhinoplasty approach was planned, making incisions in the previous columellar in an inverted-V fashion, extending to marginal on the right and rim incision on the left, elevating the nasal envelope in the subnasal SMAS plane. Dissection continued over the left lateral crus, minimally malpositioned, and freeing this, allowing more cephalic positioning. Horizontal mattress dome-shaping sutures were placed and fixed to the septal angle to restructure the tip one side to the other and gain tip support to prevent tip ptosis that was contributing to the crimping of the nasal nerves.

An incision was made in the left antihelix, elevating a subperichondrial flap to expose the concha cavum and cymba, excising a fusiform of appropriate-shaped cartilage to fit the left dome from the underlying perichondrium. The donor site was closed with interrupted and running 5-0 plain gut sutures, placing mattress sutures to close the dead space and on completion pressing an antibiotic-soaked cotton ball in this bowl to create a tamponade effect. The cartilage was further beveled, shaped, and thinned into an even graft measuring 2.5 cm × 0.5 cm.

Following the lateral crus and extending more caudally, a pocket was created in the nostril on the left to re-create the dome shape of the left nostril and brace this area. This was fixed percutaneously with mattress sutures of 4-0 plain gut suture. Bilateral Weir excisions were made 1 mm from the alar groove, excising greater floor skin on the left to create symmetry of the nostrils, anchoring the ala with 5-0 vicryl, and closing the incisions with interrupted 5-0 plain gut sutures.

The nasal envelope was then relaid and closed with interrupted 5-0 plain gut sutures. Mastisol and Steri-Strip dressing was applied, and the patient was handed over to Anesthesia for awakening and transfer to the recovery room.

SIGNED: Dr. Bob Welkins, DO

Select the appropriate codes for the case study.

1. List the ICD-10-CM code(s):

   ICD-10-CM code(s): _______________

2. List the CPT/HCPCS code(s) and any applicable modifiers:

   CPT code(s): _______________, _______________

3. List the procedure and diagnosis codes on the CMS-1500 form. Be sure to correctly link the procedure and diagnosis codes.

21. DIAGNOSIS OR NATURE OF ILLNESS OR INJURY Relate A-L to service line below (24E) ICD Ind.

A.	B.	C.	D.
E.	F.	G.	H.
I.	J.	K.	L.

22. RESUBMISSION CODE

23. PRIOR AUTHORIZATION NU

	24. A. DATE(S) OF SERVICE From MM DD YY	To MM DD YY	B. PLACE OF SERVICE	C. EMG	D. PROCEDURES, SERVICES, OR SUPPLIES (Explain Unusual Circumstances) CPT/HCPCS	MODIFIER	E. DIAGNOSIS POINTER	F. $ CHARGES	G. DAYS OR UNITS
1									
2									
3									
4									

Anesthesia and Pain Management Services

Vocabulary

Instructions: Define each of the following key terms in the space provided.

1. Acupuncture: ______________________________

____

____

2. Analgesia: ______________________________

____

____

3. Anesthesia services: ______________________________

____

____

4. Anesthesiology: ______________________________

____

____

5. ASA crosswalk: ______________________________

____

____

6. Base units: ______________________________

7. Cervicalgia: ______________________________

8. Chronic pain: ______________________________

9. Conversion factor (CF): ______________________________

10. Electrodiagnostic studies: ______________________________

11. Electromyography (EMG): ______________________________

12. Enthesopathy: ______________________________

13. Epidural steroid injection: ______________________________

14. Facet joint injection: ______________________________

15. Fibromyalgia: ______________________________

____

____

16. General anesthesia: ______________________________

____

____

17. Integrative medicine: ______________________________

____

____

18. Interventional pain procedures: ______________________________

____

____

19. Kyphoplasty: ______________________________

____

____

20. Local anesthesia: ______________________________

____

____

21. Lumbago: ______________________________

____

____

22. Moderate (conscious) sedation: ______________________________

____

____

23. Modifying factors: ______________________________

____

____

24. Monitored anesthesia care (MAC): ______________________________

25. Myalgia: ______________________________

26. Myositis: ______________________________

27. Nerve condition study (NCS): ______________________________

28. Occipital nerve block: ______________________________

29. Osteoarthritis: ______________________________

30. Pain management services: ______________________________

31. Peripheral nerve stimulation: ______________________________

32. Physical status modifier: ______________________________

33. Qualifying circumstance CPT codes: ______________________________

____

____

34. Radiculopathy: ______________________________

____

____

35. Radiofrequency nerve ablation: ______________________________

____

____

36. Regional anesthesia: ______________________________

____

____

37. Sciatica: ______________________________

____

____

38. Spinal cord stimulation (SCS): ______________________________

____

____

39. Time units: ______________________________

____

____

Multiple Choice

Instructions: Choose the best answer.

1. Which of the following medical providers is a medical doctor who provides anesthesia to patients?
a. Anesthesiology assistant
b. Certified registered nurse anesthetist
c. Anesthesiologist
d. Physician assistant

2. Which of the following produces an incomplete loss of consciousness, which allows the patient to be sedated but awake at the same time?
   a. Moderate sedation
   b. Regional anesthesia
   c. General anesthesia
   d. Local anesthesia

3. Which of the following employs an injection to block a large amount of nerves?
   a. Moderate sedation
   b. Regional anesthesia
   c. General anesthesia
   d. Local anesthesia

4. Which of the following anesthesia modifiers would be used for an anesthesia service provided by a CRNA under the medical direction of a physician?
   a. QX
   b. QZ
   c. AA
   d. QY

5. Which of the following procedures uses a controlled heat source to disable nerves as a treatment for back or neck pain?
   a. Joint injections
   b. Moderate sedation
   c. Nerve blocks
   d. Radiofrequency nerve ablation

6. Which of the following diagnosis codes would be reported if the patient has a past history of failed moderate sedation?
   a. T88.4XXA
   b. T88.51XA
   c. Z92.83
   d. Z92.84

7. Which of the following diagnosis codes would be reported if a patient presented with chronic pain caused by a malignancy in the lung?
   a. G89.12
   b. G89.18
   c. G89.29
   d. G89.3

8. Which of the following is the constant or long-term sensation of pain?
   a. Traumatic pain
   b. Nerve pain
   c. Chronic pain
   d. Postoperative pain

9. Which of the following is a medical doctor who specializes in anesthesiology?
   a. AA
   b. MD/DO
   c. CRNA
   d. PA

10. Which of the following physical status modifiers would be assigned for a patient with severe systemic disease that is not a constant threat to life?
   a. P3
   b. P4
   c. P2
   d. P5

Fill in the Blank

Instructions: Complete the following for anesthesia services.

1. ________________ units describe the relative values for anesthesia services.

2. ________________ units identify how much time was spent on an anesthesia service, from start to finish.

3. ________________ ________________ identify special circumstances of the anesthesia procedure or the health of the patient.

4. The ________________ ________________ modifier identifies the health of the patient.

5. ________________ ________________ codes identify special circumstances surrounding the anesthesia service.

6. The ________________ ________________ is the dollar amount used to calculate the charge amount for an anesthesia service.

7. Charges for anesthesia services are determined based on the following calculation:

(________________ + ________________ + ________________)

×

________________ = total charge amount

Matching

Instructions: Match the Surgery subsection with the code range for that section.

1. __________ 99100

2. __________ 99116

3. __________ 99135

4. __________ 99140

A. Anesthesia complicated by utilization of total body hypothermia

B. Anesthesia complicated by utilization of controlled hypotension

C. Anesthesia for patient of extreme age

D. Anesthesia complicated by emergency conditions

Labeling

Instructions: Complete the following anatomical diagram with the correct labels to identify the levels of the spine.

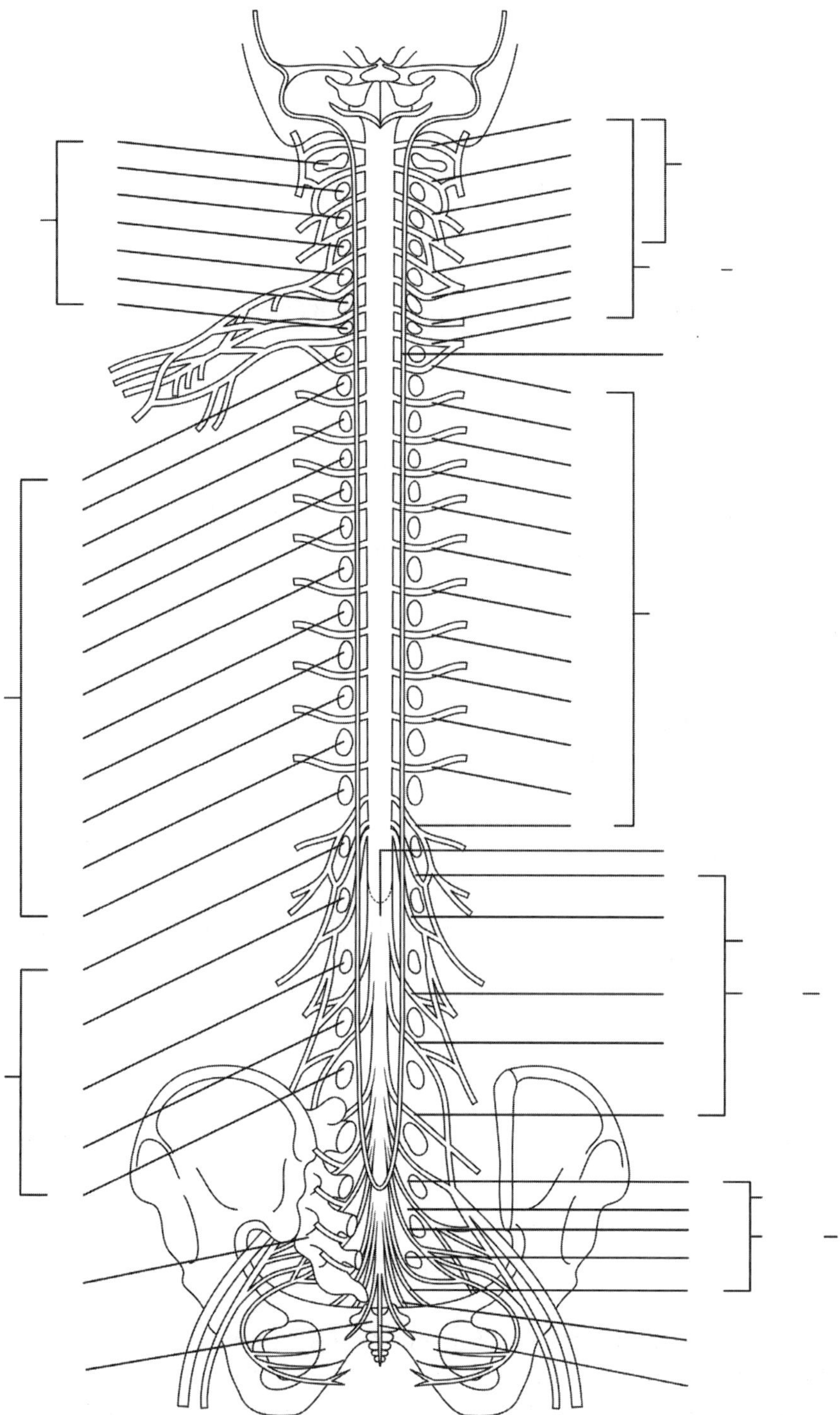

Source: ©AHIMA.

Coding

Instructions: Identify the correct CPT and ICD-10-CM codes for the following statements.

1. Anesthesia for pulmonary resection and thoracoplasty in a normal healthy patient

CPT code(s): ______________-______

2. Anesthesia for physiological support for harvesting of organs from brain-dead patient

CPT code(s): ______________-______

3. Anesthesia for repair of cleft palate in normal healthy patient, aged 3 years, with cleft hard palate

CPT code(s): ______________-______

ICD-10-CM code(s): ______________

4. Anesthesia performed for pneumocentesis for moribund patient with traumatic hemothorax; patient presented under emergency conditions after MVA

CPT code(s): ______________-______, ______________

ICD-10-CM code(s): ______________

5. 30 minutes of acupuncture with electrical stimulation performed on 42-year-old female patient with lumbago with sciatica of the right and left sides

CPT code(s): ______________, ______________

ICD-10-CM code(s): ______________, ______________

6. Fluoroscopy-guided bilateral facet joint injections of the lumbar spine at L2 and L3 for patient with lumbago

CPT code(s): ______________-______, ______________-______

ICD-10-CM code(s): ______________

7. Anesthesia for normal healthy patient with bilateral vasectomy for elective sterilization

CPT code(s): ______________-______

ICD-10-CM code(s): ______________

8. Placement of indwelling catheter for continuous administration of anesthetic substance into the interlaminar epidural into the lumbar area, with imaging guidance, for patient with chronic low back pain and left-sided sciatica

CPT code(s): ______________

ICD-10-CM code(s): ______________, ______________

9. Chemodenervation by neurolytic destruction of L4-L5, L5-L6, and L6-L7 facets joints bilaterally for patient with lumbar radiculopathy

CPT code(s): ______________, ______________-_____ (×_____)

ICD-10-CM code(s): ______________

10. Kyphoplasty of T2 and T3 vertebrae for treatment of collapsed vertebra

CPT code(s): ______________, ______________

ICD-10-CM code(s): ______________

11. Anesthesia for coronary artery bypass graft for 55-year-old female with CAD. No use of pump oxygenator.

CPT code(s): ______________

ICD-10-CM code(s): ______________

12. 40-year-old male with closed fracture of distal right radius required general anesthesia for manipulative treatment of fracture.

CPT code(s): ______________

ICD-10-CM code(s): ______________

13. Anesthesia provided to 67-year-old male undergoing radical prostatectomy for prostate cancer.

CPT code(s): ______________

ICD-10-CM code(s): ______________

14. Detailed history, problem focused examination, and moderate MDM for an established patient seen in the office setting. Patient has a long-standing history of opioid dependence due to chronic lumbar pain and sciatica.

CPT code(s): ______________

ICD-10-CM code(s): ______________, ______________, ______________

15. Electronic analysis of implanted neurostimulator pulse generator, with simple programming of an implanted spinal nerve neurostimulator pulse generator.

CPT code(s): ______________

Case Studies Anesthesia

Case Study 12.1

PATIENT: Tania Lopez

PREOPERATIVE DIAGNOSIS: Cystic lesion of right mandibular body

POSTOPERATIVE DIAGNOSIS: Traumatic bone cyst of right mandibular body

PRODECURES PERFORMED: Removal/treatment/curettage of traumatic bone cyst

ANESTHESIA: General nasoendotracheal

ASA LEVEL 1: Normal, healthy patient

ANESTHESIA TIME: Total anesthesia time 60 minutes

ESTIMATED BLOOD LOSS: 5 ml

COMPLICATIONS: None

SPECIMENS REMOVED: Wall and curettage of lesion

INDICATIONS FOR SURGERY:
The patient is a 13-year-old white female who was found to have a 1 × 1 radiolucency associated with the right body of the mandible on routine dental examination. Cone-beam CT scan of this lesion showed slight expansion of the lateral surface of the mandible and significant thinning of the cortical bone in the area between the roots of teeth #28 and #29 and extending to the lingual cortex. Due to the relatively small size of the lesion and its proximity to the mental nerve at the mental foramen, she was scheduled for outpatient excision and appropriate management.

PROCEDURE IN DETAIL:
The patient was taken to the operating room and placed in the supine position. After induction of anesthesia, nasoendotracheal intubation, she was prepped and draped in a routine fashion for intraoral surgery. A throat pack was placed, and a total of 5 ml of Xylocaine with 1:100,000 epinephrine, along with 2 ml of 0.5% Marcaine with 1:200,000 epinephrine was given to anesthetize the right side of the mandible.

An incision was made crestal from the mesial of tooth #30 forward to the distal of tooth #27, and then an angled vertical incision from this point was made down to the depth of the vestibule. A full-thickness subperiosteal dissection was carried out, and it could be seen that the bone overlying the lesion was extremely thin and had some slight expansion evident as well. An 18-gauge needle on 5-ml syringe was placed within the lesion and some blood and air were able to be suctioned from the lesion. The was not, however, evident of a potential vascular lesion. The needle was withdrawn and hand instruments were used to create a bony osteotomy through the thin outer wall of the lesion, which was placed in the specimen jar. It could soon be seen that there was no true cystic lining, and that the lesion was indeed a traumatic bone cyst. The osteotomy was enlarged to gain access both visually and with all instruments to all areas of the lesion. No evidence of cystic lining or tumor was seen. Curettage of some of the inner portions of the cystic was accomplished and, after thorough irrigation, the lesion was filled with Gelfoam to control oozing, and the incision was closed with 3-0 and 4-0 chromic suture.

The patient tolerated the procedure well.

It should be mentioned that the lesion had thinned the superior wall of the mental foramen to the point where this bone could easily be removed with a small mosquito hemostat. There was no overt injury to the mental nerve.

SIGNED: Dr. Bob Welkins, DO

Select the appropriate codes for the case study.

Note: This case was also presented in chapter 11 of this workbook. For this case study, select the appropriate codes for anesthesia billing:

1. List the ICD-10-CM code(s):

   ICD-10-CM code(s): ______________

2. List the CPT/HCPCS code(s) and any applicable modifiers:

   CPT code(s): ______________ - _____ × _____

3. List the procedure and diagnosis codes on the CMS-1500 form. Be sure to correctly link the procedure and diagnosis codes.

21. DIAGNOSIS OR NATURE OF ILLNESS OR INJURY Relate A-L to service line below (24E) ICD Ind.				22. RESUBMISSION CODE
A.	B.	C.	D.	
E.	F.	G.	H.	23. PRIOR AUTHORIZATION NU
I.	J.	K.	L.	

	24. A. DATE(S) OF SERVICE From MM DD YY	To MM DD YY	B. PLACE OF SERVICE	C. EMG	D. PROCEDURES, SERVICES, OR SUPPLIES (Explain Unusual Circumstances) CPT/HCPCS	MODIFIER	E. DIAGNOSIS POINTER	F. $ CHARGES	G. DAYS OR UNITS
1									
2									
3									
4									

Case Study 12.2

PATIENT: Jacob Marks

DATE OF PROCEDURE: 09/15/20XX

INDICATIONS:

1. Congenital cleft lip

ANESTHESIA: General nasoendotracheal

ASA LEVEL 1: Normal, healthy patient

ANESTHESIA TIME: Total anesthesia time 120 minutes

PROCEDURES PERFORMED:

1. Cleft lip rhinoplasty, secondary to congenital deformity
2. Conchal cartilage graft harvest for nasal reconstruction

DESCRIPTION OF PROCEDURE:
In the operating room, the patient was induced under general anesthesia, following which he was prepped and draped in a sterile fashion. Lidocaine 1% with 1:100,000 parts epinephrine was used for local infiltration and intraorbital foramen block.

An external right rhinoplasty approach was planned, making incisions in the previous columellar in an inverted-V fashion, extending to marginal on the right and rim incision on the left, elevating the nasal envelope in the subnasal SMAS plane. Dissection continued over the left lateral crus, minimally malpositioned, and freeing this, allowing more cephalic positioning. Horizontal mattress dome-shaping sutures were placed and fixed to the septal angle to restructure the tip one side to the other and gain tip support to prevent tip ptosis that was contributing to the crimping of the nasal nerves.

An incision was made in the left antihelix, elevating a subperichondrial flap to expose the concha cavum and cymba, excising a fusiform of appropriate-shaped cartilage to fit the left dome from the underlying perichondrium. The donor site was closed with interrupted and running 5-0 plain gut sutures, placing mattress sutures to close the dead space and on completion pressing an antibiotic-soaked cotton ball in this bowl to create a tamponade effect. The cartilage was further beveled, shaped, and thinned into an even graft measuring 2.5 cm × 0.5 cm.

Following the lateral crus and extending more caudally, a pocket was created in the nostril on the left to re-create the dome shape of the left nostril and brace this area. This was fixed percutaneously with mattress sutures of 4-0 plain gut suture. Bilateral Weir excisions were made 1 mm from the alar groove, excising greater floor skin on the left to create symmetry of the nostrils, anchoring the ala with 5-0 vicryl, and closing the incisions with interrupted 5-0 plain gut sutures.

The nasal envelope was then relaid and closed with interrupted 5-0 plain gut sutures. Mastisol and Steri-Strip dressing were applied, and the patient handed over to Anesthesia for awakening and transfer to the recovery room.

SIGNED: Dr. Bob Welkins, DO

Select the appropriate codes for the case study.

Note: This case was also presented in chapter 11 of this workbook. For this case study, select the appropriate codes for anesthesia billing.

1. List the ICD-10-CM code(s):
   ICD-10-CM code(s): ________________

2. List the CPT/HCPCS code(s) and any applicable modifiers:
   CPT code(s): ________________ - _____ × _____

3. List the procedure and diagnosis codes on the CMS-1500 form. Be sure to correctly link the procedure and diagnosis codes.

21. DIAGNOSIS OR NATURE OF ILLNESS OR INJURY Relate A-L to service line below (24E) ICD Ind.

A. ____ B. ____ C. ____ D. ____
E. ____ F. ____ G. ____ H. ____
I. ____ J. ____ K. ____ L. ____

22. RESUBMISSION CODE

23. PRIOR AUTHORIZATION NU

	24. A. DATE(S) OF SERVICE From MM DD YY	To MM DD YY	B. PLACE OF SERVICE	C. EMG	D. PROCEDURES, SERVICES, OR SUPPLIES (Explain Unusual Circumstances) CPT/HCPCS	MODIFIER	E. DIAGNOSIS POINTER	F. $ CHARGES	G. DAYS OR UNITS
1									
2									
3									
4									

Case Study 12.3

PATIENT: Lori White

DATE OF PROCEDURE: 05/21/20XX

CHIEF COMPLAINT:
The patient is a 68-year-old female referred by Dr. Susan Alameda with chief complaint of low back pain and some leg discomfort bilaterally (left leg greater than the right). She has responded beautifully to central steroids with over five months of complete relief with an injection to back one year ago. Her pain has returned with a vengeance, but there is no additional numbness or weakness nor any bowel or bladder change. We are going to reinject today. Follow up with be on a PRN basis.

Thank you once again for allowing me to participate in this nice patient's care.

PROCEDURE:
Epidural steroid injection

PERFORMING PHYSICIAN:
Dr. Bob Welkins, DO

PROCEDURE IN DETAIL:
With the patient in the prone position on the fluoroscopy table, the back is prepped and draped in a sterile fashion. All personnel and operator are wearing hat and masks, and the operator is using sterile gloves. A #20-gauge Tuohy needle is placed through a lidocaine skin wheal and, under fluoroscopic guidance, advanced interlaminar 4–5. 0.5 ml of water-soluble contrast is injected with no vascular uptake or myelographic appearance. Injection is made of 80 mg Kenalog and 1 ml Isovue-M 300. An epidurogram is produced that extends from 3–4 to 4–5. The needle is removed intact. The patient is left in the prone position in good condition. At no time was dysesthesia produced nor was CSF or blood obtained.

The patient is instructed to continue home exercise. This is intended to enhance rehabilitation.

DIAGNOSES:

1. Lumbar stenosis
2. Lumbar radiculopathy

ANESTHESIA:
Despite detailed information and counseling, the patient remained quite anxious preprocedure. In my judgment, the patient was unable to tolerate this procedure without the use of conscious sedation secondary to anxiety and low pain threshold to protect against inadvertent patient reaction or movement which could create a safety issue.

Review of patient's history revealed no contraindications for conscious sedation. An intravenous line was started to allow for intravenous medication. Vital signs including blood pressure, heart rate, and oxygen saturation were monitored and documented in the conscious sedation record by the attending RN in addition to start and stop times. The total duration of face-to-face time with Dr. Welkins of conscious sedation was 12 minutes.

The patient recovered satisfactorily from conscious sedation and was discharged to home in good condition.

SIGNED: Dr. Bob Welkins, DO

Select the appropriate codes for the case study.

Note: Select the appropriate codes for anesthesia billing only. Do not code for any imaging services or contrast materials.

1. List the ICD-10-CM code(s):

   ICD-10-CM code(s): ________________, ________________

2. List the CPT/HCPCS code(s) and any applicable modifiers:

CPT code(s): ________________, ________________

HCPCS code(s): ________________ × _____

3. List the procedure and diagnosis codes on the CMS-1500 form. Be sure to correctly link the procedure and diagnosis codes.

21. DIAGNOSIS OR NATURE OF ILLNESS OR INJURY Relate A-L to service line below (24E)			ICD Ind.	22. RESUBMISSION CODE
A.	B.	C.	D.	23. PRIOR AUTHORIZATION NU
E.	F.	G.	H.	
I.	J.	K.	L.	

	24. A. DATE(S) OF SERVICE From MM DD YY	To MM DD YY	B. PLACE OF SERVICE	C. EMG	D. PROCEDURES, SERVICES, OR SUPPLIES (Explain Unusual Circumstances) CPT/HCPCS	MODIFIER	E. DIAGNOSIS POINTER	F. $ CHARGES	G. DAYS OR UNITS
1									
2									
3									
4									

Case Study 12.4

PATIENT: Elizabeth Negroni

PREOPERATIVE DIAGNOSIS: Foreign body (FB) right nostril

POSTOPERATIVE DIAGNOSIS: FB right nostril

ANESTHESIA: General inhalant

ASA STATUS: 1, Normal healthy patient

ANESTHESIA TIME: 13 minutes

PROCEDURE NOTE:
3-year-old patient requiring general anesthesia was prepped and draped and the right nostril was examined. FB appeared to be sponge of some sort, with noted degeneration indicating that FB had been in nasal passage for some time. FB was noted and was retrieved using forceps. Saline irrigation was used to ensure all particles of the FB had been successfully removed. Patient tolerated the procedure well and was returned to the postanesthesia care unit in stable condition.

COMPLICATIONS: None, patient tolerated the procedure well

SIGNED: Dr. Bob Welkins, DO

Select the appropriate codes for the case study.

Note: This case was also presented in chapter 5 of this workbook. For this case study, select the appropriate codes for anesthesia billing:

1. List the ICD-10-CM code(s):

   ICD-10-CM code(s): ________________

2. List the CPT/HCPCS code(s) and any applicable modifiers:

   CPT code(s): ________________ - _____ × _____

3. List the procedure and diagnosis codes on the CMS-1500 form. Be sure to correctly link the procedure and diagnosis codes.

21. DIAGNOSIS OR NATURE OF ILLNESS OR INJURY Relate A-L to service line below (24E) ICD Ind.

A.	B.	C.	D.
E.	F.	G.	H.
I.	J.	K.	L.

22. RESUBMISSION CODE

23. PRIOR AUTHORIZATION NU

	24. A. DATE(S) OF SERVICE From MM DD YY	To MM DD YY	B. PLACE OF SERVICE	C. EMG	D. PROCEDURES, SERVICES, OR SUPPLIES (Explain Unusual Circumstances) CPT/HCPCS	MODIFIER	E. DIAGNOSIS POINTER	F. $ CHARGES	G. DAYS OR UNITS
1									
2									
3									
4									

Case Study 12.5

PATIENT: Jamie Bencomo

INDICATIONS: The patient presents with symptomatic gallbladder disease and will undergo laparoscopic cholecystectomy.

PREOPERATIVE DIAGNOSIS: Biliary dyskinesia

POSTOPERATIVE DIAGNOSIS: Same

ANESTHESIA: General endotracheal
ASA STATUS: 2, Patient with mild systemic disease
ANESTHESIA TIME: 42 minutes

PROCEDURE NOTE:
The risks, benefits, complications, treatment options, and expected outcomes were discussed with the patient. The possibilities of reaction to medication, pulmonary aspiration, perforation of viscus, bleeding, recurrent infection, finding a normal gallbladder, the need for additional procedures, failure to diagnosis a condition, the possible need to convert to an open procedure, and creating

a complication requiring a transfusion operation were discussed with the patient. The patient concurred with the proposed plan, giving informed consent. The patient was taken to the OR. A time-out was held and all information was verified.

Prior to the induction of general anesthesia, antibiotic prophylaxis was administered. General endotracheal anesthesia was then administered and tolerated well. After the induction, the abdomen was prepped in the usual sterile fashion. The patient was positioned in the supine position with some reverse Trendelenburg.

After injecting local anesthetic, a 5-mm incision was made in the right upper quadrant and, with the help of 5-mm Optiview trocar and a 5-mm camera, the peritoneal cavity was accessed without complications. Pneumoperitoneum was then created with CO_2 and tolerated well without any adverse changes in the patient's vital signs.

The gallbladder was identified, the fundus grasped and retracted cephalad. Adhesions were lysed bluntly and with the electrocautery where indicated, taking care not to injure any adjacent organs or viscus. The infundibulum was grasped and retracted laterally, exposing the peritoneum overlying the triangle of Calot. This was then divided and exposed in a blunt fashion. The cystic duct was clearly identified and bluntly dissected circumferentially. The junctions of the gallbladder, cystic duct, and common bile duct were clearly identified prior to the division of any linear structure.

The cystic duct was then doubly ligated with surgical clips on the patient side and singly clipped on the gallbladder side and divided. The cystic artery was identified, dissected free, ligated with clips, and divided as well.

The gallbladder was dissected from the liver bed in retrograde fashion with the electrocautery. The gallbladder was removed. The liver bed was inspected. Hemostasis was achieved with the electrocautery. No irrigation was performed.

Pneumoperitoneum was completely reduced after viewing removal of the trocars under direct supervision. The wound was thoroughly irrigated and the fascia was then closed with a figure-of-eight suture; the skin was then closed with a 4-0 Monocryl and Dermabond was applied.

Instrument, sponge, and needle counts were correct at closure and at the conclusion of the case.

FINDINGS: Biliary dyskinesia

SPECIMENS: Gallbladder

COMPLICATIONS: None; the patient tolerated the procedure well

DISPOSITION: PACU—Hemodynamically stable

CONDITION: Stable

SIGNED: Dr. Steven Ray, DO

Select the appropriate codes for the case study.

Note: This case was also presented in chapter 5 of this workbook. For this case study, select the appropriate codes for anesthesia billing.

1. List the ICD-10-CM code(s):

   ICD-10-CM code(s): ________________

2. List the CPT/HCPCS code(s) and any applicable modifiers:

   CPT code(s): ________________ - _____ × _____

3. List the procedure and diagnosis codes on the CMS-1500 form. Be sure to correctly link the procedure and diagnosis codes.

21. DIAGNOSIS OR NATURE OF ILLNESS OR INJURY Relate A-L to service line below (24E) ICD Ind.

A. ______ B. ______ C. ______ D. ______

E. ______ F. ______ G. ______ H. ______

I. ______ J. ______ K. ______ L. ______

22. RESUBMISSION CODE

23. PRIOR AUTHORIZATION NU

	24. A. DATE(S) OF SERVICE From MM	DD	YY	To MM	DD	YY	B. PLACE OF SERVICE	C. EMG	D. PROCEDURES, SERVICES, OR SUPPLIES (Explain Unusual Circumstances) CPT/HCPCS	MODIFIER	E. DIAGNOSIS POINTER	F. $ CHARGES	G. DAYS OR UNITS
1													
2													
3													
4													

CHAPTER 13

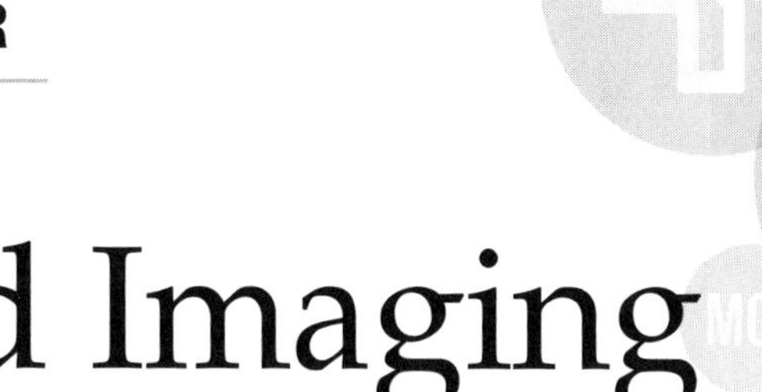

Radiology and Imaging Services

Vocabulary

Instructions: Define each of the following key terms in the space provided.

1. Anterior: ______________________________

____

____

2. Antero-posterior: ______________________________

____

____

3. Axial plane: ______________________________

____

____

4. Computed tomography (CT): ______________________________

____

____

5. Contralateral: ______________________________

____

____

6. Contrast material: ______________________________

____

____

7. Coronal plane: ______________________________

____

____

8. Distal: ______________________________

____

____

9. Doppler ultrasound: ______________________________

____

____

10. Global radiology service: ______________________________

____

____

11. Imaging services: ______________________________

____

____

12. Independent radiology and imaging center: ______________________________

____

____

13. Inferior: ______________________________

____

____

14. Ipsilateral: ______________________________

____

____

15. Lateral: ______________________________

____

____

16. Lateral (view): ______________________________

____

____

17. Magnetic resonance imaging (MRI): ______________________________

____

____

18. Mammography: ______________________________

____

____

19. Medial: ______________________________

____

____

20. Nuclear medicine: ______________________________

____

____

21. Oblique: ______________________________

____

____

22. Pleural effusion: ______________________________

____

____

23. Posterior: ______________________________

____

____

24. Postero-anterior: ______________________________

____

____

25. Professional component (PC): ______________________________

____

____

26. Projection: ______________________________

____

____

27. Proximal: ______________________________

____

____

28. Pulmonary edema: ______________________________

____

____

29. Radiologic guidance: ______________________________

____

____

30. Radiological supervision and interpretation (S&I): ______________________________

____

____

31. Radiologist: ______________________________

____

____

32. Radiology services: ______________________________

____

____

33. Sagittal plane: ______________________________

____

____

34. Superior: ______________________________

____

____

35. Technical component (TC): ______________________________

____

____

36. Transverse plane: ______________________________

____

____

37. Ultrasound: ______________________________

____

____

38. X-ray: ______________________________

____

____

Multiple Choice

Instructions: Choose the best answer.

1. Which of the following projection passes through the back to the front of the body?
a. Oblique
b. Lateral
c. Postero-anterior
d. Antero-posterior

2. Which of the following modifiers identifies the professional component of a service?
a. -26
b. -TC
c. -25
d. -RT

3. Which of the following modifiers identifies the technical component of a service?
a. -26
b. -RT
c. -LT
d. -TC

4. Radiological supervision and interpretation (S&I) is another term used for which of the following?
a. Technical component
b. Performing the imaging service
c. Professional component
d. Ordering the imaging service

5. Which of the following modifiers is reported to identify a global imaging service?
a. -26
b. -TC
c. Both -26 and -TC
d. No modifier would be used

6. Which of the following types of radiology procedures uses strong magnetic fields and radio waves to produce images of the internal structures of the body?
a. MRI
b. X-ray
c. CT
d. PET

7. Which of the following diagnostic studies uses sound waves to view a specific area of the body?
a. PET
b. Ultrasound
c. X-ray
d. Nuclear imaging

8. Which of the following mammograms is performed on a regular basis to detect early changes in the breast, which may indicate breast cancer?
a. Diagnostic
b. Therapeutic
c. Screening
d. Presumptive

9. Which of the following mammograms is performed when a patient has a clinical sign or symptom of the breast?
a. Diagnostic
b. Therapeutic
c. Screening
d. Presumptive

10. If a patient presents to the office for treatment and the provider performs an x-ray to diagnose the patient, and then the same provider performs an additional x-ray after a therapeutic service, which of the following modifiers would be used?
a. -50
b. No modifier would be used for the global service
c. -77
d. -76

Matching

Instructions: Match the terms with the appropriate description.

1. __________	Anterior	**A.** Toward the midline of the body (the belly button)
2. __________	Posterior	**B.** Situated toward the back of the body (such as the buttocks or heels)
3. __________	Superior	**C.** Away from the body (the fingertips)
4. __________	Inferior	**D.** The opposite side of the body (the right arm and the left arm)
5. __________	Medial	**E.** Situated toward the front of the body (such as the face or the breasts)
6. __________	Lateral	**F.** The same side of the body (the right upper and lower extremities)
7. __________	Proximal	**G.** Away from the midline of the body (the sides)
8. __________	Distal	**H.** Toward the top of the body (the head)
9. __________	Ipsilateral	**I.** Toward the center of the body (the upper arm)
10. __________	Contralateral	**J.** Toward the bottom of the body (the feet)

Coding

Instructions: Identify the correct CPT and ICD-10-CM codes for the following statements.

1. MRI of the kidneys and liver with contrast (4-ml octafluoropropane microspheres) in a patient with kidney failure. 2-cm mass of the liver identified.
CPT code(s): ____________________
HCPCS code(s): ____________________ × ______
ICD-10-CM code(s): ____________________, ____________________

2. X-ray of the alimentary tract (nose to rectum) in 8-year-old child who accidentally swallowed three 0.5-cm magnets. Three foreign bodies identified: one in stomach and two in small intestine.

CPT code(s): ________________

ICD-10-CM code(s): ________________, ________________

3. Transrectal ultrasound for patient with benign prostatic hyperplasia.

CPT code(s): ________________

ICD-10-CM code(s): ________________

4. Vertebral fracture assessment via dual-energy x-ray absorptiometry (DXA) in 80-year-old female patient with collapsed vertebra of the T4 and T5.

CPT code(s): ________________

ICD-10-CM code(s): ________________

5. Nuclear imaging study of the joints of the lower extremities, including hips, for patient with bilateral acute osteomyelitis of the lower legs.

CPT code(s): ________________

ICD-10-CM code(s): ________________, ________________

6. X-ray of the left hip (three views) in 75-year-old patient who suffered a fall and is now complaining of unilateral hip pain. No fractures identified.

CPT code(s): ________________

ICD-10-CM code(s): ________________

7. Complete retroperitoneal ultrasound reveals staghorn calculus of the left kidney.

CPT code(s): ________________

ICD-10-CM code(s): ________________

8. Complete osseous survey in a 20-day-old female patient.

CPT code(s): ________________

9. Fetal biophysical profile without nonstress testing completed via ultrasound on female patient with pregnancy complicated by blood clotting disease in the second trimester.

CPT code(s): ________________

ICD-10-CM code(s): ________________

10. CT colonography with and without contrast for 36-year-old obese male with intestinal adhesions with incomplete obstruction.

CPT code(s): ________________

ICD-10-CM code(s): ________________, ________________

Case Studies Radiology and Imaging

Case Study 13.1

PATIENT: Roberta Weiss

ORDERING PROVIDER: Susan Alameda, DO

XR ORTHO KNEE 4V RIGHT:

Findings: Four weight-bearing views of the right knee compared to prior study from 12/4/20XX.

Healing fracture of the proximal metaphysis of the fibula. No displacement. Joint spaces and soft tissues are unremarkable.

IMPRESSION:
Healing nondisplaced proximal fibular fracture.

SIGNED: Dr. Gene I. Kim, MD

Select the appropriate codes for the case study:

1. List the ICD-10-CM code(s):

   ICD-10-CM code(s): ________________

2. List the CPT/HCPCS code(s) and any applicable modifiers:

   CPT code(s): ________________ - _____

3. List the procedure and diagnosis codes on the CMS-1500 form. Be sure to correctly link the procedure and diagnosis codes.

21. DIAGNOSIS OR NATURE OF ILLNESS OR INJURY Relate A-L to service line below (24E) ICD Ind.

A. ____ B. ____ C. ____ D. ____
E. ____ F. ____ G. ____ H. ____
I. ____ J. ____ K. ____ L. ____

22. RESUBMISSION CODE

23. PRIOR AUTHORIZATION NU

	24. A. DATE(S) OF SERVICE From MM	DD	YY	To MM	DD	YY	B. PLACE OF SERVICE	C. EMG	D. PROCEDURES, SERVICES, OR SUPPLIES (Explain Unusual Circumstances) CPT/HCPCS	MODIFIER	E. DIAGNOSIS POINTER	F. $ CHARGES	G. DAYS OR UNITS
1													
2													
3													
4													

Case Study 13.2

PATIENT: Tyanna Markels

ORDERING PROVIDER: Susan Alameda, DO

US OB ANATOMIC STUDY: >/= 14 WKS, SINGLE FETUS

Findings: OB anatomic study. Patient had early OB ultrasound 09/06/20XX.

Single intrauterine gestation in breech presentation. The placenta is posteriorly located and is unremarkable. Normal amount of amniotic fluid. Cervical length 4.5 cm.

No intracranial anomalies. No facial anomalies. No spinal anomalies. Four-chamber heart. Heart rate 144 beats per minute. Left-sided stomach bubble. Three-vessel cord with normal insertion. The kidneys and bladder were unremarkable. Limb movement was seen on real-time exam.

Fetal measurements:
BPD: 4.4 cm = 19w3d
Head circumference: 17.14 cm = 19w5d
Abdominal circumference: 14.74 cm = 20w0d
Femur length: 3.0 cm = 19w2d
Estimated fetal weight: 306 grams (21st percentile)
Mean gestational age: 19 weeks 4 days with estimated date of confinement of 02/28/20XX

IMPRESSION:

1. Single viable intrauterine gestation at 19 weeks 4 days with an estimated date of conferment of 02/28/20XX.
2. No fetal anomalies

SIGNED: Dr. Gene I. Kim, MD

Select the appropriate codes for the case study.

1. List the ICD-10-CM code(s):
   (Hint: You will also need to add a code to identify the weeks of gestation.)
   ICD-10-CM code(s): ________________, ________________
2. List the CPT/HCPCS code(s) and any applicable modifiers:
   CPT code(s): ________________

3. List the procedure and diagnosis codes on the CMS-1500 form. Be sure to correctly link the procedure and diagnosis codes.

21. DIAGNOSIS OR NATURE OF ILLNESS OR INJURY Relate A-L to service line below (24E) ICD Ind.

A. ____ B. ____ C. ____ D. ____
E. ____ F. ____ G. ____ H. ____
I. ____ J. ____ K. ____ L. ____

22. RESUBMISSION CODE

23. PRIOR AUTHORIZATION NU

	24. A. DATE(S) OF SERVICE From MM DD YY	To MM DD YY	B. PLACE OF SERVICE	C. EMG	D. PROCEDURES, SERVICES, OR SUPPLIES (Explain Unusual Circumstances) CPT/HCPCS	MODIFIER	E. DIAGNOSIS POINTER	F. $ CHARGES	G. DAYS OR UNITS
1									
2									
3									
4									

Case Study 13.3

PATIENT: Burt Rogers

ORDERING PROVIDER: Susan Alameda, DO

FOR: Elevated PSA

US PROSTATE/TRANSRECTAL:

Findings: The patient was brought into the examination room and placed in the left lateral decubitus position. He was prepped and draped in the usual manner. The 7.5-MHz ultrasound probe was inserted into the rectum, and the prostate was imaged in the transverse and sagittal planes. Prostate volume was estimated at 26 grams with a PSA density of 1.33. No suspicious hypoechoic or hyperechoic areas were noted. The procedure was then terminated. The patient appeared to tolerate the procedure well.

SIGNED: Dr. Gene I. Kim, MD

Select the appropriate codes for the case study.

1. List the ICD-10-CM code(s):

ICD-10-CM code(s): ________________

2. List the CPT/HCPCS code(s) and any applicable modifiers:

CPT code(s): ________________

3. List the procedure and diagnosis codes on the CMS-1500 form. Be sure to correctly link the procedure and diagnosis codes.

21. DIAGNOSIS OR NATURE OF ILLNESS OR INJURY Relate A-L to service line below (24E)				ICD Ind.	22. RESUBMISSION CODE
A.	B.	C.	D.		
E.	F.	G.	H.		23. PRIOR AUTHORIZATION NU
I.	J.	K.	L.		

	24. A. DATE(S) OF SERVICE From MM DD YY	To MM DD YY	B. PLACE OF SERVICE	C. EMG	D. PROCEDURES, SERVICES, OR SUPPLIES (Explain Unusual Circumstances) CPT/HCPCS	MODIFIER	E. DIAGNOSIS POINTER	F. $ CHARGES	G. DAYS OR UNITS
1									
2									
3									
4									

Case Study 13.4

PATIENT: Joanne Stewart

ORDERING PROVIDER: Susan Alameda, DO

CTA ABDOMEN AND PELVIS WO/W CONTRAST:

Findings: The heart size is within normal limits. No pleural or pericardial effusions. Mild calcified atherosclerotic disease of the coronary arteries. Minimal atelectasis at the lung bases. There is a 6.5-cm lesion in the right lobe of the liver with peripheral puddling of contrast, which is most consistent with a giant hemangioma. There is no biliary ductal dilatation. The pancreas, spleen, and adrenal glands are normal in appearance. Mild cortical scarring of the kidneys. There is a 2-cm cyst in the upper pole of the left kidney. No pathologically enlarged lymphadenopathy.

The urinary bladder is within normal limits. Normal uterus and ovaries. No free fluid in the pelvis.

Mild fecal retention. No focal bowel wall thickening. Normal appendix. Normal small bowel.

Vasculature: There is 30–40% narrowing of the celiac axis based on NASCET criteria. Minimal poststenotic dilatation. There has been interval placement of a stent in the proximal SMA with significant improvement of flow. No definitive evidence of in-stent stenosis, although the stent is of small caliber. Mild narrowing of the right proximal renal artery. There is a 40–50% stenosis at the origin of the left renal artery. 50% stenosis of the IMA. Moderate atherosclerotic disease of the distal abdominal aorta. There are kissing bilateral iliac stents. Moderate atherosclerotic disease of the internal iliac arteries. Mild atherosclerotic disease of the external iliac arteries. Moderate disease of the common femoral arteries bilaterally. The profunda femoral arteries are mildly to moderately diseased.

Normal alignment of the lumbosacral spine with osteopenia. There is mild compression deformity of T12. Multilevel degenerative disease.

IMPRESSION:

1. Interval placement of a stent in the origin of the SMA with significant improvement of flow. No definitive evidence of in-stent stenosis.
2. 30–40% stenosis of the origin of the celiac axis
3. 40–50% stenosis at the origin of the left main renal artery
4. 50% stenosis of the origin of the IMA
5. Kissing common iliac stents with moderate atherosclerotic disease
6. Giant hemangioma in the right lobe of the liver
7. Mild chronic compression deformity of the T12 vertebral body
8. 2-cm left renal cyst

Percentages stenosis were obtained using NASCET technique of stenosis calculation.

SIGNED: Dr. Gene I. Kim, MD

Select the appropriate codes for the case study.

1. List the ICD-10-CM code(s):

   ICD-10-CM code(s): ______________, ______________, ______________, ______________, ______________, ______________, ______________, ______________

2. List the CPT/HCPCS code(s) and any applicable modifiers:

   CPT code(s): ______________

3. List the procedure and diagnosis codes on the CMS-1500 form. Be sure to correctly link the procedure and diagnosis codes.

21. DIAGNOSIS OR NATURE OF ILLNESS OR INJURY Relate A-L to service line below (24E) ICD Ind.

A.	B.	C.	D.
E.	F.	G.	H.
I.	J.	K.	L.

22. RESUBMISSION CODE

23. PRIOR AUTHORIZATION NU

	24. A. DATE(S) OF SERVICE From MM DD YY	To MM DD YY	B. PLACE OF SERVICE	C. EMG	D. PROCEDURES, SERVICES, OR SUPPLIES (Explain Unusual Circumstances) CPT/HCPCS	MODIFIER	E. DIAGNOSIS POINTER	F. $ CHARGES	G. DAYS OR UNITS
1									
2									
3									
4									

Case Study 13.5

PATIENT: Lario Robison

ORDERING PROVIDER: Susan Alameda, DO

US INGUINAL GROIN: US ABDOMINAL LIMITED

CLINICAL DATA:
59-year-old male with left lower abdominal quadrant pain

TECHNICAL DATA:
Multiple longitudinal and transverse real-time images of the left groin were performed by the ultrasound technologist.

FINDINGS:
There are no previous exams available for comparison.

Images of the left groin with and without the Valsalva maneuver demonstrate a small fat-containing left inguinal hernia with approximately 1.7 cm in greatest dimension enlarged with a left inguinal ring.

There is no evidence of a dominant mass, hypoechoic lesion, or pathologic lymphadenopathy.

IMPRESSION:
Small fat-containing left inguinal hernia as described above.

SIGNED: Dr. Gene I. Kim, MD

Select the appropriate codes for the case study.

1. List the ICD-10-CM code(s):
   ICD-10-CM code(s): ________________
2. List the CPT/HCPCS code(s) and any applicable modifiers:
   CPT code(s): ________________

3. List the procedure and diagnosis codes on the CMS-1500 form. Be sure to correctly link the procedure and diagnosis codes.

21. DIAGNOSIS OR NATURE OF ILLNESS OR INJURY Relate A-L to service line below (24E) ICD Ind.

A. ____ B. ____ C. ____ D. ____
E. ____ F. ____ G. ____ H. ____
I. ____ J. ____ K. ____ L. ____

22. RESUBMISSION CODE

23. PRIOR AUTHORIZATION NU

	24. A. DATE(S) OF SERVICE From MM	DD	YY	To MM	DD	YY	B. PLACE OF SERVICE	C. EMG	D. PROCEDURES, SERVICES, OR SUPPLIES (Explain Unusual Circumstances) CPT/HCPCS	MODIFIER	E. DIAGNOSIS POINTER	F. $ CHARGES	G. DAYS OR UNITS
1													
2													
3													
4													

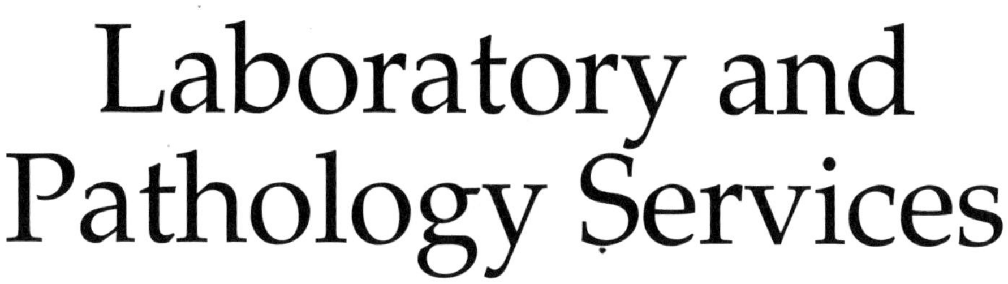

Chapter 14: Laboratory and Pathology Services

Vocabulary

Instructions: Define each of the following key terms in the space provided.

1. Bacteriology: ______________________________

____

____

2. Cytopathology: ______________________________

____

____

3. Frozen block: ______________________________

____

____

4. Frozen section: ______________________________

____

____

5. Gross examination: ______________________________

____

____

6. Independent laboratory: ______________________________

____

____

7. Laboratory and pathology services: ______________________________

____

____

8. Methicillin-resistant *Staphylococcus aureus* (MRSA): ______________________________

____

____

9. Microscopic examination: ______________________________

____

____

10. Mycology: ______________________________

____

____

11. Nonspecific test: ______________________________

____

____

12. Panel: ______________________________

____

____

13. Parasitology: ______________________________

____

____

14. Pass-through billing: ______________________________

____

____

15. Permanent block: ____________________

____

____

16. Permanent section: ____________________

____

____

17. Qualitative examination: ____________________

____

____

18. Quantitative examination: ____________________

____

____

19. Smear: ____________________

____

____

20. Specific test: ____________________

____

____

21. Specimen: ____________________

____

____

22. Virology: ____________________

____

____

Multiple Choice

Instructions: Choose the best answer.

1. In which of the following laboratories are the procedures typically low-risk, lox-complexity procedures?
a. CLIA-waived laboratories
b. Independent laboratories
c. Hospital laboratories
d. Practice-dependent laboratories

2. Which of the following would not be classified as a CLIA-waived laboratory test?
a. Mono spot
b. Strep swab
c. Gene analysis
d. Urinalysis

3. In pass-through billing, which modifier is appended to the CPT code for the laboratory service to indicate that it was performed by an independent laboratory?
a. -81
b. -90
c. -59
d. -91

4. In pass-through billing, the charges for the laboratory service are entered into which box on the CMS-1500 form?
a. Box 24.A
b. Box 90
c. Box 21
d. Box 20

5. Which of the following levels of surgical pathology procedures includes only the gross examination of a specimen?
a. Level I
b. Level II
c. Level III
d. Level IV

6. In which of the following settings would a CLIA-waived laboratory test be performed?
a. Inpatient hospital
b. Healthcare provider office
c. Certified independent laboratory
d. Imaging center

7. If the result of a test is a numerical value, what type of test is it?
a. Quantitative
b. CLIA-waived
c. Laboratory and pathology
d. Qualitative

8. Which of the following describes a specimen that has been permanently fixed in a fixative agent?
a. Frozen block
b. Smear
c. Permanent section
d. Frozen section

9. Which of the following panels consists of carbon dioxide, chloride, potassium, and sodium lab tests?
a. Basic metabolic panel
b. General health panel
c. Electrolyte panel
d. Comprehensive metabolic panel

10. What modifier would be reported for a laboratory service that had to be repeated due to an error with a lab machine?
a. Modifier -90
b. Modifier -52
c. Modifier -91
d. No modifier is applicable.

Fill in the Blank

Instructions: Complete the following statements.

1. In pass-through billing, the three things you must do on the CMS-1500 form are: change the place of service to __________; add the charges in box __________ of the CMS-1500 claim form; and append modifier __________ to the CPT code for the __________.

2. Laboratory services identify only the __________ of the specimen. CPT codes from the surgical section of the CPT code book are required to identify the __________ of the specimen.

3. After specimens are collected, they may be examined in a number of different ways. __________ is an examination of the physical characteristics of a specimen. __________ is the examination of a specimen at a microscopic level, which allows the pathologist to see the cells of the specimen. A __________ is a specimen that is submerged into liquid or a fluid substance, and then smeared onto the surface of a slide. A __________ is a small slice of a specimen that has been frozen; and a __________ is a small slice of a specimen that has been preserved in a fixative agent.

4. A __________ examination is one that examines the characteristics or properties of a specimen. A __________ examination is one that determines the amount of a substance within a specimen.

Coding

Instructions: Identify the correct CPT and ICD-10-CM codes for the following statements.

1. Collection of venous blood by venipuncture for complete blood count (automated with differential) in patient with upper respiratory infection

   CPT code(s): ______________, ______________

   ICD-10-CM code(s): ______________

2. 45-year-old established male presents to the office for routine physical examination; complete lipid panel completed in office, which revealed hypercholesterolemia

   CPT code(s): ______________, ______________

   ICD-10-CM code(s): ______________, ______________

3. HIV confirmation test on patient with recently diagnosed asymptomatic HIV status

   CPT code(s): ______________

   ICD-10-CM code(s): ______________

4. Postmortem examination of stillborn infant (including brain)

   CPT code(s): ______________

5. Pathological examination of prostatic tissue obtained from transurethral resection of the prostate, performed for benign prostatic hypertrophy

   CPT code(s): ______________

   ICD-10-CM code(s): ______________

6. Electrolyte panel completed on a patient with dehydration and electrolyte imbalance

   CPT code(s): ______________

   ICD-10-CM code(s): ______________

7. Adenovirus antibody test performed on patient with upper respiratory infection and diarrhea

   CPT code(s): ______________

   ICD-10-CM code(s): ______________, ______________

8. Serologic Rh(D) blood typing test performed on G1P0 patient at 8 weeks' gestation

CPT code(s): ______________

9. Vaginal chlamydial culture for patient who engages in high-risk heterosexual behavior, with vaginal discharge and pelvic pain confirming chlamydial vulvovaginitis

CPT code(s): ______________

ICD-10-CM code(s): ______________, ______________

10. HIV-1 antigen and HIV-2 antibody tests performed on a fully transportable testing platform confirms asymptomatic HIV status

CPT code(s): ______________-______

ICD-10-CM code(s): ______________

11. 48-hour Dexamethasone suppression panel

CPT code(s): ______________

12. Blood count with spun microhematocrit

CPT code(s): ______________

13. Quantitative examination for zinc

CPT code(s): ______________

14. Peripheral vein renin stimulation panel, including 6 individual labs for renin level

CPT code(s): ______________

15. Definitive drug class testing for 6 tricyclic antidepressants

CPT code(s): ______________

16. KOH prep for vaginal smear (wet mount)

CPT code(s): ______________

Case Studies Laboratory and Pathology

Case Study 14.1

PATIENT: Kayceon Munson

ORDERING PROVIDER: Susan Alameda, DO

FOR: Neonatal jaundice

BILIRUBIN, BLOOD, NEONATAL TOTAL:
Critical result called to Trina at pediatric clinic on 12/08/20XX

Test:
Bilirubin, neonate

Result:
17.7

Units:
mg/dl

Flag Reference Range:
HH 0.4–12.0

Select the appropriate codes for the case study.

1. List the ICD-10-CM code(s):

   ICD-10-CM code(s): ________________

2. List the CPT/HCPCS code(s) and any applicable modifiers:

   CPT code(s): ________________

3. List the procedure and diagnosis codes on the CMS-1500 form. Be sure to correctly link the procedure and diagnosis codes.

21. DIAGNOSIS OR NATURE OF ILLNESS OR INJURY Relate A-L to service line below (24E) ICD Ind.

A. ____ B. ____ C. ____ D. ____
E. ____ F. ____ G. ____ H. ____
I. ____ J. ____ K. ____ L. ____

22. RESUBMISSION CODE

23. PRIOR AUTHORIZATION NU

	24. A. DATE(S) OF SERVICE From MM DD YY	To MM DD YY	B. PLACE OF SERVICE	C. EMG	D. PROCEDURES, SERVICES, OR SUPPLIES (Explain Unusual Circumstances) CPT/HCPCS	MODIFIER	E. DIAGNOSIS POINTER	F. $ CHARGES	G. DAYS OR UNITS
1									
2									
3									
4									

Case Study 14.2

DERMATOPATHOLOGY REPORT

PATIENT: Todd Nielson

ORDERING PROVIDER: Susan Alameda, DO

FOR: Shave right proximal thigh; acrochordon with fat

CLINICAL DATA: Acrochordon vs. nevus vs. nevus lipomatosis vs. other

SPECIMEN SITE: Shave right proximal thigh

GROSS DESCRIPTION: Received in formal is a 9 mm × 7 mm × 4 mm shave specimen of skin. Bisected and submitted in one cassette.

MICROSCOPIC DESCRIPTION: The specimen is a shave biopsy of skin present as multiple H&E stained sections on one side. Sections show a pedunculated, exophytic papule demonstrating papillomatous hyperplasia of the epidermis and a central code of unremarkable connective tissue, blood vessels, and adipocytes.

SIGNED: Dr. Grace Young, MD

Select the appropriate codes for the case study.

1. List the ICD-10-CM code(s):

   ICD-10-CM code(s): ________________

2. List the CPT/HCPCS code(s) and any applicable modifiers:

   CPT code(s): ________________

3. List the procedure and diagnosis codes on the CMS-1500 form. Be sure to correctly link the procedure and diagnosis codes.

21. DIAGNOSIS OR NATURE OF ILLNESS OR INJURY Relate A-L to service line below (24E) ICD Ind.

A. ______	B. ______	C. ______	D. ______
E. ______	F. ______	G. ______	H. ______
I. ______	J. ______	K. ______	L. ______

22. RESUBMISSION CODE

23. PRIOR AUTHORIZATION NU

	24. A. DATE(S) OF SERVICE From MM DD YY	To MM DD YY	B. PLACE OF SERVICE	C. EMG	D. PROCEDURES, SERVICES, OR SUPPLIES (Explain Unusual Circumstances) CPT/HCPCS	MODIFIER	E. DIAGNOSIS POINTER	F. $ CHARGES	G. DAYS OR UNITS
1									
2									
3									
4									

Case Study 14.3

PATIENT: Eleanore Fillmore

ORDERING PROVIDER: Susan Alameda, DO

FOR: Health maintenance screening for diabetes

HGB A1c WITH eAG:

Test:
Hemoglobin A1c

Result:
6.2%

Flag Reference Range:
Patient normal 4.0–5.6%
Border line 5.7–6.4%
Diabetes ≥ 6.5%
Diabetic goal ≤ 7.0%

Test:
Mean blood glucose est.

Result:
131 mg/dl

Select the appropriate codes for the case study.

1. List the ICD-10-CM code(s):
   ICD-10-CM code(s): ________________
2. List the CPT/HCPCS code(s) and any applicable modifiers:
   CPT code(s): ________________
3. List the procedure and diagnosis codes on the CMS-1500 form. Be sure to correctly link the procedure and diagnosis codes.

21. DIAGNOSIS OR NATURE OF ILLNESS OR INJURY Relate A-L to service line below (24E) ICD Ind.

A. ______ B. ______ C. ______ D. ______
E. ______ F. ______ G. ______ H. ______
I. ______ J. ______ K. ______ L. ______

22. RESUBMISSION CODE

23. PRIOR AUTHORIZATION NU

	24. A. DATE(S) OF SERVICE From MM	DD	YY	To MM	DD	YY	B. PLACE OF SERVICE	C. EMG	D. PROCEDURES, SERVICES, OR SUPPLIES (Explain Unusual Circumstances) CPT/HCPCS	MODIFIER	E. DIAGNOSIS POINTER	F. $ CHARGES	G. DAYS OR UNITS
1													
2													
3													
4													

Case Study 14.4

PATIENT: Christina Ronson

ORDERING PROVIDER: Susan Alameda, DO

FOR: Long-term use of anticoagulants

ANTITHROMBIN III (FUNCTIONAL) A:

Test:
Antithrombin activity

Result:
84%

Flag:
None

Reference:
75–135

Note:
Direct thrombin inhibitor anticoagulants such as rivaroxaban, apixaban, and edoxaban will lead to spuriously elevated antithrombin activity levels, possibly masking a deficiency.

Select the appropriate codes for the case study.

1. List the ICD-10-CM code(s):
   ICD-10-CM code(s): ________________
2. List the CPT/HCPCS code(s) and any applicable modifiers:
   CPT code(s): ________________
3. List the procedure and diagnosis codes on the CMS-1500 form. Be sure to correctly link the procedure and diagnosis codes.

21. DIAGNOSIS OR NATURE OF ILLNESS OR INJURY Relate A-L to service line below (24E) ICD Ind.

A. ____ B. ____ C. ____ D. ____
E. ____ F. ____ G. ____ H. ____
I. ____ J. ____ K. ____ L. ____

22. RESUBMISSION CODE

23. PRIOR AUTHORIZATION NU

	24. A. DATE(S) OF SERVICE From MM DD YY	To MM DD YY	B. PLACE OF SERVICE	C. EMG	D. PROCEDURES, SERVICES, OR SUPPLIES (Explain Unusual Circumstances) CPT/HCPCS	MODIFIER	E. DIAGNOSIS POINTER	F. $ CHARGES	G. DAYS OR UNITS
1									
2									
3									
4									

Case Study 14.5

PATIENT: Carolee Campbell

ORDERING PROVIDER: Susan Alameda, DO

FOR: Screening for lipoid disorders

LIPID PROFILE-AMA: (Chol, HDL, risk ratio, trig)

Test:	**Result:**	**Flag:**	**Reference:**
Cholesterol	165 mg/dl		124–199
Triglycerides	615 mg/dl	H	40–150
HDL	35 mg/dl	L	40–150
Risk Ratio	4.8%		3.7–5.4
LDL Calc	10 mg/dl		0–129
Non-HDL Calc	133 mg/dl		

Select the appropriate codes for the case study.

1. List the ICD-10-CM code(s):

   ICD-10-CM code(s): ________________

2. List the CPT/HCPCS code(s) and any applicable modifiers:

   CPT code(s): ________________

3. List the procedure and diagnosis codes on the CMS-1500 form. Be sure to correctly link the procedure and diagnosis codes.

21. DIAGNOSIS OR NATURE OF ILLNESS OR INJURY Relate A-L to service line below (24E) ICD Ind.

A. ____ B. ____ C. ____ D. ____
E. ____ F. ____ G. ____ H. ____
I. ____ J. ____ K. ____ L. ____

22. RESUBMISSION CODE

23. PRIOR AUTHORIZATION NU

	24. A. DATE(S) OF SERVICE From MM DD YY	To MM DD YY	B. PLACE OF SERVICE	C. EMG	D. PROCEDURES, SERVICES, OR SUPPLIES (Explain Unusual Circumstances) CPT/HCPCS	MODIFIER	E. DIAGNOSIS POINTER	F. $ CHARGES	G. DAYS OR UNITS
1									
2									
3									
4									

Orthopedic Services

Vocabulary

Instructions: Define each of the following key terms in the space provided.

1. Amputation: ____

____

____

2. Arthritis: ____

____

____

3. Arthrocentesis: ____

____

____

4. Arthrodesis: ____

____

____

5. Arthropathy: ____

____

____

6. Arthroplasty: ______________________________

____

____

7. Arthroscopy: ______________________________

____

____

8. Bursa: ______________________________

____

____

9. Chiropractor: ______________________________

____

____

10. Closed fracture: ______________________________

____

____

11. Closed treatment: ______________________________

____

____

12. Comminuted fracture: ______________________________

____

____

13. Compound fracture: ______________________________

____

____

14. Compression fracture: ______________________________

____

____

15. Displaced fracture: ____

____

____

16. Fascia: ____

____

____

17. Gout: ____

____

____

18. Greenstick fracture: ____

____

____

19. Gustilo-Anderson classification: ____

____

____

20. Impacted fracture: ____

____

____

____

21. Internal fixation device: ____

____

____

22. Interspace: ____

____

____

23. Kyphosis: ____

____

____

24. Malunion: ______________________________

____

____

25. Manipulation: ______________________________

____

____

26. Monoarthritis: ______________________________

____

____

27. Musculoskeletal system: ______________________________

____

____

28. Nondisplaced fracture: ______________________________

____

____

29. Nonunion: ______________________________

____

____

30. Oblique fracture: ______________________________

____

____

31. Open fracture: ______________________________

____

____

32. Open treatment: ______________________________

____

____

33. Orthopedic services: ______________________________

____

____

34. Orthopedist: ______________________________

____

____

35. Osteoarthritis: ______________________________

____

____

36. Osteopathic manipulative treatment (OMT): ______________________________

____

____

37. Pathological fracture: ______________________________

____

____

38. Percutaneous: ______________________________

____

____

39. Percutaneous skeletal fixation: ______________________________

____

____

40. Physeal fracture: ______________________________

____

____

41. Polyarthritis: ______________________________

____

____

42. Salter-Harris classification: ______________________________

43. Scoliosis: ______________________________

44. Segment: ______________________________

45. Segmental fracture: ______________________________

46. Skeletal traction: ______________________________

47. Skin traction: ______________________________

48. Spiral fracture: ______________________________

49. Sprain: ______________________________

50. Strain: ______________________________

51. Tophus: ______________________________

____

____

52. Torus fracture: ______________________________

____

____

53. Traction: ______________________________

____

____

54. Transverse fracture: ______________________________

____

____

55. Traumatic fracture: ______________________________

____

____

Multiple Choice

Instructions: Choose the best answer.

1. Excisions of subcutaneous soft tissue tumors are for the removal of tissue:
   a. Below the skin
   b. Below the deep fascia
   c. More than one layer of tissue
   d. Of the bone

2. Which of the following types of procedures identifies the aspiration of a joint?
   a. Arthrodesis
   b. Arthrocentesis
   c. Arthritis
   d. Amputation

3. Which of the following types of traction uses straps, ropes, pulleys, and weights on the outside of the body?
   a. Skeletal
   b. Percutaneous
   c. Internal
   d. Skin

4. Which of the following types of fracture treatments involves the manual application of external forces to place the bone back to its original position?
a. Manipulation
b. Traction
c. Fixation
d. Rotation

5. Which of the following treatment types includes the incision of the skin in order to view the fracture site and/or place internal fixation devices?
a. Closed treatment
b. Percutaneous skeletal fixation
c. Open treatment
d. Internal fixation

6. In which of the following circumstances would it be appropriate to report the code for the casting of a fracture?
a. After the fracture is manipulated into place and then set
b. After the application of internal fixation devices
c. If no fracture manipulation or repair was performed
d. When the casting is an especially difficult procedure

7. Which of the following procedures involves the replacement of the knee joint?
a. Knee arthroplasty
b. Knee arthrodesis
c. Knee arthrocentesis
d. Knee amputation

8. Which of the following amputation codes would be reported to identify a midtarsal amputation?
a. 28800
b. 28805
c. 28810
d. 28820

9. Which of the following is used to identify the severity of a compound fracture?
a. Salter-Harris classification
b. Lund-Browder classification
c. Gustilo-Anderson classification
d. The rule of nines

10. Which of the following is used to identify the type of fracture that occurs on a growth plate?
a. Salter-Harris classification
b. Lund-Browder classification
c. Gustilo-Anderson classification
d. The rule of nines

Matching

Instructions: Match the fracture type with the fracture description.

1. __________ Greenstick	**A.** Fracture found in the spine when vertebrae collapse under their own pressure
2. __________ Transverse	**B.** Fracture composed of at least two fracture lines that isolate a larger section of bone
3. __________ Spiral	**C.** Fracture spirals around and extends down the bone
4. __________ Oblique	**D.** Fracture travels horizontally across the bone
5. __________ Comminuted	**E.** Ends of the bone are pushed into each other
6. __________ Segmental	**F.** Bone bends and cracks on one side
7. __________ Torus	**G.** Fracture travels diagonally across the bone
8. __________ Impacted	**H.** Fracture in which only one part of the bone buckles; occurs in children
9. __________ Compression	**I.** Fracture has more than two parts with multiple broken pieces

Labeling

Instructions: Complete the following anatomical diagram with the correct labels to identify the bones of the human body.

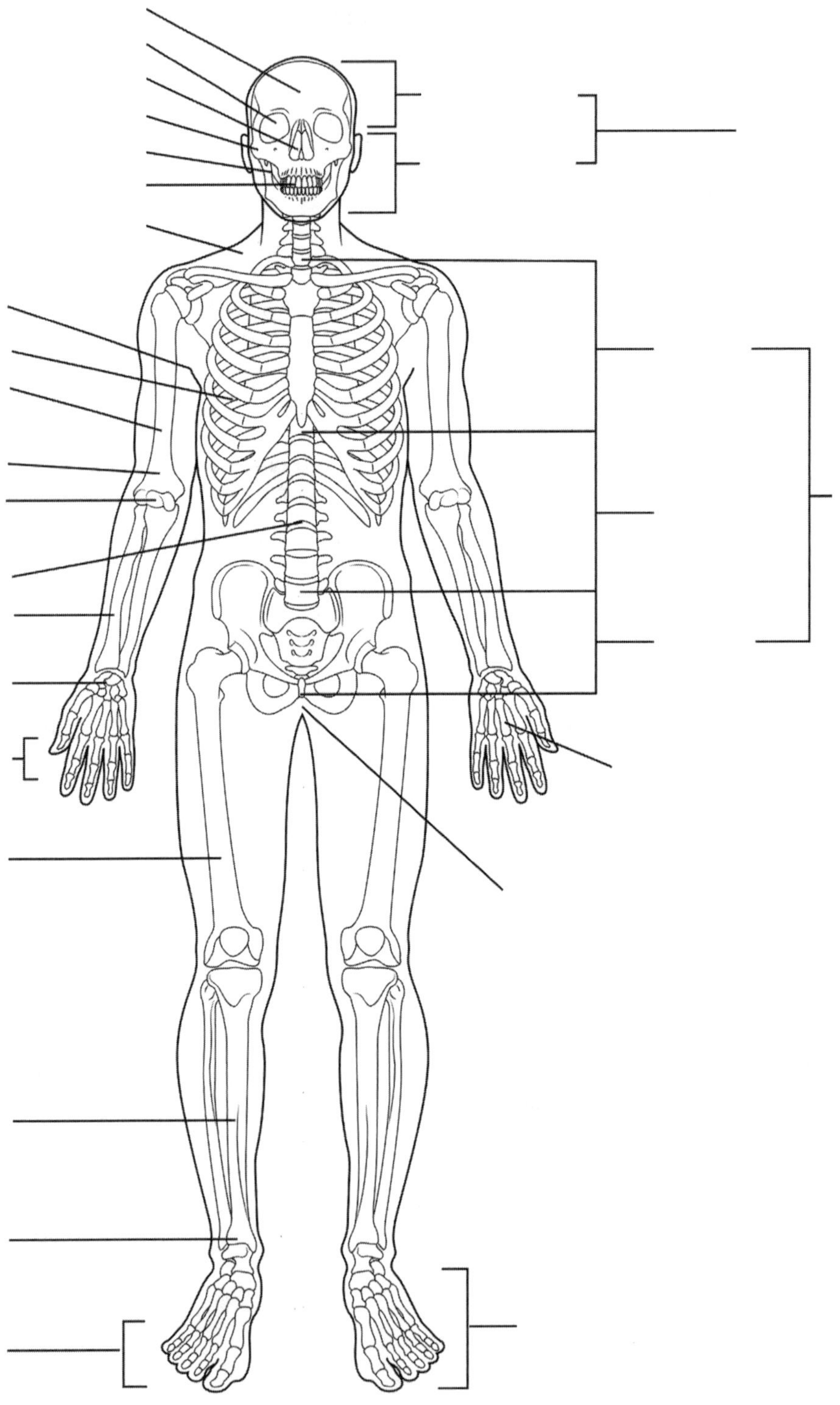

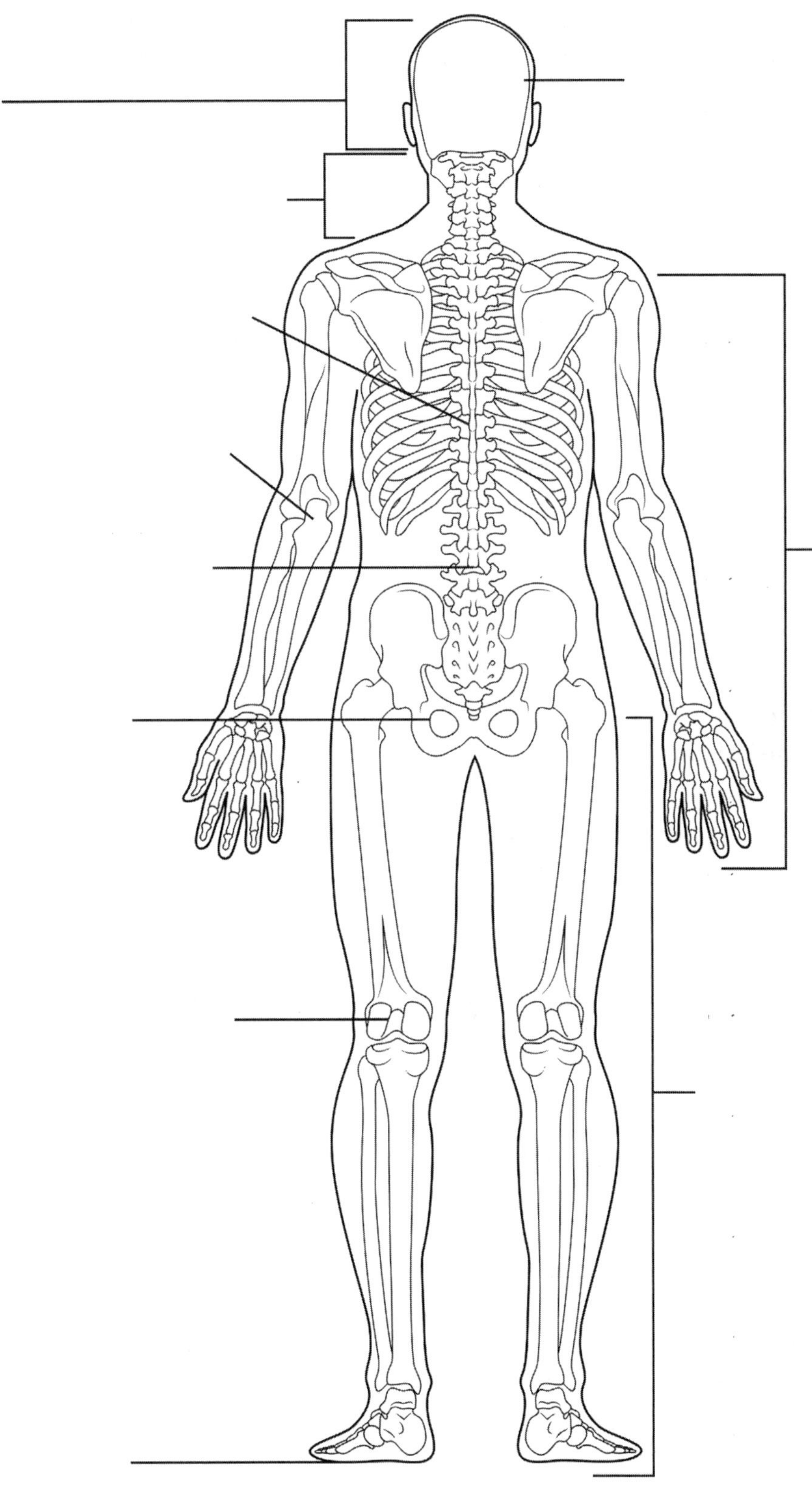

Coding

Instructions: Identify the correct CPT and ICD-10-CM codes for the following statements.

1. Report the code for a Salter-Harris type I physeal fracture of lower end of right femur, initial encounter for closed fracture.

ICD-10-CM code(s): _______________

2. Percutaneous skeletal fixation of metatarsal bone for displaced fracture of fifth metatarsal bone of the left foot. (Tip: Remember to identify the laterality of the procedure with the correct modifier.)

CPT code(s): _______________-_____

ICD-10-CM code(s): _______________

3. Patient with osteoporosis is seen for pain in right forearm after falling in her kitchen. 78-year-old female has age-related osteoporosis. X-ray of the forearm (two views) reveals nondisplaced fracture of the right radius. Static splint applied in office without manipulation for immobilization of fracture site and patient advised to return in one month for follow-up to check healing status.

CPT code(s): _______________-_____, _______________-_____

ICD-10-CM code(s): _______________

4. Release of thenar muscle of the left hand due to thumb contracture.

CPT code(s): _______________-_____

ICD-10-CM code(s): _______________

5. Metatarsal amputation of great toe of right foot due to gangrene.

CPT code(s): _______________-_____

ICD-10-CM code(s): _______________

6. 80-year-old female presents for evaluation of her senile osteoporosis. She has no current osteoporotic fractures but does have a history of healed pathological fracture of her left radius and ulna.

ICD-10-CM code(s): _______________, _______________

7. Antibiotic injection without ultrasound guidance provided to 38-year-old male patient with MSSA infectious arthritis of right knee joint.

CPT code(s): _______________-_____

ICD-10-CM code(s): _______________, _______________

8. 34-year-old male presents for a follow-up on an open (Type IIIB) displaced oblique fracture of the shaft of the right femur, which was surgically fixed and is now healing well. Cast was removed and replaced with an ambulatory long leg cast.

CPT code(s): ________________-_____

ICD-10-CM code(s): ________________

9. Incision and drainage of deep abscess of the lumbosacral spine.

CPT code(s): ________________

ICD-10-CM code(s): ________________

10. Arthrotomy of left glenohumeral joint for removal of foreign body of left shoulder remaining after a puncture wound.

CPT code(s): ________________-_____

ICD-10-CM code(s): ________________

11. Tennis elbow, right

ICD-10-CM code(s): ________________

12. Effusion of right knee

ICD-10-CM code(s): ________________

13. Plantar fasciitis

ICD-10-CM code(s): ________________

14. Acromioclavicular osteoarthritis

ICD-10-CM code(s): ________________

15. Bicipital tendinitis of the left shoulder

ICD-10-CM code(s): ________________

16. Prepatellar bursitis

ICD-10-CM code(s): ________________

17. DeQuervain's tenosynovitis

ICD-10-CM code(s): ________________

18. Trigger finger, left middle finger

ICD-10-CM code(s): ________________

19. Dupuytren's contracture

ICD-10-CM code(s): ________________

20. Rotator cuff tendinitis of the left shoulder

ICD-10-CM code(s): ______________

Case Studies Orthopedic Coding

Case Study 15.1

PATIENT: John Witte

CHIEF COMPLAINT:
60-year-old male presents with right knee injury

HISTORY OF PRESENT ILLNESS:
Right knee pain after falling while he was skiing. Pain is 1/10, denies taking anything for pain. Joint is stiff, but there is no swelling. He states that walking long distances causes a throbbing pain that radiates down the leg, causing his foot to become a little stiff. Pain is located on the medial side.

REVIEW OF SYSTEMS:
Constitutional: no chills and not feeling tired
Neurological: no difficulty walking
Musculoskeletal: no joint pain, no joint swelling, and no joint stiffness
Respiratory: no shortness of breath

PFSH:
No previous diagnosis of osteoporosis. No previous diagnosis of osteopenia. The patient has previously broken/fractured an ankle bone in 2016.
Patient drinks alcohol 1–2 times per week.
Not currently employed.

PHYSICAL EXAMINATION:
Constitutional: alert, in no acute distress. Well-developed and normal voice and communication. No injuries or skin lesions on the right upper extremity. No injuries or skin lesions on the left upper extremity. No injuries or skin lesions on the right lower extremity. No injuries or skin lesions on the left lower extremity.
Neurologic/Psychiatric: The sensory exam was normal to light touch and pinprick. Coordination was normal. Deep tendon reflexes were 2+ and symmetric. The patient was oriented to person, place, and time. Mood and affect were appropriate.
Pulmonary: no respiratory distress and normal respiratory rhythm and effort.
Musculoskeletal: right knee swelling and tenderness but no warmth, no induration, and no erythema. The appearance of the knee is normal. Range of motion: normal. Peripheral neural exam: sensation to light touch. Motor function grossly intact. Lower leg compartments are soft and without signs or symptoms of compartment syndrome.

ASSESSMENT:

1. Right knee pain

PLAN:
X-ray in office today. X-ray does not indicate that a current fracture is present.
Ordered BONE-DENSITY-DEXA
Patient take home info: Recommendation was made for patient to get bone density test done. Patient is to take vitamin D daily.

XR TIB-FIB-LOWER LEG-RIGHT:

CLINICAL DATA:
60-year-old male with proximal fibular and lateral knee pain

TECHNICAL DATA:
AP and lateral images were obtained

FINDINGS:
There is mild subcutaneous swelling involving the lateral aspect of the proximal right calf. There is cortical undulation/medullary lucency involving the posterior and medial aspect of the proximal right fibula. There is a small calcaneal spur at the Achilles tendon attachment. There is no other evidence of fracture, dislocation, joint effusion, or other significant bony or soft tissue abnormality. The joint spaces appear normal. There is normal mineralization.

IMPRESSION:

1. Probable normal cortical/medullary variation rather than a fracture involving the proximal right fibula. Clinical correlation is recommended. Total of 36 minutes was spent on the date of service in documentation and evaluation of this patient.

SIGNED: Dr. David Johnston, MD

Select the appropriate codes for the case study.

1. List the ICD-10-CM code(s):
   ICD-10-CM code(s): ________________
2. List the CPT/HCPCS code(s) and any applicable modifiers:
   CPT code(s): ________________, ________________ - _____
3. List the procedure and diagnosis codes on the CMS-1500 form. Be sure to correctly link the procedure and diagnosis codes.

21. DIAGNOSIS OR NATURE OF ILLNESS OR INJURY Relate A-L to service line below (24E) ICD Ind.

A. ______ B. ______ C. ______ D. ______
E. ______ F. ______ G. ______ H. ______
I. ______ J. ______ K. ______ L. ______

22. RESUBMISSION CODE

23. PRIOR AUTHORIZATION NU

	24. A. DATE(S) OF SERVICE From MM DD YY	To MM DD YY	B. PLACE OF SERVICE	C. EMG	D. PROCEDURES, SERVICES, OR SUPPLIES (Explain Unusual Circumstances) CPT/HCPCS	MODIFIER	E. DIAGNOSIS POINTER	F. $ CHARGES	G. DAYS OR UNITS
1									
2									
3									
4									

Case Study 15.2

PATIENT: Amanda Conner

PREOPERATIVE DIAGNOSIS:
Chronic osteomyelitis with draining sinus, right ankle and foot; transmetatarsal amputation wound dehiscence

POSTOPERATIVE DIAGNOSIS:
Chronic osteomyelitis with draining sinus, right ankle and foot; transmetatarsal amputation wound dehiscence

NAME OF OPERATION:
Right foot wound debridement with bone removal through excisional debridement

INDICATIONS:
This is a 30-year-old female patient. According to the patient, she had surgery six weeks ago but unfortunately has been unable to make any of her follow-up appointments. She says she removed her stitches herself, and unfortunately the wound opened up. Was admitted overnight with a worsening infection and is here for surgical debridement. When I saw her this morning, the foot was infected, and she has a significant wound dehiscence with bone exposure. After discussion with her, the decision was made to bring her for operative debridement.

PROCEDURE IN DETAIL:
Under mild sedation, patient was brought to the operating room and placed on the operating table in the supine position. Following general anesthesia by the anesthesiologist, the foot was scrubbed, prepped, and draped in the usual aseptic manner, and the tourniquet was inflated to 250 mmHg.

Next, the wound was debrided of all nonviable and devitalized tissue through excisional debridement. Bone was removed from the 1st, 2nd, 3rd, 4th, and 5th metatarsals, and the entire bone rack was sent for culture and sensitivity. There was an abscess of the 3rd and 2nd metatarsals, which I did irrigate and did not find any further abscess in the deep spaces of the foot. 3,000 cc of sterile normal saline with bacitracin was used to irrigate the wound. The area was then irrigated and packed open with sterile gauze. The tourniquet was deflated, and a prompt hyperemic response was noted to the plantar flap.

Following a period of postoperative monitoring, the patient will be readmitted for continuing IV antibiotics. I will see her tomorrow and change the bandages for the 1st time. Her PCP will assume normal care on Monday and decide whether or not he feels that this is a salvageable foot.

SIGNED: Dr. David Johnston, MD

Select the appropriate codes for the case study.

1. List the ICD-10-CM code(s):
ICD-10-CM code(s): ________________

2. List the CPT/HCPCS code(s) and any applicable modifiers:
CPT code(s): ________________

3. List the procedure and diagnosis codes on the CMS-1500 form. Be sure to correctly link the procedure and diagnosis codes.

21. DIAGNOSIS OR NATURE OF ILLNESS OR INJURY Relate A-L to service line below (24E) ICD Ind.

A. B. C. D.

E. F. G. H.

I. J. K. L.

22. RESUBMISSION CODE

23. PRIOR AUTHORIZATION NU

	24. A. DATE(S) OF SERVICE From MM DD YY	To MM DD YY	B. PLACE OF SERVICE	C. EMG	D. PROCEDURES, SERVICES, OR SUPPLIES (Explain Unusual Circumstances) CPT/HCPCS	MODIFIER	E. DIAGNOSIS POINTER	F. $ CHARGES	G. DAYS OR UNITS
1									
2									
3									
4									

Case Study 15.3

REPORT OF OPERATION

PATIENT: Rodrigo Gonzales

PREOPERATIVE DIAGNOSIS:
Complex tear of the medial and lateral menisci of the right knee

POSTOPERATIVE DIAGNOSIS:
Complex tear of the medial and lateral menisci of the right knee

PROCEDURE:
Arthroscopic partial medical and lateral meniscectomy with medial and lateral femoral chondroplasties

ANESTHESIA:
General endotracheal with regional nerve block

COMPLICATIONS:
None

DISPOSITION:
Stable at PACU

INDICATIONS:
This is a 44-year-old male with a history of right knee pain that has been refractory to conservative treatment. An MRI was ordered, which showed complex tears of the medial and lateral menisci of the right knee. The patient elected to undergo arthroscopic surgery after the risks were explained.

PROCEDURE IN DETAIL:
The patient was placed in the supine position on the operating table and successfully intubated. Following that, a tourniquet was placed around his leg, and the patient's leg was placed in a thigh holder. Following that, the patient was sterilely prepped and draped in the usual manner, and then a standard timeout took place noting the corrective operative site, side, and procedure.

The tourniquet was then placed at 20 mmHg with the use of an Esmarch device. A standard lateral parapatellar incision was then created, and a diagnostic arthroscopy took place at that time. The patient was noted to have moderate arthritis tricompartmentally with some full-thickness chondral changes in the medial compartment. A medical parapateller portal was created under direct visualization with a spinal needle. Following that, a probe was the introduced into the knee. The medical compartment was noted to have pretty significant chondrosis of the medial femoral condyle. Even gentle probing of the medial femoral condyle dislodged loose pieces of cartilage, and grade III changes were noted on the medial femoral condyle. Following that, there was noted to be a complex tear of the posterior horn of the medial meniscus. With the combination of a straight biter and shaver, a stable meniscal rim was created. The arthroscope was then introduced in the lateral compartment and probed, and there was noted to be a pretty significant complex tear of the posterior horn of the meniscus, extending into the lateral body. With the use of the biter and shaver, a partial medical meniscectomy took place. It was noted that, at the posterior horn, there was a very little meniscal rim tissue remaining after the meniscectomy. A limited chondroplasty then took place of the lateral femoral condyle. Following that, a limited chondroplasty of the backside of the patella was undertaken, and then the arthroscope was taken of the knee. The portals were then closed with 3-0 Monocryl in buried fashion, and then the incisions were dressed and Xeroform, 4×4s, ABD, and Ace wrap.

The tourniquet was then taken down, and the patient was then taken back to PACU and notes to be in stable condition.

SIGNED: Dr. David Johnston, MD

Select the appropriate codes for the case study.

1. List the ICD-10-CM code(s):

   ICD-10-CM code(s): _______________, _______________

2. List the CPT/HCPCS code(s) and any applicable modifiers:

   CPT code(s): _______________

3. List the procedure and diagnosis codes on the CMS-1500 form. Be sure to correctly link the procedure and diagnosis codes.

21. DIAGNOSIS OR NATURE OF ILLNESS OR INJURY Relate A-L to service line below (24E) ICD Ind.

A. ____ B. ____ C. ____ D. ____
E. ____ F. ____ G. ____ H. ____
I. ____ J. ____ K. ____ L. ____

22. RESUBMISSION CODE

23. PRIOR AUTHORIZATION NU

	24. A. DATE(S) OF SERVICE From MM DD YY	To MM DD YY	B. PLACE OF SERVICE	C. EMG	D. PROCEDURES, SERVICES, OR SUPPLIES (Explain Unusual Circumstances) CPT/HCPCS	MODIFIER	E. DIAGNOSIS POINTER	F. $ CHARGES	G. DAYS OR UNITS
1									
2									
3									
4									

Case Study 15.4

PATIENT: Kevin Lutz

CHIEF COMPLAINT:
35-year-old male presents for follow-up on knee MRI

HISTORY OF PRESENT ILLNESS:
Sharp pain at the anterior knee along proximal patellar tendon with activity. Pain level is 2/10, 6–7/10 at worst. Pain meds: IBU. Pain with stairs and full extension. Patient is unable to run.

CURRENT MEDS:
Glucosamine TABS

ALLERGY:
No known drug allergies (NKDA)

PHYSICAL EXAMINATION:
Constitutional: alert and in no acute distress. No injuries or skin lesions on the right upper, left upper, right lower, or left lower extremities.
Neurological/Psychiatrics: the sensory examination was normal to light touch and pinprick. Coordination was normal. Deep tendon reflexes were 2+ and symmetric. The patient was oriented to person, place, and time. Mood and affect were appropriate.
Pulmonary: No respiratory distress.

ASSESSMENT:

1. Patellar tendon avulsion, left. Unfortunately, he has had a setback in his recovery and remains significantly symptomatic and functionally disabled. He would like to proceed with surgical debridement and repair. Would like to coordinate diagnostic arthroscopy in conjunction with this to make sure there is nothing interarticularly that is related to his continued pain, and we'll plan for open repair and debridement. Surgical booking slip was submitted today.

RESULTS/DATA:
Recent films pertinent to today's visit were reviewed. I concur with report findings. MRI demonstrated hyperintense signal with avulsion of deep fibers of the patellar tendon of the inferior pole of the patella. At least 50% of the tendon is involved.

SIGNED: Dr. David Johnston, MD

Select the appropriate codes for the case study.

1. List the ICD-10-CM code(s):
   ICD-10-CM code(s): ________________
2. List the CPT/HCPCS code(s) and any applicable modifiers:
   CPT code(s): ________________ - ____

3. List the procedure and diagnosis codes on the CMS-1500 form. Be sure to correctly link the procedure and diagnosis codes.

21. DIAGNOSIS OR NATURE OF ILLNESS OR INJURY Relate A-L to service line below (24E) ICD Ind.

A. ______ B. ______ C. ______ D. ______
E. ______ F. ______ G. ______ H. ______
I. ______ J. ______ K. ______ L. ______

22. RESUBMISSION CODE

23. PRIOR AUTHORIZATION NU

	24. A. DATE(S) OF SERVICE From MM DD YY	To MM DD YY	B. PLACE OF SERVICE	C. EMG	D. PROCEDURES, SERVICES, OR SUPPLIES (Explain Unusual Circumstances) CPT/HCPCS	MODIFIER	E. DIAGNOSIS POINTER	F. $ CHARGES	G. DAYS OR UNITS
1									
2									
3									
4									

Physical, Occupational, and Speech Therapy Services

Vocabulary

Instructions: Define each of the following key terms in the space provided.

1. 8-minute rule: ______________________________

____

____

2. Amputation: ______________________________

____

____

3. Amputee: ______________________________

____

____

4. Amyotrophic lateral sclerosis (ALS): ______________________________

____

____

5. Aphonia: ______________________________

6. Augmentative and alternative communication (AAC): ______________________________

7. Cognitive communication disorder: ______________________________

8. Constant attendance code: ______________________________

9. Dominant side: ______________________________

10. Dyslexia: ______________________________

11. Dysphagia: ______________________________

12. Electrical stimulation: ______________________________

13. Habilitative services: ______________________________

14. Hubbard tank: ____________________

15. Hypernasality: ____________________

16. Iontophoresis: ____________________

17. Language disorder: ____________________

18. Multiple sclerosis (MS): ____________________

19. Occupational therapist (OT): ____________________

20. Occupational therapy services: ____________________

21. Physical therapist (PT): ____________________

22. Physical therapy services: ____________________

23. Rehabilitative services: ____________________

____

____

24. Service-based code: ____________________

____

____

25. Social communication disorder: ____________________

____

____

26. Speech-language pathologist (SLP): ____________________

____

____

27. Speech therapy services: ____________________

____

____

28. Therapy services: ____________________

____

____

29. Time-based code: ____________________

____

____

30. Traumatic brain injury (TBI): ____________________

____

____

31. Treatment modality: ____________________

____

____

32. Vasopneumatic device: ____

____

____

Multiple Choice

Instructions: Choose the best answer.

1. Which of the following therapy types provides noninvasive treatments to alleviate pain and improve and restore functionality?
a. Physical
b. Occupational
c. Speech

2. Which of the following therapy types helps adults and children improve their communication skills?
a. Physical
b. Occupational
c. Speech

3. Which of the following therapy types helps patients improve fine motor skills?
a. Physical
b. Occupational
c. Speech

4. Which of the following parties provides the advanced beneficiary notice?
a. The provider performing the service
b. The patient receiving the service
c. The insurance expected to pay for the service
d. The insurance expected to not pay for the service

5. Which of the following modifiers identifies that the ABN is on file at the provider's office?
a. GX
b. GA
c. GY
d. GZ

6. Which of the following types of practitioners would most likely treat a patient with dysphasia?
a. SLP
b. NP
c. PT
d. OT

7. Which of the following types of practitioners would most likely treat a patient with limitation in walking?
   a. SLP
   b. CRNA
   c. PT
   d. OT

8. Which of the following types of practitioners would most likely treat a patient with difficulty holding eating utensils?
   a. PT
   b. SLP
   c. PA
   d. OT

9. Which of the following modifiers would be used to identify that a therapeutic service was provided to restore a patient to their normal functioning?
   a. -97
   b. -57
   c. -96
   d. -53

10. Which of the following modifiers would be used to identify that a therapeutic service was provided to allow a patient with a congenital deformity to function?
   a. -97
   b. -96
   c. -78
   d. -24

Matching

Instructions: Match the disorder or healthcare condition with its description.

1. ________	Language disorder	**A.** Excessive nasal tone to the voice
2. ________	Hypernasality	**B.** Difficulty organizing thoughts, remembering, paying attention, and planning
3. ________	Social communication disorder	**C.** Difficulty in understanding or producing oral speech
4. ________	Aphonia	**D.** Difficulty reading
5. ________	Cognitive communication disorder	**E.** Loss of voice

6. __________ Dyslexia

F. Difficulty understanding social cues and nonverbal communication

7. __________ Dysphagia

G. Difficulty swallowing

8. __________ Dysphasia

H. Difficulty speaking

Coding

Instructions: Identify the correct procedure and diagnosis codes for the following statements.

1. Low-complexity physical therapy evaluation for a 53-year-old female with bilateral knee osteoarthritis

CPT code(s): ______________

ICD-10-CM code(s): ______________

2. Application of hot pack to right shoulder followed by 30 minutes of range of motion, strength, and flexibility therapy for patient with incomplete tear of rotator cuff of right shoulder

CPT code(s): ______________, ______________ × ______

ICD-10-CM code(s): ______________

3. Repair of augmentative and alternative communication (AAC) device for patient with aphonia

HCPCS code(s): ______________

ICD-10-CM code(s): ______________

4. Individual treatment of speech and language for patient with articulation disorder due to bilateral conductive hearing loss

CPT code(s): ______________

ICD-10-CM code(s): ______________, ______________

5. Assessment of tinnitus in 55-year-old male with bilateral tinnitus

CPT code(s): ______________

ICD-10-CM code(s): ______________

6. 45 minutes of direct therapeutic activities, including the use of dynamic activities to improve the functional performance of a 4-year-old male patient with congenital deformities of bilateral hands

CPT code(s): ______________-______ (× ______)

ICD-10-CM code(s): ______________

7. 30 minutes of therapeutic exercises, focused on range of motion and flexibility of the right knee, status post tear of anterior cruciate ligament of right knee (subsequent encounter)

CPT code(s): ______________-______ (× ______)

ICD-10-CM code(s): ______________

8. Dysphagia, oropharyngeal phase, as a sequela of subarachnoid hemorrhage

ICD-10-CM code(s): ______________, ______________

9. 8-year-old male with autism spectrum disorder and inattentive-type ADHD presents for OT services.

ICD-10-CM code(s): ______________, ______________

10. 45-year-old male with a history of smoking two packs per day (no longer a smoker), status posthemiglossectomy due to malignant neoplasm of the left border of the tongue, presents for fitting of speech augmentation device. Patient is still undergoing chemo and radiation therapy for the neoplasm.

ICD-10-CM code(s): ______________, ______________

11. Speech therapy services provided to a 32-year-old female with recent apraxia of speech.

ICD-10-CM code(s): ______________

12. Occupational therapy evaluation with moderate MDM

CPT code(s): ______________

13. Physical therapy re-evaluation of plan of care with low MDM

CPT code(s): ______________

14. Physical therapeutic modalities employing dynamic activities to improve the ambulation of a 42-year-old male patient with right BKA after traumatic injury (30 minutes total). Patient's functional limitation includes difficulty walking due to lower leg prosthetic.

CPT code(s): ______________-______ (× ______)

ICD-10-CM code(s): ______________, ______________, ______________

15. 30 minutes of occupational therapy employing sensory integrative techniques to enhance patient processing of sensory demands for 3-year-old female with sensory conversion disorder.

CPT code(s): ______________-______ (× ______)

ICD-10-CM code(s): ______________

Case Studies Physical Therapy

Case Study 16.1

Physical Therapy Treatment Log

PATIENT: Manuel Rockford

Chief Complaint (C/C):
A 70-year-old male patient, status postbilateral knee replacements, presents for physical therapy. Today's goals are endurance, flexibility, and increased range of motion (ROM) for both knees. He is not currently experiencing any functional limitations and is walking without the use of a cane or walker.

Daily Treatment Log:
Initiated training session with 15 minutes on a stationary training bike to increase flexion of both knees as well as to increase endurance with continued flexing and strength of both knees and leg musculature.

After bike session was complete, patient was guided through isokinetic exercises to further increase ROM and flexibility of the bilateral knees. This required a total time of 10 minutes with the patient.

Before today's physical therapy treatment session in clinic, ROM for the right knee was 50 degrees, and after treatment was 55 degrees. Prior ROM of the left knee was 55 degrees and was increased to approximately 65 degrees post-therapy. He is due to return to the clinic in one week, at which time we will focus on increasing the ROM for the right knee to equal that of the left knee to improve stability and gait symmetry.

SIGNED: Santosh Ashokprabhu, PT

Select the appropriate codes for the case study.

1. List the ICD-10-CM code(s):
   ICD-10-CM code(s): ________________
2. List the CPT/HCPCS code(s) and any applicable modifiers:
   CPT code(s): ________________ - _____ (× _____)
3. List the procedure and diagnosis codes on the CMS-1500 form. Be sure to correctly link the procedure and diagnosis codes.

21. DIAGNOSIS OR NATURE OF ILLNESS OR INJURY Relate A-L to service line below (24E) ICD Ind.

A. ______ B. ______ C. ______ D. ______
E. ______ F. ______ G. ______ H. ______
I. ______ J. ______ K. ______ L. ______

22. RESUBMISSION CODE

23. PRIOR AUTHORIZATION NU

	24. A. DATE(S) OF SERVICE From MM DD YY	To MM DD YY	B. PLACE OF SERVICE	C. EMG	D. PROCEDURES, SERVICES, OR SUPPLIES (Explain Unusual Circumstances) CPT/HCPCS	MODIFIER	E. DIAGNOSIS POINTER	F. $ CHARGES	G. DAYS OR UNITS
1									
2									
3									
4									

Case Study 16.2

Physical Therapy Treatment Log

PATIENT: Adella Weiss

Chief Complaint (C/C):
Patient is a 35-year-old female who suffered a traumatic head injury in a car accident six months ago. She is experiencing benign paroxysmal positional vertigo of the left side. She commonly experiences loss of balance and dizziness and has fallen two times within the last three weeks due to her dizziness. Today she states that her dizziness is not as bad, and she feels confident that she can complete therapy exercises. She has not experienced any syncope or collapse.

Daily Treatment Log:
Began therapy session with two individual sessions of canalith repositioning to clear any canaliths within the vestibular canals that may be contributing her to her symptoms. We then initiated 15 minutes of gaze stabilization exercises to increase balance coordination. After completing the first exercise, Adella experienced a dizzy spell, which made her unable to complete the remaining therapy session. Therapist completed an additional canalith repositioning employing a different technique and left the patient to rest for 20 minutes until the dizziness had completely passed. A ride was called, and patient was picked up from the clinic by a family member.

SIGNED: Santosh Ashokprabhu, PT

Select the appropriate codes for the case study.

1. List the ICD-10-CM code(s):

   ICD-10-CM code(s): ________________, ________________

2. List the CPT/HCPCS code(s) and any applicable modifiers:

   CPT code(s): ________________ - _____, ________________ - _____

3. List the procedure and diagnosis codes on the CMS-1500 form. Be sure to correctly link the procedure and diagnosis codes.

21. DIAGNOSIS OR NATURE OF ILLNESS OR INJURY Relate A-L to service line below (24E) ICD Ind.

A. ____ B. ____ C. ____ D. ____
E. ____ F. ____ G. ____ H. ____
I. ____ J. ____ K. ____ L. ____

22. RESUBMISSION CODE

23. PRIOR AUTHORIZATION NU

	24. A. DATE(S) OF SERVICE From MM DD YY	To MM DD YY	B. PLACE OF SERVICE	C. EMG	D. PROCEDURES, SERVICES, OR SUPPLIES (Explain Unusual Circumstances) CPT/HCPCS	MODIFIER	E. DIAGNOSIS POINTER	F. $ CHARGES	G. DAYS OR UNITS
1									
2									
3									
4									

Obstetrics and Gynecology Services

Vocabulary

Instructions: Define each of the following key terms in the space provided.

1. Abortion: ____

____

____

2. Antepartum: ____

____

____

3. Bartholin's glands: ____

____

____

4. Birthing center: ____

____

____

5. Cerclage: ____

____

____

6. Certified nurse midwife (CNM): ______

7. Cervix uteri: ______

8. Cesarean delivery: ______

9. Conization: ______

10. Corpus uteri: ______

11. Diaphragm: ______

12. Endocervical curettage (ECC): ______

13. External os: ______

14. Fallopian tubes: ______

15. Gestation: ______________________________

____

____

16. Gestational condition: ______________________________

____

____

17. Gravida: ______________________________

____

____

18. Gynecologists: ______________________________

____

____

19. Incidental pregnancy: ______________________________

____

____

20. Internal os: ______________________________

____

____

21. Intrauterine device (IUD): ______________________________

____

____

22. Introitus: ______________________________

____

____

23. Labia majora: ______________________________

____

____

24. Labia minora: ____________________

____

____

25. Last menstrual period (LMP): ____________________

____

____

26. Loop electrosurgical excision procedure (LEEP): ____________________

____

____

27. Marsupialization: ____________________

____

____

28. Maternal fetal medicine (MFM) specialist: ____________________

____

____

29. Maternity services: ____________________

____

____

30. Nonobstetric: ____________________

____

____

31. Nuchal cord: ____________________

____

____

32. Nulligravida: ____________________

____

____

33. Nulliparous: ____

____

____

34. Obstetric: ____

____

____

35. Obstetricians: ____

____

____

36. Obstetrics and gynecology services: ____________________________

____

____

37. Outcome of delivery code: ________________________________

____

____

38. Ovaries: ____

____

____

39. Oviducts: ____

____

____

40. Parity (or para): ______________________________________

____

____

41. Perinatal: ____

____

____

42. Perinatologist: ______________________________

43. Perineum: ______________________________

44. Peripartum: ______________________________

45. Pessary: ______________________________

46. Postpartum: ______________________________

47. Products of conception (POC): ______________________________

48. Puerperium: ______________________________

49. Reproductive endocrinology and infertility (REI) specialist: ______________________________

50. Reproductive surgery: ______________________________

51. Sequencing priority: ____

____

52. Sexually transmitted infection (STI): ______________________________

____

____

53. Trimesters: ____

____

____

54. Uterus: ____

____

____

55. Vagina: ____

____

____

56. Vaginal birth after cesarean (VBAC): ______________________________

____

____

57. Vaginectomy: ____

____

____

58. Vulva: ____

____

____

Multiple Choice

Instructions: Choose the best answer.

1. Which of the following providers specialize in the health of pregnant patients?
a. Gynecologists
b. Obstetricians
c. Primary care physicians
d. Female wellness practitioners

2. Which of the following providers is a mid-level provider who specializes in the health of pregnant females and in obstetric care?
a. Certified nurse midwife
b. Obstetrician
c. Maternal fetal medicine specialist
d. Gynecologist

3. Which of the following place of service codes would be used for services performed in the labor and delivery (maternity) unit of a hospital facility?
a. 24
b. 11
c. 21
d. 23

4. How many times has a G3P1 patient been pregnant?
a. 3
b. 1
c. 4
d. Cannot determine from this information

5. Which of the following terms refers to a patient who has never been pregnant?
a. Multiparous
b. Multigravida
c. Gravidanulla
d. Nulligravida

6. If a patient is at 24 weeks, 3 days' gestation, in which trimester is she?
a. First
b. Second
c. Third

7. Which of the following codes identifies a pregnancy for a patient at 15 weeks' gestation?
a. O30.892
b. O30.899
c. O30.093
d. O30.099

8. Vulvectomy codes are based on which of the two following principles?
a. Obstetric and nonobstetric
b. Depth and size
c. Extent and depth
d. Trimester and gravida status

9. Which of the following devices is used as a barrier birth control method?
a. Cerclage
b. IUD
c. Diaphragm
d. Pessary

10. Which of the following is not included in the global maternity service?
a. Delivery
b. Routine antepartum visits
c. Sick visits
d. Postpartum visit

Matching

Instructions: Match the female anatomical structure with the code range for procedures on that area.

1. ________ Vulva, perineum, and introitus	**A.** 58800 to 58960
2. ________ Vagina	**B.** 58600 to 58770
3. ________ Cervix uteri	**C.** 58100 to 58579
4. ________ Corpus uteri	**D.** 57452 to 57800
5. ________ Oviduct/Ovary	**E.** 57000 to 57426
6. ________ Ovary	**F.** 56405 to 56821

Instructions: Match the type of delivery with its description.

7. ________ Vaginal	**G.** Birth through the natural birth canal after previous surgically assisted birth
8. ________ Cesarean	**H.** Birth through the natural birth canal

Matching continued on next page

(Continued)

9. ________	Vaginal birth after cesarean	**I.** Surgically assisted birth in which the infant is delivered through an incision in the lower abdomen
10. ________	Cesarean following attempted VBAC	**J.** Surgically assisted birth after attempted birth through the natural birth canal after previous surgically-assisted birth

Labeling

Instructions: Complete the following anatomical diagrams with the correct labels to identify the anatomy of the external female genitalia.

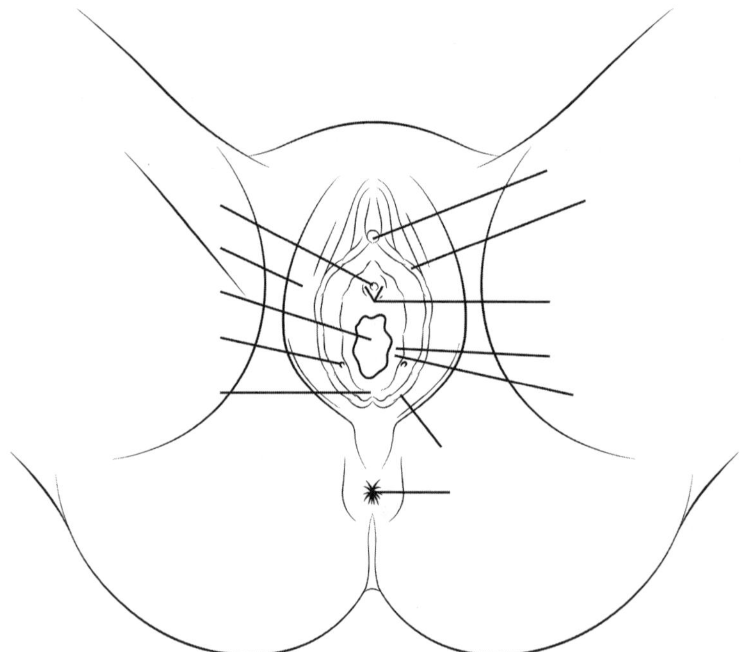

Source: ©AHIMA.

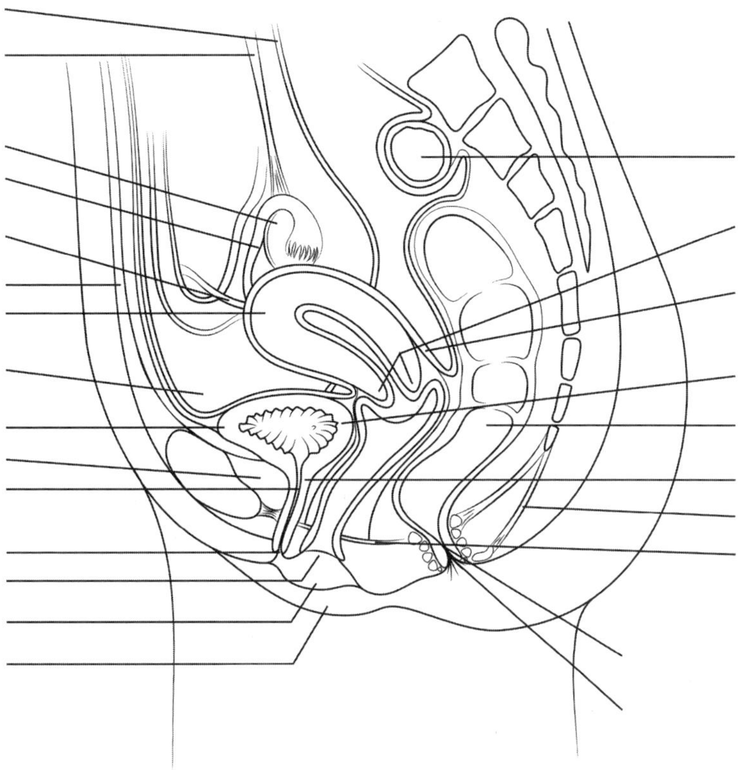

Source: ©AHIMA.

Coding

Instructions: Assign the correct CPT and ICD-10-CM codes for the following.

1. Patient at 30 weeks' gestation presents with polyhydramnios of twin A (fetus 1) in twin gestation.

ICD-10-CM code(s): ________________, ________________, ________________

2. Patient at 38 weeks' gestation and no complications presented to the delivery unit in labor. After 6 hours of natural labor, patient delivered a single, healthy female infant vaginally, without instrumentation, forceps, or episiotomy. OB who performed the delivery is billing for the global maternity service.

CPT code(s): ________________

ICD-10-CM code(s): ________________, ________________, ________________

3. G2P2 female presents for delivery at 34 weeks' gestation, and subsequently delivers single liveborn female in breech presentation vaginally. Patient suffered second-degree perineal laceration during delivery. (Provide the procedure code for the delivery only.)

CPT code(s): ________________

ICD-10-CM code(s): ________________, ________________, ________________,
________________, ________________

4. Removal of impacted vaginal foreign body, not requiring general anesthesia. Established patient had a tampon that was she was unable to remove herself. OB/GYN removed the FB without incident from the vagina and performed a detailed history and examination with low-complexity MDM.

CPT code(s): ______________

ICD-10-CM code(s): ______________

5. Gonorrhea causing pelvic inflammatory disease (PID) in 23-year-old female patient who commonly engages in high-risk heterosexual behavior. OB/GYN provided a detailed history and examination of this new patient and then spent 30 minutes counseling the patient in ways to reduce chances of obtaining sexually transmitted infections and safe sex techniques. Total time spent on the encounter was 45 minutes. Female also suffers from depression and anxiety and states that sexual deviation is related to these mental health issues.

CPT code(s): ______________

ICD-10-CM code(s): ______________, ______________, ______________, ______________

6. Code for the delivery of a single live-born infant born at 38 weeks' gestation after failed attempted VBAC (infant was born via cesarean section). Previous cesarean was completed with a low transverse incision. (Code for the delivery only.)

CPT code(s): ______________

ICD-10-CM code(s): ______________, ______________, ______________, ______________

7. Elective cesarean delivery completed without complications, resulting in a single, live-born female infant at 40 weeks' gestation. OB provided global care for the delivery.

CPT code(s): ______________

ICD-10-CM code(s): ______________, ______________, ______________

8. Gynecologist performed dilation of urethral stricture under general anesthesia for post-traumatic urethral stricture in a 30-year-old female patient, caused by childbirth.

CPT code(s): ______________

ICD-10-CM code(s): ______________

9. Surgical treatment of incomplete septic abortion due to group A streptococcus.

CPT code(s): ______________

ICD-10-CM code(s): ______________, ______________

10. Marsupialization of cyst of Bartholin's gland.

CPT code(s): ______________

ICD-10-CM code(s): ______________

Case Studies Obstetrics and Gynecology

Case Study 17.1

PATIENT: Susan Aldrich

DATE OF PROCEDURE: 02/19/20XX

PREOPERATIVE DIAGNOSIS: Symptomatic uterine fibroids

POSTOPERATIVE DIAGNOSIS: Same

ANESTESIA: General endotracheal

OPERATION: Robotic hysterectomy, bilateral salpingectomy, right ovarian cystectomy

FINDINGS: Enlarged fibroid uterus weighing 224 g; simple right ovarian cyst and endometriotic implants in the posterior pelvis and near the bladder.

ESTIMATE BLOOD LOSS: Less than 100 ml

COMPLICATIONS: None; patient tolerated the procedure well.

PROCEDURE IN DETAIL:
The patient was seen in the holding room. The risks, benefits, complications, treatment options, and expected outcomes were discussed with the patient. The patient concurred with the proposed plan, giving informed consent. The patient was taken to the operating room, and the procedure was verified as robotic hysterectomy with bilateral salpingectomy. A time-out was performed, and the above information was confirmed.

After induction of anesthesia, the patient was placed in lithotomy position and prepped and draped in the usual sterile manner. Foley catheter was placed. A VCare uterine manipulator was introduced into the endometrial cavity and secured.

An incision was made above the umbilicus, and a 5-mm port introduced. Confirmation of abdominal placement was made with laparoscope. Two additional 8-mm ports were placed in the right and left lower abdomen under direct visualization. The midline incision was extended for a 12-mm port, and a 5-mm port was introduced in the nipple line on the left, just below the ribs.

The robot was docked, and attention was turned to the console.

The uterus was found to be enlarged with multiple fibroids, and the ovaries were normal with a simple cyst and a hemorrhagic cyst on the right.

The ureters were identified and noted to be away from the surgical field. The Fallopian tubes were identified, grasped, and followed to the fimbriated ends. They were dissected from their surrounding tissue with harp dissection and cautery. The cyst on the right ovary was dissected from the ovary and removed. The round ligaments were identified, cauterized with bipolar cautery, and cut. The anterior peritoneal reflection was incised, and the bladder was dissected off the lower uterine segment. Hemostasis was observed. The uterine vessels were skeletonized, then clamped and cauterized. Using the VCare as a guide, a posterior colpotomy was made. A circumferential incision was made around the cervix, and the uterus, cervix, and tubes were delivered through the vagina. Vaginal cuff angles as well as the remainder of the vaginal cuff were closed using a V-Loc suture, incorporating the utero-sacral ligaments for support. Lavage was carried out until clear. Hemostasis was observed.

Interceed was placed in the pelvis due to endometriosis being noted.

The robot was undocked, and all instruments were removed from the abdomen and vagina. The midline fascial incision was closed with 0-Vicryl suture, and all skin incisions were closed with 4-0 Vicryl.

Instrument, sponge, and needle counts were correct prior to abdominal closure and at the conclusion of the case.

SIGNED: Dr. Jordan Cole, MD

Select the appropriate codes for the case study.

1. List the ICD-10-CM code(s):

   ICD-10-CM code(s): ________________, ________________, ________________

2. List the CPT/HCPCS code(s) and any applicable modifiers:

   CPT code(s): ________________, ________________ - _____

3. List the procedure and diagnosis codes on the CMS-1500 form. Be sure to correctly link the procedure and diagnosis codes.

21. DIAGNOSIS OR NATURE OF ILLNESS OR INJURY Relate A-L to service line below (24E)			ICD Ind.	22. RESUBMISSION CODE
A.	B.	C.	D.	
E.	F.	G.	H.	23. PRIOR AUTHORIZATION NU
I.	J.	K.	L.	

	24. A. DATE(S) OF SERVICE From MM DD YY	To MM DD YY	B. PLACE OF SERVICE	C. EMG	D. PROCEDURES, SERVICES, OR SUPPLIES (Explain Unusual Circumstances) CPT/HCPCS	MODIFIER	E. DIAGNOSIS POINTER	F. $ CHARGES	G. DAYS OR UNITS
1									
2									
3									
4									

Case Study 17.2

Vaginal Delivery Note

PATIENT: May Kasen

DATE OF PROCEDURE: 10/06/20XX

COMPLICATIONS OF CURRENT PREGNANCY:

1. Precipitous delivery en route

Delivering provider: Dr. Judith Allen, MD
Pain control: None
Description of delivery: I was called to the patient's room by the RN after the patient was transferred via EMS. She had delivered her viable/healthy female infant precipitously in the vehicle while en route to the hospital. The placenta was in situ, but there was no active bleeding. The cord had been clamped and cut by EMS in the field. Cord gasses were not obtained.

Using IV placed by ENS, Pitocin was bloused per protocol. The placenta was delivered within minutes, Schultz, with intact membranes. Uterus was massaged to firm and was at the umbilicus.

The perineum and vagina were inspected for lacerations.

Lacerations were as follows:

Perineal:	None
Labial:	None
Sulcal/vaginal:	None
Cervical:	None

EBL: 50cc
Instrument, sharps, and sponge count correct × 2

Mother and infant were both stable and in good condition when I left the room.

SIGNED: Dr. Judith Allen, MD

Select the appropriate codes for the case study.

1. List the ICD-10-CM code(s):
   ICD-10-CM code(s): ________________, ________________, ________________
2. List the CPT/HCPCS code(s) and any applicable modifiers:
   CPT code(s): ________________

3. Link the procedure and diagnosis codes on the CMS-1500 form. Be sure to correctly link the procedure and diagnosis codes.

21. DIAGNOSIS OR NATURE OF ILLNESS OR INJURY Relate A-L to service line below (24E) ICD Ind.

A. ____ B. ____ C. ____ D. ____
E. ____ F. ____ G. ____ H. ____
I. ____ J. ____ K. ____ L. ____

22. RESUBMISSION CODE

23. PRIOR AUTHORIZATION NU

	24. A. DATE(S) OF SERVICE From MM DD YY	To MM DD YY	B. PLACE OF SERVICE	C. EMG	D. PROCEDURES, SERVICES, OR SUPPLIES (Explain Unusual Circumstances) CPT/HCPCS	MODIFIER	E. DIAGNOSIS POINTER	F. $ CHARGES	G. DAYS OR UNITS
1									
2									
3									
4									

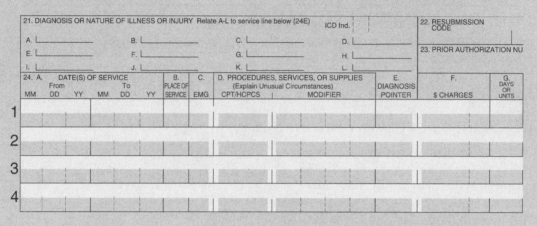

Case Study 17.3

Subsequent Hospital Care:

PATIENT: May Kasen

DATE OF PROCEDURE: 10/07/20XX

HISTORY:
23-year-old G2P2 s/p NSVD, PPD #1. Patient is ambulating, voiding, tolerating po with + flatus. She will be ready for d/c in a.m.

EXAMINATION/VITALS:
BP Min: 89/52 Max: 118/79
Temp Min: 36.5°C/97.7°F Max: 36.8°C/98.3°F
Pulse Min: 68 Max: 85
Resp Min: 16 Max: 18
SpO2 min: 95% Max: 98%

Abdomen: Soft FF at U-1

PLAN:
Routine postpartum care
Plan to d/c in a.m.

SIGNED: Signed by: Dr. Judith Allen, MD

Select the appropriate codes for the case study.

1. List the ICD-10-CM code(s):

   ICD-10-CM code(s): ________________, ________________

2. List the CPT/HCPCS code(s) and any applicable modifiers:

   CPT code(s): ________________

3. List the procedure and diagnosis codes on the CMS-1500 form. Be sure to correctly link the procedure and diagnosis codes.

21. DIAGNOSIS OR NATURE OF ILLNESS OR INJURY Relate A-L to service line below (24E) ICD Ind.

A.	B.	C.	D.
E.	F.	G.	H.
I.	J.	K.	L.

22. RESUBMISSION CODE

23. PRIOR AUTHORIZATION NU

	24. A. DATE(S) OF SERVICE From MM	DD	YY	To MM	DD	YY	B. PLACE OF SERVICE	C. EMG	D. PROCEDURES, SERVICES, OR SUPPLIES (Explain Unusual Circumstances) CPT/HCPCS	MODIFIER	E. DIAGNOSIS POINTER	F. $ CHARGES	G. DAYS OR UNITS
1													
2													
3													
4													

Case Study 17.4

Hospital Discharge:

PATIENT: May Kasen

DATE OF DISCHARGE: 10/08/20XX

ADMISSION DATE: 10/06/20XX
DISCHARGE DATE: 10/08/20XX

ADMITTING PROVIDER: Dr. Judith Allen, MD
DISCHARGING PROVIDER: Dr. Judith Allen, MD

DISCHARGE DIAGNOSES:

1. Normal delivery
2. Single live birth

STATUS:
Doing well.

HISTORY:
Interval complaints: None. The patient denies any significant pain at the present.

ACTIVE PROBLEMS:
None

PLAN:
Discharge home. Follow up in clinic in six weeks or prn. Instructions given to patient.

DETAILS OF HOSPITAL STAY:
Hospital Course:
Patient admitted for labor. No complications through hospital stay.

DISCHARGE CONDITION:
Good

VITALS:
BP Min: 89/52 Max: 118/79
Temp Min: 36.5°C/97.7°F Max: 36.8°C/98.3°F
Pulse Min: 68 Max: 85
Resp. Min: 16 Max: 18
SpO2 min: 95% Max: 98%
No intake or output data in the last 24 hours

PHYSICAL EXAMINATION:
Patient is alert and oriented, in no apparent distress.
Abdomen soft, NT, ND
Fundus firm, nt

SIGNED: Dr. Judith Allen, MD

Select the appropriate codes for the case study.

1. List the ICD-10-CM code(s):
   ICD-10-CM code(s): ________________, ________________
2. List the CPT/HCPCS code(s) and any applicable modifiers:
   CPT code(s): ________________
3. List the procedure and diagnosis codes on the CMS-1500 form. Be sure to correctly link the procedure and diagnosis codes.

21. DIAGNOSIS OR NATURE OF ILLNESS OR INJURY Relate A-L to service line below (24E) ICD Ind.

A.	B.	C.	D.
E.	F.	G.	H.
I.	J.	K.	L.

22. RESUBMISSION CODE

23. PRIOR AUTHORIZATION NU

	24. A. DATE(S) OF SERVICE From MM	DD	YY	To MM	DD	YY	B. PLACE OF SERVICE	C. EMG	D. PROCEDURES, SERVICES, OR SUPPLIES (Explain Unusual Circumstances) CPT/HCPCS	MODIFIER	E. DIAGNOSIS POINTER	F. $ CHARGES	G. DAYS OR UNITS
1													
2													
3													
4													

Case Study 17.5

PATIENT: Valeria Schmidt

DATE OF SERVICE: 08/19/20XX

CHIEF COMPLAINT:
LEEP in clinic today

HISTORY OF PRESENT ILLNESS:
Patient here for LEEP. Has CIN 2 and h/o of LEEP. Not planning future fertility.
Menstrual history: LMP: 07/29/20XX. Not using a subdermal contraceptive implant. Not using transdermal contraceptive patch. The patient is on an oral contraceptive pill. The patient does not receive injection. History of abnormal Pap smear. Reports a history of sexually transmitted disease.
Pregnancy history: Prior pregnancies: G1 and living 1

PROCEDURE: COLPOSCOPY WITH LOOP ELECTROD EXCISION OF THE CERVIX
Indication: moderate cervical dysplasia/CIN II (Cervical intraepithelial neoplasia II)
Risks, benefits, and alternatives were discussed with the patient. We discussed possible complications, including infection, bleeding, allergic reaction, and pregnancy complications. The patient was counseled regarding nothing per vagina for two weeks. Calling the office if she is experiencing heavy bleeding and calling the office if she is experiencing severe abdominal pain or fever. Written consent was obtained prior to the procedure. Verbal consent was obtained prior to the procedure.
The patient was premedicated with ibuprofen 800 mg.
The cervix was prepped with Lugol's.
Anesthesia: a paracervical block was performed, and endocervical block was performed using 10 ml of lidocaine injected 1% with epinephrine, using 10 ml of lidocaine injected 1% without epinephrine of lidocaine.
Procedure note:
Vaginal vault: no abnormalities seen
Vulva: no abnormalities seen
LEEP: a cone biopsy was performed using a loop electrode. The endocervix was excised to a depth of 1 cm. The blend setting was 60 watts. Hemostasis was obtained using ball electrode using coagulation and Monsel's solution. The coagulation setting was 60 watts. A total of two specimens were excised. The excised lesions were placed in buffered formalin and sent for pathology.
Patient status: the patient tolerated the procedure well.
Complications: There were no complications.

SIGNED: Dr. Jordan Cole, MD

Select the appropriate codes for the case study.

1. List the ICD-10-CM code(s):

   ICD-10-CM code(s): ________________

2. List the CPT/HCPCS code(s) and any applicable modifiers:

   CPT code(s): ________________

3. List the procedure and diagnosis codes on the CMS-1500 form. Be sure to correctly link the procedure and diagnosis codes.

21. DIAGNOSIS OR NATURE OF ILLNESS OR INJURY Relate A-L to service line below (24E) ICD Ind.

A. ____ B. ____ C. ____ D. ____

E. ____ F. ____ G. ____ H. ____

I. ____ J. ____ K. ____ L. ____

22. RESUBMISSION CODE

23. PRIOR AUTHORIZATION NU

	24. A. DATE(S) OF SERVICE From MM	DD	YY	To MM	DD	YY	B. PLACE OF SERVICE	C. EMG	D. PROCEDURES, SERVICES, OR SUPPLIES (Explain Unusual Circumstances) CPT/HCPCS	MODIFIER	E. DIAGNOSIS POINTER	F. $ CHARGES	G. DAYS OR UNITS
1													
2													
3													
4													

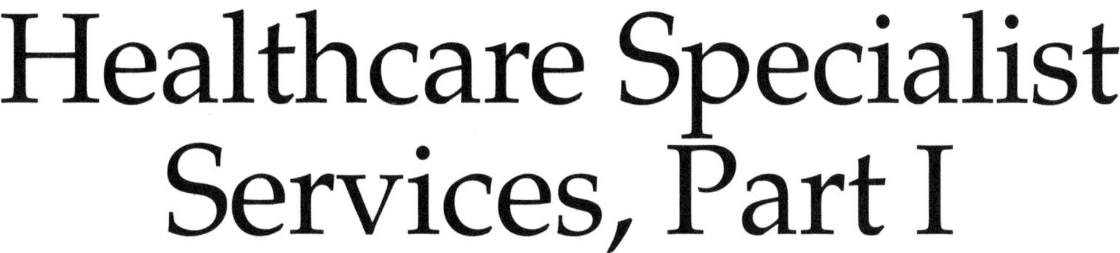

Healthcare Specialist Services, Part I

Vocabulary

Instructions: Define each of the following key terms in the space provided.

1. Alzheimer's disease: ______________________________

____

____

2. Anemia: ______________________________

____

____

3. Benign prostatic hyperplasia (BPH): ______________________________

____

____

4. Brachytherapy: ______________________________

____

____

5. Catheterizations: ______________________________

____

____

6. Central nervous system (CNS): ______________________

7. Cerebrospinal fluid (CSF) shunt: ______________________

8. Chemodenervation: ______________________

9. Chemotherapy: ______________________

10. Circumcision: ______________________

11. Consultation: ______________________

12. Corpora cavernosa: ______________________

13. Corpora spongiosum: ______________________

14. Craniectomy: ______________________

15. Craniotomy: ____

____

____

16. Dementia: ____

____

____

17. Dialysis: ____

____

____

18. Dosimetry: ____

____

____

19. Electroencephalogram (EEG): ______________________________

____

____

20. Electronic brachytherapy: ______________________________

____

____

21. Epididymis: ____

____

____

22. Epilepsy: ____

____

____

23. Extracorporeal shock wave lithotripsy (ESWL): ____________________

____

____

24. Hematologist: ____________________

25. Hemodialysis: ____________________

26. Hydration: ____________________

27. Hydrocele: ____________________

28. Infusion: ____________________

29. Injection: ____________________

30. Intensity Modulated Radiation Treatment Delivery (IMRT): ____________________

31. Interstitial brachytherapy: ____________________

32. Intracavitary brachytherapy: ____________________

33. Intractable condition: ______________________________

____

____

34. Kidney: ______________________________

____

____

35. Lower urinary tract symptoms (LUTS): ______________________________

____

____

36. Nephrolithiasis: ______________________________

____

____

37. Nephrolithotomy: ______________________________

____

____

38. Nephrologist: ______________________________

____

____

39. Neurologist: ______________________________

____

____

40. Neuropsychiatry: ______________________________

____

____

41. Neurosurgery: ______________________________

____

____

42. Oncologist: ______________________________

____

____

43. Orchiopexy: ______________________________

____

____

44. Parkinson's disease: ______________________________

____

____

45. Penis: ______________________________

____

____

46. Peripheral nervous system (PNS): ______________________________

____

____

47. Peritoneal dialysis: ______________________________

____

____

48. Prostate: ______________________________

____

____

49. Push: ______________________________

____

____

50. Radiation oncologist: ______________________________

____

____

51. Scrotum: ____

____

____

52. Seminal vesicles: ____

____

____

53. Spermatic cord: ____

____

____

54. Staghorn calculus: ____

____

____

55. Status epilepticus: ____

____

____

56. Status migrainosus: ____

____

____

57. Stereotactic body radiation treatment (SBRT): ______________________________

____

____

58. Stereotactic radiosurgery (SRS): ______________________________________

____

____

59. Testes: ____

____

____

60. Transurethral resection of the prostate (TURP): ______________________________

61. Tunica vaginalis: ______________________________

62. Ureters: ______________________________

63. Urethra: ______________________________

64. Urinary bladder: ______________________________

65. Urodynamics: ______________________________

66. Urologist: ______________________________

67. Vas deferens: ______________________________

68. Vasectomy: ______________________________

Fill in the Blank

Instructions: Complete the following statements.

1. List and describe the three Rs of consultations.

a. ______________________: ______________________________

____

b. ______________________: ______________________________

____

c. ______________________: ______________________________

____

2. If a patient's third-party payer, such as Medicare, does not cover consultation services, then the service provided should be reported with the appropriate ______________________ code (for either the inpatient or outpatient office setting).

3. A ______________________ is a medical professional who specializes in the diagnosis and treatment of diseases of the blood.

4. A ______________________ is a medical professional who specializes in the diagnosis and treatment of malignant neoplasms and tumors.

5. A ______________________ is a medical professional who specializes in the diagnosis and treatment of neurological disorders.

6. A ______________________ is a medical professional who specializes in the diagnosis and treatment of conditions of the urinary system as well as the male and female genital systems.

7. A ______________________ is a medical professional who specializes in the diagnosis and treatment of conditions affecting the kidneys.

8. In radiation oncology treatments, ______________________ is the term used for the calculation of the correct dose amount.

9. The ______________________ nervous system is composed of the nerves of the brain and the spinal cord, and the ______________________ nervous system is composed of the nerves throughout the rest of the body.

10. A ______________________ is a procedure in which a piece of the skull is removed and then replaced, whereas a ______________________ is a procedure in which a piece of the skull is removed and not replaced.

Matching

Instructions: Match the terms with the appropriate descriptions.

1. ________ Chemotherapy

2. ________ Brachytherapy

3. ________ Radiation oncology

4. ________ Surgical excision

A. Cancer treatment that involves the insertion of radioactive seeds into body tissues

B. Involves the removal of malignant tissue

C. The infusion of chemical substances to treat a malignancy

D. Treatment of malignant neoplasm that involves the use of radioactive treatments

Multiple Choice

Instructions: Choose the best answer.

1. Which of the following identifies the administration of a therapeutic, prophylactic, or diagnostic substance via an IV line, which occurs in 15 minutes or less?
a. Push
b. Infusion
c. Injection
d. Hydration

2. Which of the following identifies the administration of a therapeutic, prophylactic, or diagnostic substance via an IV line, which occurs in 15 minutes or more?
a. Push
b. Infusion
c. Injection
d. Hydration

3. Which of the following is the last part of the urinary system, through which urine is eliminated from the body?
a. Ureter
b. Urether
c. Urethra
d. Ureteral sphincter

4. Which of the following terms identifies a kidney stone?
a. Renal calculi
b. Nephrolithotomy
c. Hepatolithiasis
d. Cholelithiasis

5. Which of the following involves the provider sending a written letter containing findings from a consultation to the requesting provider?
a. Request
b. Render
c. Report
d. Consultation

6. Which of the following is a description of the "render" portion of a consultation?
a. The consulting provider creates a report of his or her findings.
b. The consulting provider performs the requested service.
c. The requesting provider gives a final diagnosis.
d. The consulting provider completes a request for additional services.

7. A PCP requests that his patient receive an MRI before undergoing surgery. Prior to the MRI, his office may complete paperwork with the insurance company to ensure that the cost of the MRI will be covered. Which of the following *best* describes this scenario?
a. Consultation
b. Prior authorization
c. Referral
d. Prior registration

8. A surgical specialist performs a consultation for a new patient in the office setting with a comprehensive history, comprehensive examination, and moderate MDM. Which of the following codes would be reported?
a. 99243
b. 99245
c. 99254
d. 99244

9. A hematologist provides a consultation for an inpatient suffering from sickle cell anemia. She provides an expanded problem-focused history, a problem-focused examination, and straightforward MDM. Which of the following codes would be reported?
a. 99251
b. 99252
c. 99241
d. 99242

10. A urologist performs a surgical consultation to a Medicare new patient in the clinic setting. He spends a total time of 30 minutes counseling the patient on the risks, benefits, and possible complications of surgical intervention for recurrent kidney stones. Which of the following codes would be reported?
a. 99242
b. 99251
c. 99243
d. 99203

Labeling

Instructions: Complete the following anatomical diagrams with the correct labels to identify the anatomy of the male genital system.

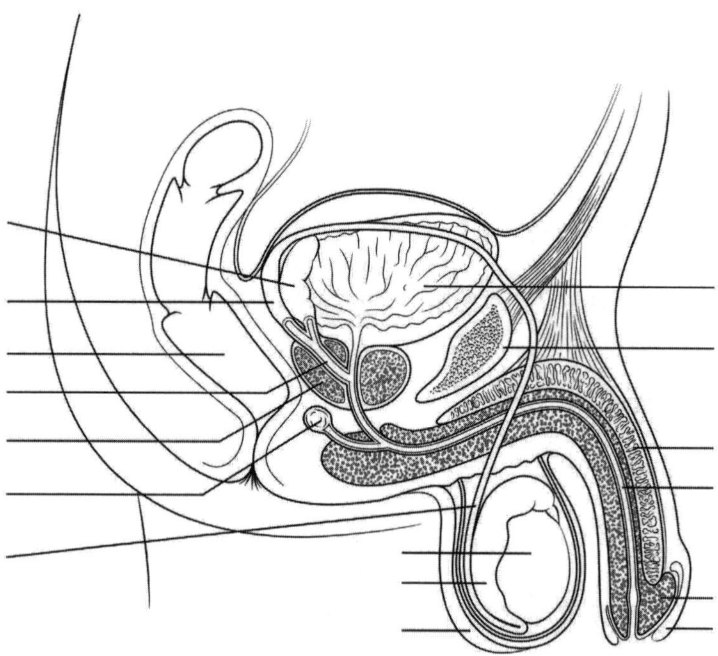

Source: ©AHIMA.

Coding

Instructions: Report all applicable ICD-10-CM and CPT codes for the following statements.

1. Intermediate proton treatment delivery
CPT code(s): ________________

2. Radiation treatment management involving four treatments
CPT code(s): ________________

3. Complex IMRT delivery
CPT code(s): ________________

4. Complex intracavitary application of brachytherapy source for 65-year-old male patient with prostate cancer that has metastasized to the bladder sphincter

ICD-10-CM code(s): ________________, ________________

CPT code(s): ________________

5. Code for 6 hours and 15 minutes of hydration service via IV line

CPT code(s): ________________, ________________ × _____

6. Consultation provided to a patient in the inpatient setting, moderate complexity MDM with detailed history and examination

CPT code(s): ________________

7. Patient presents for the administration of chemotherapy for metastatic liver cancer

ICD-10-CM code(s): ________________, ________________

8. Creation of subarachnoid/subdural-auricular shunt for patient with obstructive hydrocephalus

ICD-10-CM code(s): ________________

CPT code(s): ________________

9. Percutaneous stereotactic stimulation of the spinal cord for patient with neoplasm of uncertain behavior

ICD-10-CM code(s): ________________

CPT code(s): ________________

10. Extradural laminectomy and excision of neoplasm of the lumbar spinal cord

ICD-10-CM code(s): ________________

CPT code(s): ________________

11. Digital analysis of EEG for patient with absence epilepsy, intractable, with status epilepticus

ICD-10-CM code(s): ________________

CPT code(s): ________________

12. Laparoscopic pyeloplasty in 45-year-old male with chronic obstructive pyelonephritis

ICD-10-CM code(s): ________________

CPT code(s): ________________

13. Transvesical ureterolithotomy for patient with ureteral calculus

ICD-10-CM code(s): ________________

CPT code(s): ________________

14. Transurethral resection of the prostate due to residual regrowth of prostatic tissue; patient has BPH with the following LUTS: urinary hesitancy, urinary retention, and weak urinary stream

ICD-10-CM code(s): ________________, ________________,

________________, ________________

CPT code(s): ________________

15. Linear-based stereotactic radiosurgery (SRS), one session

CPT code(s): ________________

16. Simple intracavitary radiation source application for patient with prostate cancer

ICD-10-CM code(s): ________________

CPT code(s): ________________

17. Infratemporal suture of facial nerve without grafting for a laceration of the nerve of the left cheek

ICD-10-CM code(s): ________________

CPT code(s): ________________

18. Replacement of spinal neurostimulator receiver with direct coupling

CPT code(s): ________________

19. Complicated cystorrhaphy for nontraumatic bladder rupture

ICD-10-CM code(s): ________________

CPT code(s): ________________

20. Marsupialization of male urethral diverticulum

ICD-10-CM code(s): ________________

CPT code(s): ________________

Case Studies Healthcare Specialist Services—Part I

Case Study 18.1

PATIENT: Jerry McClelland

DATE OF SERVICE: 09/02/20XX

CHIEF COMPLAINT:
81-year-old male established patient presents for six-month follow-up from prostate cancer with Lupron injection

HISTORY OF PRESENT ILLNESS:
This 81-year-old male patient was referred for an elevated PSA. He had a PSA of 8.7 ng/ml last year and was seen by Dr. Kennedy. Free PSA was 0.8 mg/ml and % Free PSA was 9%, correlating to a .56% chance of having prostate cancer. The patient does not remember having a digital rectal exam. He was told that a biopsy was not recommended and that a repeat PSA should be performed. He had another PSA on 02/08/20XX, which had increased to 12.3 ng/ml. Patient discussed the rise in PSA with his PCP and desired a second opinion regarding the elevation of the PSA. Patient has a family history of prostate cancer and his father died of prostate cancer at age 87. He voids 1–2 times per night and does report some bothersome hesitancy.

He opted for a TRUS prostate biopsy, which was completed on 04/11/20XX without complication. Volume estimated to 28 grams. All 12 cores were positive for adenocarcinoma of the prostate. 6 cores were positive for Gleason 6, 4 cores were positive for Gleason 3+4=7, and 2 cores were positive for Gleason 9 (right apex and right lateral apex).

Patient completed radiation therapy on 12/31/20XX. He does report less energy, diarrhea, fecal incontinence when urinating and increased urinary frequency, and nocturia since starting androgen deprivation therapy and radiation. He does report that some of his symptoms are improving since the completion of the radiation therapy. He also reports some nausea after eating. He is currently voiding every 2 hours during the daytime and 4–5 times per night when, prior to treatment, he was urinating 2–3 times per night. He is scheduled to see his oncologist in approximately 10 days to follow up with some of his acute side effects from the radiation and androgen deprivation therapy.

His PSA is 0.043 ng/ml.

PHYSICAL EXAM:
Constitutional: the patient appeared to be in no acute distress, is well nourished and well developed.
Head and face: the head and face were normal in appearance.
Eyes: the sclera and conjunctiva were normal. Extraocular movements were intact. No strabismus was seen.
ENT: the ears and nose were normal in appearance.
Neck: no neck mass was observed, the thyroid was not enlarged, and there were no palpable thyroid nodules. The appearance of the neck was normal. The neck demonstrated no decrease in suppleness. There was no jugular-venous distention.
Pulmonary: no respiratory distress and no accessory muscle use.

Cardiovascular: no peripheral edema The radial pulses were normal. No varicosities.
Abdomen: no CVA tenderness. The abdomen was nondistended. The abdomen was soft. No masses were palpated. The abdomen was nontender. No hernias were palpable. No hepatosplenomegaly noted. The liver was not enlarged. Not tender. The spleen was not enlarged.
Lymphatics: the supraclavicular and axillary nodes were normal in size and not tender.
Musculoskeletal: the thoracolumbar spine had a normal appearance, the patient had a normal gait, and muscle strength and tone were normal. No involuntary movements were seen. Normal range of motion.
Neurological: no disturbance of coordination.
Psychiatric: oriented to person, place, and time. Insight and judgment were intact, and the mood was normal.
Skin: normal skin color and pigmentation. No rash and no lesions.

ASSESSMENT:

1. Prostate cancer
2. Androgen deprivation therapy
3. Urinary frequency
4. Nocturia

DISCUSSION/SUMMARY:
Medications were reviewed and reconciled. Allergies were reviewed and reconciled.

PLAN:

1. Prostate cancer. Administered Lupron Depot (6-Month) 45 mg intramuscularly in office. Patient is having some mild acute side effects from the radiation therapy and androgen deprivation therapy. He is scheduled to see his oncologist in approximately 10 days. Will follow up with him regarding the bowel symptoms as well as the urinary symptoms. If the patient continues to have worsening urinary frequency and nocturia, a cystoscopy can be performed to rule out stricture or significant urinary obstruction from the prostate. We discussed the option of starting medications for his urinary symptoms, and the patient wishes to hold off for now. We did discuss the option of this continuing androgen deprivation therapy due to the fatigue and hot flashes. The patient does wish to continue to androgen deprivation therapy given the clinical benefit of treating the prostate cancer. Patient received an injection of Lupron 45 mg intramuscularly today and will return to clinic in 6 months with a PSA prior.

SIGNED: Dr. Alexander Miller, MD

Select the appropriate codes for the case study.

1. List the ICD-10-CM code(s):
   ICD-10-CM code(s): ________________, ________________, ________________, ________________
2. List the CPT/HCPCS code(s) and any applicable modifiers:
   CPT code(s): ________________, ________________, ________________ × _____

3. List the procedure and diagnosis codes on the CMS-1500 form. Be sure to correctly link the procedure and diagnosis codes.

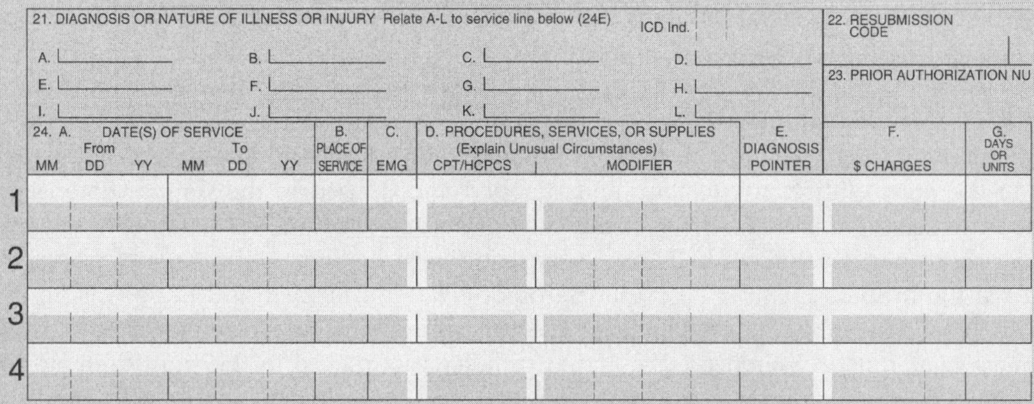

21. DIAGNOSIS OR NATURE OF ILLNESS OR INJURY Relate A-L to service line below (24E) ICD Ind.

A. B. C. D.
E. F. G. H.
I. J. K. L.

22. RESUBMISSION CODE

23. PRIOR AUTHORIZATION NU

	24. A. DATE(S) OF SERVICE From MM DD YY To MM DD YY	B. PLACE OF SERVICE	C. EMG	D. PROCEDURES, SERVICES, OR SUPPLIES (Explain Unusual Circumstances) CPT/HCPCS MODIFIER	E. DIAGNOSIS POINTER	F. $ CHARGES	G. DAYS OR UNITS
1							
2							
3							
4							

Case Study 18.2

OPERATIVE NOTE:

PATIENT: Betsy Shoemaker

DATE OF SERVICE: 01/11/20XX

PREOPERATIVE DIAGNOSIS: Right distal ureteral stone and possible urinary tract infection

POSTOPERATIVE DIAGNOSIS: Same

OPERATION/PROCEDURE PERFORMED: Cystoscopy, right retrograde pyelogram, right ureteral stent placement

ANESTHESIA: General anesthesia

COMPLICATIONS: None

FINDINGS: Right distal ureteral stone with hydronephrosis

ESTIMATED BLOOD LOSS: 0 ml

ANTIBIOTICS: Rocephin

SPECIMENS: Urine culture following stent placement

DRAINS: Right-sided 6-French × 24-cm JJ ureteral stent with string off

INDICATION FOR SURGERY: 75-year-old female who presented to the ER with right-sided flank pain. She was found to have a 4-mm right distal ureteral stone on CT. There was a concern for a urinary tract infection since her UA was positive for nitrites and leukocyte esterase. She opted for cystoscopy and right ureteral stent placement.

DESCRIPTION OF SURGERY:
The patient was brought to the operating room and received general anesthesia. The patient was placed in the dorsal lithotomy position and prepped and draped in the standard sterile fashion. The patient received antibiotics prior to the start of surgery. A time-out was held, and all in the operating room participated. A 30-degree cystoscope with 21-French sheath was placed into the urethra via the urethral meatus. A cystourethroscopy was performed and there was no evidence of any neoplastic or inflammatory changes, and the ureteral orifices were of normal location and appearance bilaterally. A 5-French open-ended catheter was placed in the right ureteral orifice. A retrograde ureteropyelogram was performed on that side. A Sensor guidewire was then advanced through the catheter and proper placement of the wire was confirmed with fluoroscopy. Over the wire and through the cystoscope, a 6-French × 24-cm double-J ureteral stent was placed, and proper placement was confirmed with fluoroscopy and with direct visualization using the cystoscope. A urine specimen was then obtained for culture. The bladder was then emptied through the cystoscope sheath. The patient was extubated and taken to the PACU in stable condition.

SIGNED: Dr. Alexander Miller, MD

Select the appropriate codes for the case study.

1. List the ICD-10-CM code(s):

ICD-10-CM code(s): ________________

2. List the CPT/HCPCS code(s) and any applicable modifiers:

CPT code(s): ________________ - _____, ________________

3. List the procedure and diagnosis codes on the CMS-1500 form. Be sure to correctly link the procedure and diagnosis codes.

21. DIAGNOSIS OR NATURE OF ILLNESS OR INJURY Relate A-L to service line below (24E)			ICD Ind.	22. RESUBMISSION CODE
A.	B.	C.	D.	
E.	F.	G.	H.	23. PRIOR AUTHORIZATION NU
I.	J.	K.	L.	

	24. A. DATE(S) OF SERVICE From MM DD YY	To MM DD YY	B. PLACE OF SERVICE	C. EMG	D. PROCEDURES, SERVICES, OR SUPPLIES (Explain Unusual Circumstances) CPT/HCPCS	MODIFIER	E. DIAGNOSIS POINTER	F. $ CHARGES	G. DAYS OR UNITS
1									
2									
3									
4									

Case Study 18.3

PATIENT: Amy Hall

DATE OF SERVICE: 05/15/20XX

PREOPERATIVE DIAGNOSIS: Left ureteral stone

POSTOPERATIVE DIAGNOSIS: Left ureteral stone

PROCEDURE: Cystoscopy, left retrograde pyelogram, left ureteroscopy, laser lithotripsy, basket extraction of stone fragments, left ureteral stent placement

ANESTHESIA: General

INDICATIONS FOR SURGERY: The patient is a 79-year-old female who was evaluated for left flank pain. A CT scan was performed, and this showed a 6-mm stone in the distal left ureter and a 5-cm stone at the left ureteropelvic junction. She has had minimal symptoms, but over the past few days they have been increasing. She is now brought to the operating room for further treatment.

DESCRIPTION OF OPERATION: The patient was brought to the operating room and placed in the supine position. After satisfactory laryngeal mask anesthesia was achieved, she was placed in the lithotomy position and prepped and draped in the usual sterile manner. The 21-French cystoscope sheath with obturator was inserted into the urethral meatus and advanced into the bladder without difficulty. The obturator was removed with good return of urine. The bladder was inspected in all quadrants. No masses, tumors, or other abnormalities were found. The ureteral orifices were identified bilaterally. A flexible-tipped Teflon-coated guidewire was passed through the working port of the cystoscope and inserted into the left ureteral orifice. The guidewire was then advanced into the distal left ureter where the stone was impacted. I was unable to pass the wire more proximally. A 5-French open-ended ureteral catheter was passed over the guidewire, but even using this for manipulation, I was unable to pass either the catheter or the wire. Accordingly, the guidewire was left in place adjacent to the stone. The 6.9-French semirigid ureteroscope was inserted into the urethral meatus and advanced into the bladder under direct visualization. The ureteroscope was inserted into the left ureteral orifice and advanced into the distal left ureter where the stone was identified. A 200-micron quartz laser fiber was passed through the working port of the ureteroscope, and the holmium laser at a setting of 0.8 joules and 8 pulses per second was used to break up the stone into smaller fragments. A Nitinol basket was used to capture the fragments, and these were sent to pathology for biochemical analysis. At this point, I was able to advance the guidewire up the left ureter so that the proximal top was in the left renal pelvis. The ureteral catheter was advanced over the wire into the left renal pelvis as well. The guidewire was removed. Several milliliters of 50% contrast were injected through the ureteral catheter to obtain a retrograde pyelogram. This showed good filling of a dilated renal pelvis and collecting system. The stone, which had previously been at the ureteropelvic junction, had migrated into a lower pole calyx. The cystoscope and ureteral catheter were withdrawn. A 10-French dual-lumen catheter was passed over the wire and advanced up unto the left renal pelvis. A second guidewire was passed through the second lumen, and this was also advanced into the left renal pelvis. The dual-lumen catheter was removed, and one of the guidewires was set aside to act as a safety wire. The 7.5-French flexible ureteroscope was passed over the second wire and advanced into the left renal pelvis. The second guidewire was then removed to allow for better visibility. I was able to visualize the stone in a lower pole calyx using the flexible scope; however, because of angulation, I was unable to visualize the stone if either a laser fiber or a Nitinol basket was passed through the working port of the ureteroscope. Accordingly, the ureteroscope was withdrawn. The remaining guidewire was backloaded through the cystoscope, which was reinserted through the bladder. A 6-French multilength stent was loaded over the wire and advanced up the left ureter under fluoroscopic guidance until the proximal end of the stent was curled in the left renal pelvis. The guidewire was then withdrawn, allowing the distal tip of the stent to curl freely within the bladder. Proper positioning was confirmed cystoscopically and fluoroscopically. The bladder was drained through the cystoscope sheath, which was then withdrawn. The procedure was terminated, and the patient was transferred to the recovery room in satisfactory condition.

PROCEDURAL FINDINGS: Impacted 6-mm stone in the distal left ureter broken up with holmium laser and fragments removed. 5-mm stone, which had been at left UPJ, migrated into lower pole calyx and could be visualized with flexible ureteroscope but, because of angulation, could not be treated with laser lithotripsy nor repositioned with basket. 6-French stent placed.

ESTIMATED BLOOD LOSS: Minimal

COMPLICATIONS: There were no complications. The patient appeared to tolerate the procedure well.

SIGNED: Dr. Alexander Miller, MD

Select the appropriate codes for the case study.

1. List the ICD-10-CM code(s):

   ICD-10-CM code(s): ________________

2. List the CPT/HCPCS code(s) and any applicable modifiers:

   CPT code(s): ________________ - _____, ________________

3. List the procedure and diagnosis codes on the CMS-1500 form. Be sure to correctly link the procedure and diagnosis codes.

21. DIAGNOSIS OR NATURE OF ILLNESS OR INJURY Relate A-L to service line below (24E) ICD Ind.

A. ______ B. ______ C. ______ D. ______
E. ______ F. ______ G. ______ H. ______
I. ______ J. ______ K. ______ L. ______

22. RESUBMISSION CODE

23. PRIOR AUTHORIZATION NU

	24. A. DATE(S) OF SERVICE From MM DD YY	To MM DD YY	B. PLACE OF SERVICE	C. EMG	D. PROCEDURES, SERVICES, OR SUPPLIES (Explain Unusual Circumstances) CPT/HCPCS	MODIFIER	E. DIAGNOSIS POINTER	F. $ CHARGES	G. DAYS OR UNITS
1									
2									
3									
4									

Case Study 18.4

Neurology Office Consult

PATIENT: Marie Wilson

DATE OF SERVICE: 03/04/20XX

REFERRAL SOURCE: Dr. Kennedy

CHIEF COMPLAINT:
Reason for referral: Small fiber neuropathy

HISTORY OF PRESENT ILLNESS:
Marie is a 61-year-old pleasant female patient who is referred to neurological consultation regarding suspected small fiber neuropathy with symptoms that began two years ago. She comes into the examination today unaccompanied.

Marie indicated that her symptoms began about two years ago with itching involving the left axilla. Subsequent to that, she developed left arm pain and noted some color change in the left hand. She indicates that her initial evaluation included a mammogram and ultrasound, and that was unremarkable. She had had swelling and itching and pain, which have recurred every three to four months since. Sometime later she developed similar symptoms in the right axilla, and ultimately, she underwent an evaluation by her PCP, who suggested that she may have diminished sensation in the toes and suspected peripheral neuropathy. Marie indicated that she subsequently developed numbness and tingling in the extremities in a more generalized fashion superimposed upon the aforementioned symptoms. She indicated that she underwent an MRI study of the brain, which was reported to be unremarkable. Ultimately, she was started on gabapentin and takes 100 mg every four hours with significant relief of her symptoms. Additionally, she has noticed some twitching, or what I would assume are fasciculations. She developed these in her right elbow and her left hand and has a video of the latter. She indicated that, for the past 18 months or so, she has been getting some hot flashes with sweating at night.

Currently, she does still get the itching in the axillary regions. She experiences numbness and tingling in her arms, legs, and face. Her arms are affected more than her legs. She frequently can get cramps. They occur about three times per week and can be anywhere. They are most frequent in the legs. She does experience pain in the extensor left forearm surface if she does not take the gabapentin.

PSFH: Remote tobacco use, no longer a smoker. Drinks a couple of glasses of wine per night. Notable family history of peripheral neuropathy. Both of her parents suffer from dementia.

REVIEW OF SYSTEMS:
As outlined above, otherwise as follows:
Constitutional: reports some weight loss, otherwise negative
HEENT: reports some imbalance in the past, otherwise negative
Cardiovascular: negative
Pulmonary: negative
GI: reports reflux and does get some fecal soiling at times
Genitourinary: negative
Musculoskeletal: has noticed some joint swelling and pain in her left hand and knee.

Neurologic: as above
Dermatologic: negative
Psychiatric: reports a tendency to worry and feel anxious
Endocrinologic: negative
Hematologic: diagnosed with left leg phlebitis 13 years ago.

PHYSICAL EXAMINATION:

Neurological examination: Height 159.5 cm, weight 66.9 kg, temperature 36.8 centigrade, heart rate 73, blood pressure 129/84. Speech, language, and mental status examination was normal to conversation. Manual muscle strength was normal in the upper and lower extremities. Deep tendon reflexes were intact, normal, and symmetric. Plantar responses were flexor bilaterally. The sensory examination was entirely normal. This included sensation in the upper extremities. There was a subjective diminution to temperature from the knees out distally, but this was pretty modest.

IMPRESSION/REPORT/PLAN:

1. Sensory symptoms consistent with peripheral neuropathy. It is an interesting history with upper extremity predominant sensory symptoms and axillary region pruritus and left extensor forearm pain. I wonder if this might not be something akin to brachioradial pruritus with a superimposed small fiber peripheral neuropathy.

I have recommended laboratory studies, EMG, autonomic reflex screen, and an epidermal skin punch biopsy provided the electrodiagnostic studies are negative. I will plan on visiting back with Marie following completion of this testing.

Report of findings copied to PCP.

SIGNED: Dr. April Goodman, MD

Select the appropriate codes for the case study.

1. List the ICD-10-CM code:

   ICD-10-CM code(s): ________________

2. List the CPT/HCPCS code(s) and any applicable modifiers:

   CPT code(s): ________________

3. List the procedure and diagnosis codes on the CMS-1500 form. Be sure to correctly link the procedure and diagnosis codes.

21. DIAGNOSIS OR NATURE OF ILLNESS OR INJURY Relate A-L to service line below (24E) ICD Ind.

A. ______ B. ______ C. ______ D. ______
E. ______ F. ______ G. ______ H. ______
I. ______ J. ______ K. ______ L. ______

22. RESUBMISSION CODE

23. PRIOR AUTHORIZATION NU

	24. A. DATE(S) OF SERVICE From MM	DD	YY	To MM	DD	YY	B. PLACE OF SERVICE	C. EMG	D. PROCEDURES, SERVICES, OR SUPPLIES (Explain Unusual Circumstances) CPT/HCPCS	MODIFIER	E. DIAGNOSIS POINTER	F. $ CHARGES	G. DAYS OR UNITS
1													
2													
3													
4													

Case Study 18.5

PATIENT: Marie Wilson

DATE OF SERVICE: 03/05/20XX

ELECTROMYOGRAPHY REPORT:
CLINICAL: The electrodiagnostic consultant reviewed the patient's available pertinent medical records, including history and examination notes, and/or performed a focused history and physical examination prior to completing the electrodiagnostic studies.

INDICATIONS: Small fiber peripheral neuropathy

STIMULAE	AMPLITUDE	VELOCITY	DISTAL LATENCY
	Normal	Normal	Normal
Fibular (peroneal) motor (EDB)	4.1 (≥1.9)	52 (≥41)	4.2 (≤5.0)
Tibial, motor (and hal)	15.6 (≥2.7)	49 (≥41)	3.9 (≤5.0)
Sural sensory (B point malleolus)	8.3 (≥2.8)		3.5 (≤4.4)
Medial, plantar, sensory, sole (ankle)	10.2 (≥0)		2.6 (≤3.9)
Median, sensory (index)	30.1 (≥15.9)	61 (≥51)	2.8 (≤3.7)

SUMMARY: Nerve conduction studies and needle examination of the left upper and left lower limb were normal.

INTERPRETATION: Normal study. There is no electrodiagnostic evidence of a large fiber peripheral neuropathy or of a left cervical radiculopathy.

SIGNED: Dr. April Goodman, MD

Select the appropriate codes for the case study.

1. List the ICD-10-CM code(s):
   ICD-10-CM code(s): ________________
2. List the CPT/HCPCS code(s) and any applicable modifiers:
   CPT code(s): ________________

3. List the procedure and diagnosis codes on the CMS-1500 form. Be sure to correctly link the procedure and diagnosis codes.

21. DIAGNOSIS OR NATURE OF ILLNESS OR INJURY Relate A-L to service line below (24E)			ICD Ind.	22. RESUBMISSION CODE
A.	B.	C.	D.	
E.	F.	G.	H.	23. PRIOR AUTHORIZATION NU
I.	J.	K.	L.	

	24. A. DATE(S) OF SERVICE From MM DD YY	To MM DD YY	B. PLACE OF SERVICE	C. EMG	D. PROCEDURES, SERVICES, OR SUPPLIES (Explain Unusual Circumstances) CPT/HCPCS	MODIFIER	E. DIAGNOSIS POINTER	F. $ CHARGES	G. DAYS OR UNITS
1									
2									
3									
4									

Chapter 19

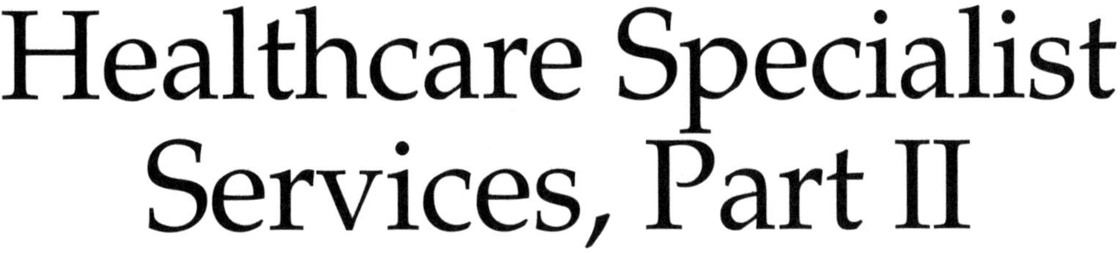

Healthcare Specialist Services, Part II

Vocabulary

Instructions: Define each of the following key terms in the space provided.

1. Abdominal aortic aneurysm (AAA): ______________________________

____

____

2. Aneurysm: ______________________________

____

____

3. Angiography: ______________________________

____

____

4. Atherosclerosis: ______________________________

____

____

5. Bariatric surgery: ______________________________

____

____

6. Cardiac electrophysiology: ______________________________

____

____

7. Cardiologist: ______________________________

____

____

8. Cardiopulmonary bypass (CPB): ______________________________

____

____

9. Cardiothoracic surgery: ______________________________

____

____

10. Central venous access devices (CVAD): ______________________________

____

____

11. Colonoscopy: ______________________________

____

____

12. Colorectal surgery: ______________________________

____

____

13. Coronary artery bypass grafts (CABG): ______________________________

____

____

14. Coronary artery disease: ______________________________

____

____

15. Deep vein thrombosis (DVT): ______________________________

____

____

16. Dissecting aneurysm: ______________________________

____

____

17. Diverticulitis: ______________________________

____

____

18. Diverticulosis: ______________________________

____

____

19. Embolus: ______________________________

____

____

20. Endoscopic retrograde cholangiopancreatography (ERCP): ______________________________

____

____

21. Endovascular procedure: ______________________________

____

____

22. Esophagogastroduodenoscopy (EGD): ______________________________

____

____

23. Fundoplasty: ______________________________

____

____

24. Gastric bypass: ______________________________

25. Gastroenterologist: ______________________________

26. Gastro-esophageal reflux disease (GERD): ______________________________

27. Hemorrhoids: ______________________________

28. Implantable cardiac defibrillator (ICD): ______________________________

29. Nonruptured aneurysms: ______________________________

30. Pacemaker: ______________________________

31. Percutaneous transluminal coronary angioplasty (PTCA): ______________________________

32. Pericardium: ______________________________

33. Proctosigmoidoscopy: ____

____

____

34. Pulmonary embolism: ____

____

____

35. Ruptured aneurysm: ____

____

____

36. Sigmoidoscopy: ____

____

____

37. Thrombosis: ____

____

____

38. Transluminal procedure: ____

____

____

39. Varicose vein: ____

____

____

Matching

Instructions: Match the type of pacemaker and implantable cardioverter-defibrillator with its description.

1. ________ Single chamber

2. ________ Dual chamber

A. Leads are placed into the right atrium, left ventricle, and right ventricle

B. Leads are placed into the right atrium and the right ventricle

Matching continued on next page

(Continued)

3. ________ Biventricular pacing — **C.** Includes a pulse generator and one electrode, placed into the atrium or the ventricle

Instructions: Match the word or term with its description.

4. ________ Patient-activated cardiac event recorder — **D.** Procedure in which a catheter is inserted into the body, means "inside the vessel"

5. ________ Coronary artery bypass graft — **E.** X-ray examination of the blood vessels after the administration of a contrast material

6. ________ Endovascular procedure — **F.** Implanted device that records the electrical activity of the heart when activated by the patient

7. ________ Angioplasty — **G.** Procedure in which a small piece of vessel is used to bypass a coronary artery

8. ________ Angiography — **H.** Procedure in which a catheter is inserted into the body, and a balloon is inserted inside the vessel

Multiple Choice

Instructions: Choose the best answer.

1. Which of the following healthcare specialists would perform a heart and lung transplant?
a. Cardiologist
b. Gastroenterologist
c. Cardiothoracic surgeon
d. Pulmonologist

2. Which of the following healthcare specialists would perform a routine screening colonoscopy, including biopsy of colonic polyps?
a. Gastroenterologist
b. Bariatric surgeon
c. Cardiologist
d. Urologist

3. A Roux-en-Y procedure is which of the following types of procedures?
a. Esophagoscopy
b. Colonoscopy
c. Intestinal resection
d. Gastric bypass

4. A screening colonoscopy found a number of small polyps in a patient's transverse colon and a biopsy of the polyps was performed. How should this service be reported?
a. 45378
b. 45380
c. 45378, 45380
d. 45385

5. Which of the following codes identifies diverticulosis that is occurring in only the small intestine?
a. K57.12
b. K57.30
c. K57.50
d. K57.10

6. Which of the following diagnosis codes would be used to report atherosclerosis of a native coronary artery of a transplanted heart with angina pectoris?
a. I25.750
b. I25.759
c. I25.758
d. I25.751

7. An endoscope was passed through the oral cavity and extended to the esophagus. How would this procedure be described?
a. Esophagogastroscopy
b. Esophagogastroduodenoscopy
c. Esophagoscopy
d. Tracheoscopy

8. A patient was diagnosed with hemorrhoids that prolapse out of the anal canal with straining but retract spontaneously. Which of the following codes would identify this condition?
a. K64.4
b. K64.8
c. K64.2
d. K64.1

9. Which of the following procedures is an open surgical treatment that can use a small selection of the patient's vein to go around a clogged artery of the heart?
a. Varicose vein
b. Atherectomy
c. Coronary artery bypass graft
d. Percutaneous coronary angioplasty

10. A patient presented for an endoscopic examination of the entire colon due to blood in the stool. During the procedure, a biopsy of a polyp was taken. Which of the following CPT codes would be most appropriate?
    a. 45378
    b. 45379
    c. 45384
    d. 45380

Coding

Instructions: Report the CPT and ICD-10-CM code(s) from the following diagnostic statements. Pay attention to sequencing conventions and instructions in the Tabular List to ensure that multiple codes are sequenced correctly.

1. Cervical esophagotomy with removal of foreign body due to puncture wound of cervical esophagus, initial encounter

   CPT code(s): _______________

   ICD-10-CM code(s): _______________

2. Diagnostic flexible transoral esophagoscopy for patient with GERD and esophagitis; multiple biopsies of esophageal tissues were obtained during the procedure

   CPT code(s): _______________

   ICD-10-CM code(s): _______________

3. Laparoscopic removal of adjustable gastric restrictive device in patient with moderate protein-calorie malnutrition

   CPT code(s): _______________

   ICD-10-CM code(s): _______________

4. Enterolysis for adhesions with partial obstruction

   CPT code(s): _______________

   ICD-10-CM code(s): _______________

5. Proctosigmoidoscopy with decompression of volvulus

   CPT code(s): _______________

   ICD-10-CM code(s): _______________

6. Hartmann type (partial) open colectomy for patient with diverticulitis of colon with perforation and abscess with bleeding

   CPT code(s): _______________

   ICD-10-CM code(s): _______________

7. Pericardiotomy for removal of intracardiac thrombosis

CPT code(s): ________________

ICD-10-CM code(s): ________________

8. Insertion of dual transvenous electrodes for implantable defibrillator due to documented nonreversible symptomatic bradycardia due to second degree atrioventricular block

CPT code(s): ________________

ICD-10-CM code(s): ________________, ________________

9. Operative ablation of supraventricular arrhythmogenic pathway for Wolff-Parkinson-White syndrome, without cardiopulmonary bypass

CPT code(s): ________________

ICD-10-CM code(s): ________________

10. Konno procedure replacement of aortic valve for rheumatic aortic stenosis with insufficiency

CPT code(s): ________________

ICD-10-CM code(s): ________________

11. CABG utilizing one arterial graft

CPT code(s): ________________

12. CABG utilizing four venous grafts harvested from the saphenous vein

CPT code(s): ________________

13. Combined coronary artery bypass graft utilizing three venous grafts harvested from the saphenous vein and one arterial graft harvested from the radial artery; patient has atherosclerotic heart disease with angina and is currently dependent on cigarettes, and is also morbidly obese due to excess calories with a BMI of 40.1

CPT code(s): ________________, ________________, ________________

ICD-10-CM code(s): ________________

14. Abdominal aortography (S&I only) shows dissection of abdominal aorta

CPT code(s): ________________

ICD-10-CM code(s): ________________

15. PTCA of left anterior descending artery and left anterior descending diagonal branch in patient with atherosclerosis of native coronary artery of transplanted heart

CPT code(s): ________________, ________________

ICD-10-CM code(s): ________________

Case Studies Healthcare Specialist Services—Part II

Case Study 19.1

PATIENT: Sylvia Gomez

DATE OF SERVICE: 10/10/20XX

PROCEDURE: Colonoscopy

INDICATIONS: Screening for malignant neoplasm of the colon

PATIENT PROFILE: Last colonoscopy: none. The patient's first colonoscopy is today.

MEDICINES: General anesthesia

COMPLICATIONS: No immediate complications

PROCEDURE:
Preanesthesia assessment: prior to the procedure, a history and physical were performed, and patient medications and allergies were reviewed. The patient is competent. The risks and benefits of the procedure and the sedation options and risks were discussed with the patient. All questions were answered, and informed consent was obtained. Patient identification and proposed procedure were verified by the physician.
Mental status examination: alert and oriented
Airway examination: normal oropharyngeal airway and neck mobility
Respiratory examination: clear to auscultation
CV examination: normal
Prophylactic antibiotics: the patient does not require prophylactic antibiotics
Prior anticoagulants: the patient has taken no previous anticoagulant or antiplatelet agents
ASA grade assessment: per anesthesia
After reviewing the risks and benefits, the patient was deemed in satisfactory condition to undergo the procedure. The anesthesia plan was to use monitored anesthesia care (MAC). Immediately prior to administration of medications, the patient was reassessed for adequacy to receive sedatives. The heart rate, respiratory rate, oxygen saturations, blood pressure, adequacy of pulmonary ventilation, and response to care were monitored throughout the procedure. The physical status of the patient was re-assessed after the procedure. After I obtained informed consent, the scope was passed under direct vision. Throughout the procedure, the patient's blood pressure, pulse, and oxygen saturations were monitored continuously. The colonoscope was introduced through the anus and advanced to the cecum, identified by appendiceal orifice and ileocecal valve. The colonoscopy was performed without difficulty. The patient tolerated the procedure well. The quality of the bowel preparation was adequate.

FINDINGS: Nonbleeding internal hemorrhoids were found during the retroflexion. The hemorrhoids were moderate, medium-sized, and grade II (internal hemorrhoids that prolapse but reduce spontaneously).

IMPRESSION:

1. Nonbleeding internal hemorrhoids
2. The examination was otherwise normal
3. No specimens collected

RECOMMENDATION:

1. To make sure that the risk of developing colon cancer remains low, the next colonoscopy should be performed in 10 years.
2. Please check for blood in stool with an annual FIT starting in 5 years, as this has shown to pick up both interval polyps and colon cancer at a higher rate.
3. Follow up with this office in 2–4 weeks to discuss hemorrhoid therapies.

SIGNED: Dr. Lukasz Podniesinski, MD

Select the appropriate codes for the case study.

1. List the ICD-10-CM code(s):

   ICD-10-CM code(s): ________________, ________________

2. List the CPT/HCPCS code(s) and any applicable modifiers:

   CPT code(s): ________________

3. List the procedure and diagnosis codes on the CMS-1500 form. Be sure to correctly link the procedure and diagnosis codes.

21. DIAGNOSIS OR NATURE OF ILLNESS OR INJURY Relate A-L to service line below (24E) ICD Ind.

A. ______ B. ______ C. ______ D. ______
E. ______ F. ______ G. ______ H. ______
I. ______ J. ______ K. ______ L. ______

22. RESUBMISSION CODE

23. PRIOR AUTHORIZATION NU

	24. A. DATE(S) OF SERVICE From MM DD YY	To MM DD YY	B. PLACE OF SERVICE	C. EMG	D. PROCEDURES, SERVICES, OR SUPPLIES (Explain Unusual Circumstances) CPT/HCPCS	MODIFIER	E. DIAGNOSIS POINTER	F. $ CHARGES	G. DAYS OR UNITS
1									
2									
3									
4									

Case Study 19.2

PATIENT: Padraig O'Shea

DATE OF SERVICE: 02/07/20XX

CHIEF COMPLAINT:
74-year-old male here for one-year CAD follow up

HISTORY OF PRESENT ILLNESS:

1. Coronary artery disease. Hx NSTEMI 08/XX and had CABG × 3 with LIMA to LAD, SVG to OM, SVG to dRCA. Since surgery, has had constant left-sided chest pain. Bengay helps. Symptoms: denies chest pain when at rest, denies exertional chest pain, stable shortness of breath and having incisional and left upper chest/LIMA site chest pain, nonangina.
2. Dylipidemia. Stable on atorvastatin 40 mg.
   Symptoms: no muscle pain, no muscle weakness, and no leg claudication.
3. Hypertension. A little elevated here today. And has been running 140s to 150s consistently. He has agreed to start lisinopril 5 mg daily. I have also asked him to check his blood pressure more regularly.
4. Atrial fibrillation. AF post CABG 08/XX. Afib persisted in hospital until POD 5 converted to normal amiodarone.
   Symptoms: denies palpitations, denies dyspnea on exertion, denies dizziness but stable chest pain. The patient is currently asymptomatic.
5. Mitral valve disease. MR-echo-02/11/XX with mild MR. He had mild regurgitation.
   Symptoms: no shortness of breath, not feeling tired, and no palpitations.
6. Peripheral vascular disease. Carotid artery disease 50–69% stenosis of the right internal carotid artery. There is a 90–95% stenosis of the right external carotid artery and a 70–89% stenosis of the left extrarenal carotid artery. Bilateral antegrade vertebral arteries; carotid artery disease, 50–69% stenosis in the right internal carotid artery. There is a 90–95% stenosis of the right external carotid artery and a 70–89% stenosis of the left extrarenal carotid artery. Bilateral antegrade vertebral arteries. Carotid ultrasound 11/XX. Right: 16–49% moderate stenosis of the right internal carotid artery Left: 16–49% of moderate stenosis in the left internal carotid artery. He has peripheral vascular disease of the carotids.
7. Pulmonary hypertension. 2/11/XX echo with wild TR and RVSP 46 mmHg. Continue using O_2 at night. Titrate use of O_2 during the day to maintain sats 90% or above.
8. COPD. On O_2 continuously since CABG. Prior smoker quit with MI 08/XX. Recently spent week at sea level and felt better; didn't need O_2 during the day. Has ordered concentrator for portable use when out and about. We discussed ordering a sleep study, and he is not interested at this time. He has secondary pulmonary hypertension.

PHYSICAL EXAMINATION:
Constitutional: well developed, well nourished, alert, and in no acute distress
HEENT: jugular vein pressure normal
Respiratory: unlabored breathing, no respiratory distress, the lungs were clear to auscultation bilaterally, no wheezing and no rales
Cardiovascular: heart rate and rhythm were normal, no murmurs, and no edema
Musculoskeletal: normal gait, no assistive device needed for ambulation

Psychiatric: oriented, appropriate mood, and the affect was normal
Skin: normal skin color and pigmentation

ASSESSMENT:

1. Coronary artery disease. 08/XX cath after STEMI. Severe multivessel involving left main, LAD, LCx, and RCA. Hx CABG. No angina-sounding chest pain. Continue aggressive risk factor modification.
2. Carotid artery disease. 08/XX ultrasound moderate to severe calcific plaquing bilateral carotids—left greater than right, no hemodynamically significant stenosis.
3. Hypertension. Blood pressure elevated here today and historically is averaging in the 140s to 150s. I have asked him to start lisinopril 5 mg daily. We will recheck labs one week after starting the medication. Will follow up in two weeks with blood pressure logs. Continue weight loss efforts with diet and exercise.
4. Hyperlipidemia. Managed by PCP. Tolerating atorvastatin. Continue without change.
5. Secondary pulmonary hypertension
6. COPD
7. Atrial fibrillation s/p CABG

RESULTS/DATA: ECG performed in office today

ECG INTERPRETATION: Axis: left axis deviation. Comparison to prior ECGs: Sinus bradycardia, 59 bpm, left axis deviation, no change from January 20XX. No interval change.

SIGNED: Dr. Campbell Brodie, MD

Select the appropriate codes for the case study.

1. List the ICD-10-CM code(s):

   ICD-10-CM code(s): ________________, ________________, ________________,
   ________________, ________________, ________________, ________________,
   ________________, ________________

2. List the CPT/HCPCS code(s) and any applicable modifiers:

   CPT code(s): ________________ - _____, ________________

3. List the procedure and diagnosis codes on the CMS-1500 form. Be sure to correctly link the procedure and diagnosis codes.

21. DIAGNOSIS OR NATURE OF ILLNESS OR INJURY Relate A-L to service line below (24E) ICD Ind.

A. ______ B. ______ C. ______ D. ______
E. ______ F. ______ G. ______ H. ______
I. ______ J. ______ K. ______ L. ______

22. RESUBMISSION CODE

23. PRIOR AUTHORIZATION NU

	24. A. DATE(S) OF SERVICE From MM DD YY	To MM DD YY	B. PLACE OF SERVICE	C. EMG	D. PROCEDURES, SERVICES, OR SUPPLIES (Explain Unusual Circumstances) CPT/HCPCS	MODIFIER	E. DIAGNOSIS POINTER	F. $ CHARGES	G. DAYS OR UNITS
1									
2									
3									
4									

Case Study 19.3

PATIENT: Gail Turner

DATE OF SERVICE: 01/29/20XX

COMMON CAROTID ARTERY INTIMA-MDEIA THICKNESS (IMT) SCAN REPORT:

SUMMARY

	COMBINED		
	Ave	Min	Max
Mean IMT	0.778	0.640	1.036
Max Region IMT	0.989	0.743	1.124
Plaque	6.300	4.900	7.700

	RIGHT			**LEFT**		
	Ave	Min	Max	Ave	Min	Max
Mean IMT	0.761	0.650	0.952	0.794	0.640	1.036
Max Region IMT	1.009	0.839	1.122	0.970	0.743	1.124
Plaque	6.300	4.900	7.700	0.000	0.000	0.000

AVERAGE CCA MEAN IMT: Average of individual mean IT measurements:
0.778 mm

AVERAGE CCA MAX REGION IMT: Average of individual 1-mm max region measurements:
0.998 mm

COMMENTS:
Screening

SIGNED: Dr. Campbell Brodie, MD

Select the appropriate codes for the case study.

1. List the ICD-10-CM code(s):
   ICD-10-CM code(s): ________________
2. List the CPT/HCPCS code(s) and any applicable modifiers:
   CPT code(s): ________________

3. List the procedure and diagnosis codes on the CMS-1500 form. Be sure to correctly link the procedure and diagnosis codes.

21. DIAGNOSIS OR NATURE OF ILLNESS OR INJURY Relate A-L to service line below (24E) ICD Ind.

A. B. C. D.

E. F. G. H.

I. J. K. L.

22. RESUBMISSION CODE

23. PRIOR AUTHORIZATION NU

	24. A. DATE(S) OF SERVICE From MM DD YY	To MM DD YY	B. PLACE OF SERVICE	C. EMG	D. PROCEDURES, SERVICES, OR SUPPLIES (Explain Unusual Circumstances) CPT/HCPCS	MODIFIER	E. DIAGNOSIS POINTER	F. $ CHARGES	G. DAYS OR UNITS
1									
2									
3									
4									

Case Study 19.4

PATIENT: Dave Duers

DATE OF SERVICE: 09/26/20XX

PROCEDURES PERFORMED:

1. Left heart catheterization
2. Right coronary angiography
3. Left coronary angiography
4. Diagnostic coronary flow reserve
5. PTCA right coronary artery (RCA)
6. Intervention on proximal RCA: drug-eluting stent

SUMMARY:
CORONARY CIRCULATION:
Proximal RCA: There was a 70% stenosis. There was TIMI grade 3 flow through the vessel (brisk flow). Mid RCA: There was a 50% stenosis. The lesion was ulcerated, with visible filling defect.

FIRST LESION INTERVENTIONS:
A successful drug-eluting stent was performed on the 50% lesion in the proximal RCA. Following intervention, there was an excellent angiographic appearance with a 0% residual stenosis. A XIENCE Alpine RC 3.25 mm × 23 mm everolimus-eluting stent at a maximum inflation pressure and mean distal coronary pressures were then obtained at maximum hyperemia. FFR was calculated to be 0.78. Based on the results, the lesion was judged to be significant, and an intervention was performed.

SIGNED: Dr. Campbell Brodie, MD

Select the appropriate codes for the case study.

1. List the ICD-10-CM code(s):

   ICD-10-CM code(s): ________________

2. List the CPT/HCPCS code(s) and any applicable modifiers:

   CPT code(s): ________________, ________________

3. List the procedure and diagnosis codes on the CMS-1500 form. Be sure to correctly link the procedure and diagnosis codes.

21. DIAGNOSIS OR NATURE OF ILLNESS OR INJURY Relate A-L to service line below (24E)			ICD Ind.	22. RESUBMISSION CODE
A.	B.	C.	D.	
E.	F.	G.	H.	23. PRIOR AUTHORIZATION NU
I.	J.	K.	L.	

	24. A. DATE(S) OF SERVICE From MM DD YY	To MM DD YY	B. PLACE OF SERVICE	C. EMG	D. PROCEDURES, SERVICES, OR SUPPLIES (Explain Unusual Circumstances) CPT/HCPCS	MODIFIER	E. DIAGNOSIS POINTER	F. $ CHARGES	G. DAYS OR UNITS
1									
2									
3									
4									

Case Study 19.5

PATIENT: Henrietta Potts

DATE OF SERVICE: 04/22/20XX

US CAROTID-DOPPLER:
Result annotations: NP/carotid artery US shows atherosclerosis with 50–69% blockage. Kidney function is decreased and a1c is up to 8.5. Recommend f/u with PCP to review results in detail.

Test: US CAROTID DOPPLER BILATERAL:
Bilateral duplex Doppler imaging was performed of the carotid systems.

Findings:
Right: Minimal intimal thickening within the right common carotid artery. There is moderate to severe soft and proximal and calcified plaque in the carotid bulb with extension into the proximal internal carotid artery. There is no significant turbulent flow. Peak systolic velocities are as follows: ICA 172.1cm/sec, CCA 44.3 cm/sec, ECA 160.1 cm/sec for a corresponding ICA/CCA ratio 3.9. Antegrade vertebral artery. Percentage stenosis of the ICS 50–59%

Left: Mild intimal thickening within the left common carotid artery. There is mild focal calcified and soft plaque at the carotid bulb with extension into the proximal ICA. Peak systolic velocities are as follows: ICD 63.9 cm/sec, CCA 51.0 cm/sec, ECA 98.9 cc/sec for a corresponding ICD/CCA ratio 1.3. Antegrade left vertebral artery. Percentage stenosis of the ICD 0–49%

IMPRESSION:

1. 50–69% stenosis with the right internal carotid artery. There are also elevated velocities in the right external carotid artery suggesting a 50–69% stenosis. This is not significantly changed when compared to previous study from 2013.
2. Bilateral antegrade vertebral arteries.

SIGNED: Dr. Campbell Brodie, MD

Select the appropriate codes for the case study.

1. List the ICD-10-CM code(s):

   ICD-10-CM code(s): ________________

2. List the CPT/HCPCS code(s) and any applicable modifiers:

   CPT code(s): ________________

3. List the procedure and diagnosis codes on the CMS-1500 form. Be sure to correctly link the procedure and diagnosis codes.

21. DIAGNOSIS OR NATURE OF ILLNESS OR INJURY Relate A-L to service line below (24E) ICD Ind.

A. ________ B. ________ C. ________ D. ________

E. ________ F. ________ G. ________ H. ________

I. ________ J. ________ K. ________ L. ________

22. RESUBMISSION CODE

23. PRIOR AUTHORIZATION NU

	24. A. DATE(S) OF SERVICE From MM	DD	YY	To MM	DD	YY	B. PLACE OF SERVICE	C. EMG	D. PROCEDURES, SERVICES, OR SUPPLIES (Explain Unusual Circumstances) CPT/HCPCS	MODIFIER	E. DIAGNOSIS POINTER	F. $ CHARGES	G. DAYS OR UNITS
1													
2													
3													
4													

Inpatient Hospital Services

Vocabulary

Instructions: Define each of the following key terms in the space provided.

1. Alteration: ____

____

____

2. Approach: ____

____

____

3. Bypass: ____

____

____

4. Change: ____

____

____

5. Character: ____

____

____

6. Code table: ______________________________

____

____

7. Complication/Comorbidity (CC): ______________________________

____

____

8. Control: ______________________________

____

____

9. Creation: ______________________________

____

____

10. Delivery: ______________________________

____

____

11. Destruction: ______________________________

____

____

12. Detachment: ______________________________

____

____

13. Device: ______________________________

____

____

14. Diagnosis-related groups (DRGs): ______________________________

____

____

15. Dilation: ______________________________

____

____

16. Division: ______________________________

____

____

17. Drainage: ______________________________

____

____

18. Excision: ______________________________

____

____

19. Extirpation: ______________________________

____

____

20. Extraction: ______________________________

____

____

21. Fragmentation: ______________________________

____

____

22. Fusion: ______________________________

____

____

23. Hospital-acquired condition (HAC): ______________________________

____

____

24. Inpatient prospective payment system (IPPS): ______________________________

____

____

25. Insertion: ______________________________

____

____

26. Inspection: ______________________________

____

____

27. Major complication/comorbidity (MCC): ______________________________

____

____

28. Map: ______________________________

____

____

29. Multiaxial structure: ______________________________

____

____

30. Occlusion: ______________________________

____

____

31. Prospective payment system (PPS): ______________________________

____

____

32. Qualifier: ______________________________

____

____

33. Reattachment: ____

____

____

34. Release: ____

____

____

35. Removal: ____

____

____

36. Repair: ____

____

____

37. Replacement: ____

____

____

38. Reposition: ____

____

____

39. Resection: ____

____

____

40. Restriction: ____

____

____

41. Revision: ____

____

____

42. Root operation: ____

____

____

43. Supplement: ____

____

____

44. Transfer: ____

____

____

45. Transplantation: ____

____

____

46. UB-04: ____

____

____

47. Uniform Hospital Discharge Data Set (UHDDS): ______________________

____

____

Matching

Instructions: Match the type of ICD-10-PCS section with its description.

1. ________ Medical and Surgical	**A.** Invasive and noninvasive procedures performed on patients, and compiles the vast majority of procedures reported with PCS codes
2. ________ Obstetrics	**B.** Procedures that are not classified elsewhere in the ICD-10-PCS code set and that identify procedures that utilize a new device substance or technology
3. ________ Placement	**C.** Procedures aimed at eliminating substance use, abuse, and dependence, and includes detoxification services and individual counseling

4. _______ Administration	**D.** Procedures that are focused on treating the emotional and behavioral health of the patient, and include crisis intervention and educational and vocational counseling
5. _______ Measurement and Monitoring	**E.** Procedures that identify physical, occupational, and speech language pathology services
6. _______ Extracorporeal Assistance and Performance	**F.** Procedures that utilize radiation to treat cancerous disorders (radiation oncology)
7. _______ Extracorporeal Therapies	**G.** Procedures that introduce radioactive material into the patient in order to create an image of the patient's anatomical structures, such as PET
8. _______ Osteopathic	**H.** Procedures that involve creating images of the patient's anatomical structures, including plain radiography (x-ray), fluoroscopy, CT, MRI, and ultrasound
9. _______ Other Procedures	**I.** Procedures that involve a direct thrust to a joint for the purpose of moving it as a therapeutic treatment
10. _______ Chiropractic	**J.** A miscellaneous range of procedures that do not fall into any other section, including acupuncture, in vitro fertilization, and suture removal
11. _______ Imaging	**K.** Procedures that involve the manual treatment of alleviating somatic dysfunction and related disorders
12. _______ Nuclear Medicine	**L.** Procedures that utilize equipment outside of the body for therapeutic purposes that do not assist or perform a physiological function
13. _______ Radiation Therapy	**M.** Procedures that utilize equipment outside of the body to assist or perform a physiological function
14. _______ Physical Rehabilitation and Diagnostic Audiology	**N.** Procedures that determine the level of a physical or physiological function
15. _______ Mental Health	**O.** Procedures that involve putting in or on a substance used as a therapeutic, diagnostic, nutritional, physiological, or prophylactic
16. _______ Substance Abuse	**P.** Procedures that involve placing an external device in or on a body part in order to protect, immobilize, stretch, compress, or for packing purposes
17. _______ New Technology	**Q.** Procedures performed on the products of conception only, including the fetus, amnion, umbilical cord, and placenta

Short Answer

Instructions: Using the given code table, answer the questions that follow.

Section	**0**	**Medical and Surgical**
Body System	**D**	**Gastrointestinal System**
Operation	**T**	**Resection:** Cutting out or off, without replacement, all of a body part

Body Part (4th)	Approach (5th)	Device (6th)	Qualifier (7th)
1 Esophagus, Upper **2** Esophagus, Middle **3** Esophagus, Lower **4** Esophagogastric Junction **5** Esophagus **6** Stomach **7** Stomach, Pylorus **8** Small Intestine **9** Duodenum **A** Jejunum **B** Ileum **C** Ileocecal Valve **E** Large Intestine **F** Large Intestine, Right **H** Cecum **J** Appendix **K** Ascending Colon **P** Rectum **Q** Anus	**0** Open **4** Percutaneous Endoscopic **7** Via Natural or Artificial Opening **8** Via Natural or Artificial Opening Endoscopic	**Z** No Device	**Z** No Qualifier
G Large Intestine, Left **L** Transverse Colon **M** Descending Colon **N** Sigmoid Colon	**0** Open **4** Percutaneous Endoscopic **7** Via Natural or Artificial Opening **8** Via Natural or Artificial Opening Endoscopic **F** Via Natural or Artificial Opening With Percutaneous Endoscopic Assistance	**Z** No Device	**Z** No Qualifier
R Anal Sphincter **U** Omentum	**0** Open **4** Percutaneous Endoscopic	**Z** No Device	**Z** No Qualifier

Source: Casto 2022.

1. What does the fifth character identify? ____________________

2. What body part does the character "U" identify? ____________________

3. How many different approaches are possible options for the anal sphincter and omentum? ____________________

4. What character is used to identify the left large intestine? ____________________

5. What code would be assigned for the resection of the sigmoid colon via an open approach?

____

Fill in the Blank

Instructions: Complete the following statements regarding ICD-10-PCS codes.

1. The first character identifies the ____________________, which is the general type of procedure.

2. The second character identifies the ___________________, which is the general physiological or anatomical region on which the procedure is performed.

3. The third character identifies the ___________________, which is the type and objective of the procedure.

4. The fourth character identifies the ___________________, which is the specific organ or anatomical region involved in the procedure.

5. The fifth character identifies the ___________________ to the procedure, which is the technique used to gain access to the surgical site.

6. The sixth character identifies the ___________________ that was used in the procedure, which is any material or appliance that remains after the procedure is performed.

7. The seventh character identifies the ___________________ for the procedure, which identifies any additional attributes of why or how the procedure was performed.

Coding

Instructions: Report the ICD-10-PCS code(s) from the following statements.

1. Pedicle skin graft transfer including subcutaneous tissue and upper dermal layer performed on the right upper thigh

   ICD-10-PCS code(s): ________________

2. Percutaneous insertion of spacer into right carpometacarpal joint

   ICD-10-PCS code(s): ________________

3. Percutaneous biopsy of the left common iliac artery

   ICD-10-PCS code(s): ________________

4. Allogeneic heart transplant

   ICD-10-PCS code(s): ________________

5. Complete removal of right kidney via open incision

   ICD-10-PCS code(s): ________________

6. Repair of a stab wound on the abdominal wall. Stitches were placed in the dermal and epidermal layers on a 3-cm wound.

   ICD-10-PCS code(s): ________________

7. Routine vaginal delivery
   ICD-10-PCS code(s): _______________

8. Low cervical cesarean section delivery
   ICD-10-PCS code(s): _______________

9. Mechanically assisted chiropractic manipulation of the thoracic and lumbar areas of the spine
   ICD-10-PCS code(s): _______________, _______________

Case Studies Inpatient Hospital Coding

Case Study 20.1

PATIENT: Elizabeth Negroni

PREOPERATIVE DIAGNOSIS: Foreign body (FB) right nostril

POSTOPERATIVE DIAGNOSIS: FB right nostril

ANESTHESIA: General inhalant

PROCEDURE NOTE:
3-year-old patient requiring general anesthesia was prepped and draped, and the right nostril was examined. FB appeared to be sponge of some sort, with noted degeneration indicating that FB had been in nasal passage for some time. FB was noted and was retrieved using forceps. Saline irrigation used to ensure all particles of the FB had been successfully removed. Patient tolerated the procedure well and was returned to the postanesthesia care unit in stable condition.

COMPLICATIONS: None, patient tolerated the procedure well

SIGNED: Dr. Susan Alameda, DO

Select the appropriate code(s) for the case study. Note that this case was presented in a previous chapter of this workbook. For this exercise, select only the applicable PCS code(s).

1. List the ICD-10-PCS code(s):
   ICD-10-PCS code(s): _______________

Case Study 20.2

PATIENT: Roger Roberts

DATE OF PROCEDURE: 09/19/20XX

TIME: 1550

INDICATIONS: Primary open-angle glaucoma of both eyes, severe stage. Left eye more severe. Treatment today aimed at left eye only.

PROCEDURE: SELECTIVE LASER TRABECULOPLASTY
Eye treated: Left eye
Power: 0.9–1.0
Bursts: 100
Lens Used: 360°
Comments: Patient tolerated the procedure well. No complications.

Laser post-procedure orders:

1. Rinse eye if Goniosol is used
2. Take postoperative vitals
3. Meds: none
4. There should not be much, if any, pain
5. If there is intense pain, or for other concerns, please call the eye clinic during the day. In emergencies or after hours, please call the after-hours provider line.
6. Follow-up appointment on 11/06/20XX

SIGNED: Dr. Hugh C. Mee, MD

Select the appropriate code(s) for the case study. Note that this case was presented in a previous chapter of this workbook. For this exercise, select only the applicable PCS code(s).

1. List the ICD-10-PCS code(s):
   ICD-10-PCS code(s): _______________

Case Study 20.3

Urgent Care Office Visit Summary

PATIENT: Jorge Canales

DATE OF SERVICE: 02/17/20XX

SUBJECTIVE:
23-year-old male was working in a crane and attempted to throw an empty glass bottle out of the cab. Bottle hit the door frame and shattered. A piece of glass cut his right thumb. Tetanus UTD.

OBJECTIVE:
Distal phalanx (R thumb) volar surface with deep avulsion-type laceration. No pulsatile bleeding.

WOUND REPAIR:
Wound exploration: Administered anesthesia with total 8 cc 1% lidocaine / 0.25% Marcaine. Wound explored to subcutaneous fat layer.
Wound repair: Additional anesthesia of 3 cc used. Irrigated with 1000 cc of sterile saline. Sutured with eight 5.0 nylon sutures on one layer. No complications. Bacitracin with tube gauze applied. Approx. 2.5 wound repaired.

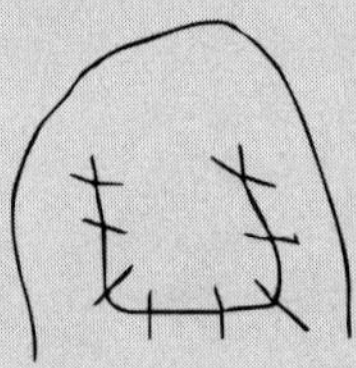

X-RAY:
Right thumb (2 views), no foreign body particles seen.

ASSESSMENT and PLAN:

1. Laceration right thumb. Return in one week for suture removal. If otherwise sick, call clinic. Gave patient wound instruction sheet.

SIGNED: Dr. Alejandro Jaramillo, MD

Select the appropriate code(s) for the case study. Note that this case was presented in a previous chapter of this workbook. For this exercise, select only the applicable PCS code(s).

1. List the ICD-10-PCS code(s):

   ICD-10-PCS code(s): ______________

Case Study 20.4

PATIENT: Tania Lopez

PREOPERATIVE DIAGNOSIS: Cystic lesion of right mandibular body

POSTOPERATIVE DIAGNOSIS: Traumatic bone cyst of right mandibular body

PRODECURES PERFORMED: Removal/treatment/curettage of traumatic bone cyst

ANESTHESIA: General nasoendotracheal

ESTIMATED BLOOD LOSS: 5 ml

COMPLICATIONS: None

INDICATIONS FOR SURGERY:
The patient is a 13-year-old white female who was found to have a 1×1 radiolucency associated with the right body of the mandible on routine dental examination. Cone-beam CT scan of this lesion showed slight expansion of the lateral surface of the mandible and significant thinning of the cortical bone in the area between the roots of teeth #28 and #29 and extending to the lingual cortex. Due to the relatively small size of the lesion and its proximity to the mental nerve at the mental foramen, she was scheduled for outpatient excision and appropriate management.

PROCEDURE IN DETAIL:
The patient was taken to the operating room, placed in the supine position. After induction of anesthesia, nasoendotracheal intubation, she was prepped and draped in a routine fashion for intra-oral surgery. A throat pack was placed, and a total of 5 ml of Xylocaine with 1:100,000 epinephrine, along with 2 ml of 0.5% Marcaine with 1:200,000 epinephrine, were given to anesthetize the right side of the mandible.

An incision was made crestal from the mesial of tooth #30 forward to the distal of tooth #27, and then an angled vertical incision from this point was made down to the depth of the vestibule. A full-thickness subperiosteal dissection was carried out, and it could be seen that the bone overlying the lesion was extremely thin and had some slight expansion evident as well. An 18-gauge needle on 5-ml syringe was placed within the lesion, and some blood and air were able to be suctioned from the lesion. There was not, however, evidence of a potential vascular lesion. The needle was withdrawn, and hand instruments were used to create a bony osteotomy through the thin outer wall of the lesion, which was placed in the specimen jar. It could soon be seen that there was no true cystic lining and that the lesion was indeed a traumatic bone cyst. The osteotomy was enlarged to gain access both visually and with all instruments to all areas of the lesion. No evidence of cystic lining or tumor was seen. Curettage of some of the inner portions of the cystic was accomplished; and, after thorough irrigation, the lesion was filled with Gelfoam to control oozing, and the incision was closed with 3-0 and 4-0 chromic sutures.

The patient tolerated the procedure well.

It should be mentioned that the lesion had thinned the superior wall of the mental foramen to the point where this bone could easily be removed with a small mosquito hemostat. There was no overt injury to the mental nerve.

SIGNED: Dr. Bob Welkins, DO

Select the appropriate code(s) for the case study. Note that this case was presented in a previous chapter of this workbook. For this exercise, select only the applicable PCS code(s).

1. List the ICD-10-PCS code(s):

ICD-10-PCS code(s): ______________

Case Study 20.5

PATIENT: Lario Robison

ORDERING PROVIDER: Susan Alameda, DO

US INGUINAL GROIN: US ABDOMINAL LIMITED

CLINICAL DATA:
59-year-old male with left lower abdominal quadrant pain

TECHNICAL DATA:
Multiple longitudinal and transverse real-time images of the left groin were performed by the ultrasound technologist.

FINDINGS:
There are no previous exams available for comparison.

Images of the left groin with and without the Valsalva maneuver demonstrate a small fat-containing left inguinal hernia with an approximately 1.7 cm in greatest dimension enlarged with a left inguinal ring.

There is no evidence of a dominant mass, hypoechoic lesion, or pathologic lymphadenopathy.

IMPRESSION:
Small fat-containing left inguinal hernia as described above.

SIGNED: Dr. Gene I. Kim, MD

Select the appropriate code(s) for the case study. Note that this case was presented in a previous chapter of this workbook. For this exercise, select only the applicable PCS code(s).

1. List the ICD-10-PCS code(s):

ICD-10-PCS code(s): ______________

Case Study 20.6

PATIENT: Amanda Conner

PREOPERATIVE DIAGNOSIS:
Chronic osteomyelitis with draining sinus, right ankle and foot; transmetatarsal amputation wound dehiscence

POSTOPERATIVE DIAGNOSIS:
Chronic osteomyelitis with draining sinus, right ankle and foot; transmetatarsal amputation wound dehiscence

NAME OF OPERATION: Right foot wound debridement with bone removal through excisional debridement

INDICATIONS:
This is a 30-year-old female patient. According to the patient, she had surgery six weeks ago but unfortunately has been unable to make any of her follow-up appointments. She says she removed her stitches herself, and unfortunately the wound opened up. Was admitted overnight with a worsening infection and is here for surgical debridement. When I saw her this morning, the foot was infected, and she has a significant wound dehiscence with bone exposure. After discussion with her, the decision was made to bring her for operative debridement.

PROCEDURE IN DETAIL:
Under mild sedation, patient was brought into the operating room and placed on the operating table in the supine position. Following general anesthesia by the anesthesiologist, the foot was scrubbed, prepped, and draped in the usual aseptic manner, and the tourniquet was inflated to 250 mmHg.

Next, the wound was debrided of all nonviable and devitalized tissue through excisional debridement. Bone was removed from the 1st, 2nd, 3rd, 4th, and 5th metatarsals, and the entire bone rack was sent for culture and sensitivity. There was an abscess of the 3rd and 2nd metatarsals, which I did irrigate and did not find any further abscess in the deep spaces of the foot. 3000 cc of sterile normal saline with bacitracin was used to irrigate the wound. The area was then irrigated and packed open with sterile gauze. The tourniquet was deflated, and a prompt hyperemic response was noted to the plantar flap.

Following a period of postoperative monitoring, the patient will be readmitted for continuing IV antibiotics. I will see her tomorrow and change the bandages for the first time. Her PCP will assume normal care on Monday and decide whether or not he feels that this is a salvageable foot.

SIGNED: Dr. David Johnston, MD

Select the appropriate code(s) for the case study. Note that this case was presented in a previous chapter of this workbook. For this exercise, select only the applicable PCS code(s).

1. List the ICD-10-PCS code(s):

ICD-10-PCS code(s): ________________

Case Study 20.7

Vaginal Delivery Note

PATIENT: May Kasen

DATE OF PROCEDURE: 10/06/20XX

COMPLICATIONS OF CURRENT PREGNANCY:

1. Precipitous delivery en route

Delivering provider: Dr. Judith Allen, MD
Pain control: None
Description of delivery: I was called to the patient's room by the RN after the patient was transferred via EMS. She had delivered her viable/healthy female infant precipitously in the vehicle while en route to the hospital. The placenta was in situ, but there was no active bleeding. The cord had been clamped and cut by EMS in the field. Cord gasses were not obtained.

Using IV placed by ENS, Pitocin was bloused per protocol. The placenta was delivered within minutes, Schultz, with intact membranes. Uterus was massaged to firm and was at the umbilicus.

The perineum and vagina were inspected for lacerations.

Lacerations were as follows:

Perineal:	None
Labial:	None
Sulcal/vaginal:	None
Cervical:	None

EBL: 50 cc
Instrument, sharps, and sponge count correct × 2

Mother and infant were both stable and in good condition when I left the room.

SIGNED: Dr. Judith Allen, MD

Select the appropriate code(s) for the case study. Note that this case was presented in a previous chapter of this workbook. For this exercise, select only the applicable PCS code(s).

1. List the ICD-10-PCS code(s):
   ICD-10-PCS code(s): ______________

Case Study 20.8

OPERATIVE NOTE:

PATIENT: Betsy Shoemaker

DATE OF SERVICE: 01/11/20XX

PREOPERATIVE DIAGNOSIS: Right distal ureteral stone and possible urinary tract infection

POSTOPERATIVE DIAGNOSIS: Same

OPERATION/PROCEDURE PERFORMED: Cystoscopy, right retrograde pyelogram, right ureteral stent placement

ANESTHESIA: General anesthesia

COMPLICATIONS: None

FINDINGS: Right distal ureteral stone with hydronephrosis

ESTIMATED BLOOD LOSS: 0 ml

ANTIBIOTICS: Rocephin

SPECIMENS: Urine culture following stent placement

DRAINS: Right-sided 6-French × 24-cm JJ ureteral stent with string off

INDICATION FOR SURGERY: 75-year-old female who presented to the ER with right-sided flank pain. She was found to have a 4-mm right distal ureteral stone on CT. There was a concern for a urinary tract infection since her UA was positive for nitrites and leukocyte esterase. She opted to cystoscopy and right ureteral stent placement.

DESCRIPTION OF SURGERY:
The patient was brought to the operating room and received general anesthesia. The patient was placed in the dorsal lithotomy position and prepped and draped in the standard sterile fashion. The patient received antibiotics prior to the start of surgery. A time-out was held, and all in the operating room participated. A 30-degree cystoscope with 21-French sheath was placed into the urethra via the urethral meatus. A cystourethroscopy was performed, and there was no evidence of any neoplastic or inflammatory changes, and the ureteral orifices were of normal location and appearance bilaterally. A 5-French open-ended catheter was placed in the right ureteral orifice. A retrograde ureteropyelogram was performed on that side. A Sensor guidewire was then advanced through the catheter, and proper placement of the wire was confirmed with fluoroscopy. Over the wire and through the cystoscope, a 6-French × 24-cm double-J ureteral stent was placed, and proper placement was confirmed with fluoroscopy and with direct visualization using the cystoscope. A urine specimen was then obtained for culture. The bladder was then emptied through the cystoscope sheath. The patient was extubated and taken to the PACU in stable condition.

SIGNED: Dr. Alexander Miller, MD

Select the appropriate code(s) for the case study. Note that this case was presented in a previous chapter of this workbook. For this exercise, select only the applicable PCS code(s).

1. List the ICD-10-PCS code(s):

ICD-10-PCS code(s): ________________, ________________

Case Study 20.9

PATIENT: Sylvia Gomez

DATE OF SERVICE: 10/10/20XX

PROCEDURE: Colonoscopy

INDICATIONS: Screening for malignant neoplasm of the colon

PATIENT PROFILE: Last colonoscopy: none. The patient's first colonoscopy is today.

MEDICINES: General anesthesia

COMPLICATIONS: No immediate complications

PROCEDURE:
Preanesthesia assessment: prior to the procedure, a history and physical was performed, and patient medications and allergies were reviewed. The patient is competent. The risks and benefits of the procedure and the sedation options and risks were discussed with the patient. All questions were answered, and informed consent was obtained. Patient identification and proposed procedure were verified by the physician.
Mental status examination: alert and oriented
Airway examination: normal oropharyngeal airway and neck mobility
Respiratory examination: clear to auscultation
CV examination: normal
Prophylactic antibiotics: the patient does not require prophylactic antibiotics
Prior anticoagulants: the patient has taken no previous anticoagulant or antiplatelet agents
ASA grade assessment: per anesthesia
After reviewing the risks and benefits, the patient was deemed in satisfactory condition to undergo the procedure. The anesthesia plan was to use monitored anesthesia care (MAC). Immediately prior to administration of medications, the patient was reassessed for adequacy to receive sedatives. The heart rate, respiratory rate, oxygen saturations, blood pressure, adequacy of pulmonary ventilation, and response to care were monitored throughout the procedure. The physical status of the patient was reassessed after the procedure. After I obtained informed consent, the scope was passed under direct vision. Throughout the procedure, the patient's blood pressure, pulse, and oxygen saturations were monitored continuously. The colonoscope was introduced through the anus and advanced to the cecum, identified by appendiceal orifice and ileocecal valve. The colonoscopy was performed without difficulty. The patient tolerated the procedure well. The quality of the bowel preparation was adequate.

FINDINGS: Nonbleeding internal hemorrhoids were found during the retroflexion. The hemorrhoids were moderate, medium-sized, and grade II (internal hemorrhoids that prolapse but reduce spontaneously).

IMPRESSION:

1. Nonbleeding internal hemorrhoids
2. The examination was otherwise normal
3. No specimens collected

RECOMMENDATION:

1. To make sure that the risk of developing colon cancer remains low, the next colonoscopy should be performed in 10 years.
2. Please check for blood in stool with an annual FIT starting in 5 years, as this has shown to pick up both internal polyps and colon cancer at a higher rate.
3. Follow up with this office in 2–4 weeks to discuss hemorrhoid therapies.

SIGNED: Dr. Lukasz Podniesinski, MD

Select the appropriate code(s) for the case study. Note that this case was presented in a previous chapter of this workbook. For this exercise, select only the applicable PCS code(s).

1. List the ICD-10-PCS code(s):

   ICD-10-PCS code(s): ________________

Reference

Casto, A.B. 2021. *2022 ICD-10-PCS Code Book*. Chicago: AHIMA.

Appendix A: Student Workbook Answer Key

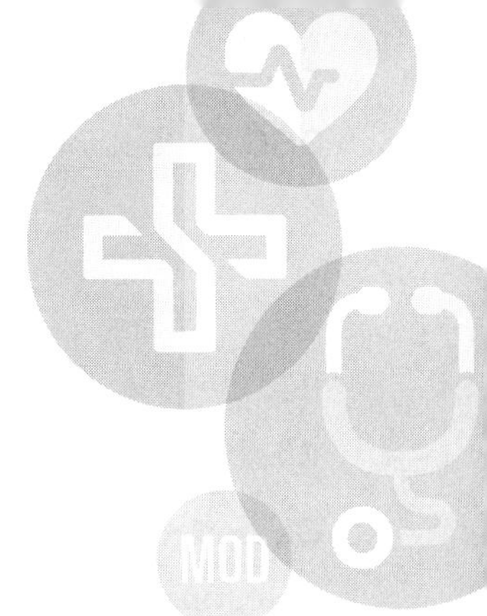

CHAPTER 1

Answers to the vocabulary section should be checked using the Medical Coding in the Real World, *Third Edition, textbook glossary.*

Matching

1. H
3. G
5. B
7. K
9. R
11. M
13. P
15. N
17. S
19. Q
21. W
23. T
25. X
27. BB
29. A
31. CC

True/False

1. True
3. True
5. False. If you work in a small clinic, you are likely to have to perform multiple responsibilities throughout the clinic.
7. True
9. True

Multiple Choice

1. D
3. B
5. C
7. B
9. B
11. B
13. D
15. A

CHAPTER 2

Answers to the vocabulary section should be checked using the Medical Coding in the Real World, *Third Edition, textbook glossary.*

True/False

1. True
3. True
5. False. The UB-04 form is used for inpatient facility billing and may also be used to bill for services performed in the outpatient facility setting. The CMS-1500 form is used for outpatient professional billing.
7. True
9. False. Capitation is a form of reimbursement that is based on a per-member per-month payment to the healthcare provider.

Multiple Choice

1. A
3. C
5. B
7. C

9. A

11. B

13. C

15. B

Case Study

Category III CPT code(s):

1123F (The documentation indicates that an advance directive was discussed and is documented in the medical record.)

1159F, 1160F (Both the medication list and a statement documenting medication review are documented in the medical record.)

1170F (The documentation includes at least five ADLs, including: dressing, using the toilet, personal hygiene, taking prescription medications, managing money, and transportation.)

CHAPTER 3

Answers to the vocabulary section should be checked using the Medical Coding in the Real World, *Third Edition, textbook glossary.*

True/False

1. False. Healthcare codes are the numeric or alphanumeric translation of all of the services, supplies, treatments, diagnoses, conditions, and other reasons for healthcare treatments.

3. True

5. False. ICD-10-CM and PCS manuals are published on October 1st of each year.

7. False. Code linkage is linking the diagnosis and procedure code together to identify the medical necessity for the services provided.

9. False. Coding guidelines are the rules that specify what codes to use in which situations, how to sequence them, which modifiers to use, and how to combine them with other codes.

Multiple Choice

1. A

3. C

5. A

7. B

9. A

11. A

13. A

15. C

Short Answer

1. Procedure: Colonoscopy with the removal of two polyps
Diagnosis: Benign colonic polyps

3. Procedure: Vaginal delivery of newborn
Diagnosis: 38 weeks' gestation of pregnancy in active labor

5. Procedure: Well-child examination, bilirubin lab test
Diagnosis: Well-child examination, neonatal jaundice

7. Because claims are billed to health insurance companies, it is important to understand the many regulations and guidelines that must be followed in order for coders to correctly sequence and report healthcare codes. If the claim is not coded correctly according to the requirements of the third-party payer, then the service may not be reimbursed.

Code Linkage:

1. Box 24.E Line 1: A
Line 2: B
Line 3: B

3. Box 24.E Line 1: A, B
Line 2: C

5. Box 24.E Line 1: A, B
Line 2: A

Case Study

1. Wellness examination
Cryotherapy of wart
Cryotherapy of six actinic keratoses
Note: Although the provider did order a colonoscopy at this encounter, it is not a procedure that the provider actually performed at this visit.

2. Encounter for preventive health examination
Abdominal aortic aneurysm (AAA) without rupture
Benign essential hypertension
Mixed hyperlipidemia
Patellofemoral syndrome of right knee
Common wart, left foot
Overweight (BMI 25.0–29.9)
Actinic keratosis

3.

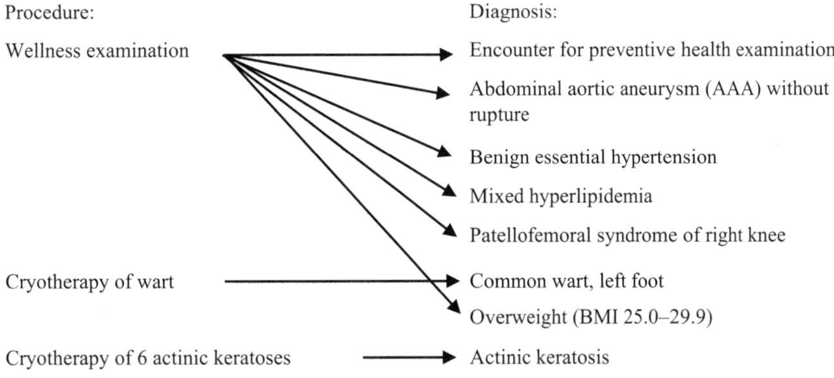

CHAPTER 4

Answers to the vocabulary section should be checked using the Medical Coding in the Real World, *Third Edition, textbook glossary.*

Fill in the Blank

1. etiology

3. combination

5. not otherwise specified

7. Table of Drugs and Chemicals

9. Table of Neoplasms

11. essential

13. Excludes2

15. Acute

17. Injury mechanism

19. Activity

21. Tabular List

Matching

1. G

3. A

5. D

7. B

9. H

11. I

13. F

Coding

Instructions: Using the ICD-10-CM code book, identify the main terms for the following diagnostic statements.

1. Senile cataract
Main term: cataract

3. Bladder hypotonicity
Main term: Hypotonicity

5. Third-degree burn of left thigh
Main term: Burn

Instructions: Essential versus nonessential modifiers: Look up the following terms in the Main Index and identify if the modifier listed is either essential or nonessential

	Main term	Modifier	Essential or nonessential
7.	Contusion	Arm	*essential*
9.	Hyperthyroidism	with goiter	*essential*

11. Moderate persistent asthma, uncomplicated
ICD-10-CM code: J45.40

13. Sore throat, fever
ICD-10-CM code: J02.9, R50.9

15. ICD-10-CM codes: K85.90, K86.1

17. ICD-10-CM code: A24.0

19. ICD-10-CM code: Q80.9

21. ICD-10-CM code: J60

23. ICD-10-CM code: C61, D63.0

25. ICD-10-CM code: B85.0

27. ICD-10-CM codes: T51.2X1A, R07.1

29. ICD-10-CM code: T45.526D

31. ICD-10-CM codes: K50.812

33. ICD-10-CM code: K71.51

35. ICD-10-CM code: J03.90, J35.01

37. ICD-10-CM code: E13.9, Z79.4

39. ICD-10-CM code: J13, J85.1

Answers to questions 41 through 44 must be found by looking up the code descriptions in an ICD-10-CM code book to identify the missing detail.

41. 15-year-old patient presents for a follow-up on her ***simple chronic*** bronchitis. She is feeling better, is less short of breath, and the medications prescribed by the doctor have been helping.

43. 62-year-old male presents with superficial foreign body in his ***left index*** finger, ***initial encounter***.

45. Complete ICD-10-CM code: I25.760

47. Complete ICD-10-CM code: S85.512A

49. Complete ICD-10-CM code: H02.121

Case Studies

Case Study 4.1

1. a. A skin lesion, also referred to as a *solar keratosis*, which develops from exposure to ultraviolet rays and is often considered pre-cancerous (Skin Cancer Foundation 2019).
b. Pain and stiffness in the front of the knee around the patella, or kneecap (AAOS 2015).

2. Encounter for preventive health examination
Abdominal aortic aneurysm (AAA) without rupture
Benign essential hypertension
Mixed hyperlipidemia
Patellofemoral syndrome of right knee
Common wart, left foot
Overweight (BMI 25.0–29.9)
Actinic keratosis

3. Z00.00, Encounter for preventive health examination
I71.4, Abdominal aortic aneurysm (AAA) without rupture
I10, Benign essential hypertension
E78.2, Mixed hyperlipidemia
M22.2X1, Patellofemoral syndrome of right knee
B07.9, Common wart, left foot
E66.3, Overweight (BMI 25.0–29.9)
L57.0, Actinic keratosis

Case Study 4.3

1. a. The need to wake up more than once per night to void urine (Weiss 2012).
b. Swelling of the extremities, especially the arms and legs.

2. Hyperlipidemia
Hypertension
Benign prostatic hyperplasia with LUTS

3. E78.5, Hyperlipidemia, unspecified
I10, Essential (primary) hypertension
N40.1, Benign prostatic hyperplasia with lower urinary tract symptoms
R35.1, Nocturia

Case Study 4.5

1. a. Nonsteroidal anti-inflammatory drugs (NSAIDs) are a class of medications that are often used to control pain, decrease fever, and decrease inflammation.
b. Otherwise known as a varicose vein, a condition that is a result of an insufficiency in the valves of the lower veins to push blood upward toward the heart, causing a buildup of blood.

2. Wrist pain
Elevated blood pressure
Stage 3 CKD
Venous stasis

3. M52.532, Pain in left wrist
R03.0, Elevated blood-pressure reading, without diagnosis of hypertension
N18.3, Chronic kidney disease, stage 3 (moderate)
I87.8, Other specified disorders of veins

CHAPTER 5

Answers to the vocabulary section should be checked using the Medical Coding in the Real World, *Third Edition, textbook glossary.*

Fill in the Blank

1. 99201–99499

3. 90281–99199, 99500–99607

5. Urinary

7. 61000; 64999

9. Subsection

11. Category

Matching

1. D
3. C
5. G
7. E
9. H
11. M
13. L
15. K

Multiple Choice

1. A
3. C
5. D
7. A
9. C

Coding

1. CPT code(s): 65091
3. CPT code(s): 60520
5. CPT code(s): 92230
7. CPT code(s): 0210T
9. CPT code(s): 15786, 15787
11. CPT code(s): 81402
13. CPT code(s): 53250
15. CPT code(s): 55970
17. CPT code(s): 78803
19. HCPCS code(s): G0442
21. HCPCS code(s): J9027
23. HCPCS code(s): J3060 × 2
25. HCPCS code(s): E0205
27. HCPCS code(s): P9032 × 5

Case Studies

Case Study 5.1

1. Subluxation of the radial head, or partial dislocation of the elbow.

2. Nursemaid's elbow

3. ICD-10-CM code(s): S53.031A, Nursemaid's elbow, right elbow, initial encounter

4. Reduction of nursemaid's elbow

5. CPT code(s): 24640-RT, Closed treatment of radial head subluxation in child, nursemaid elbow, with manipulation, right side

6.

21. DIAGNOSIS OR NATURE OF ILLNESS OR INJURY Relate A-L to service line below (24E) ICD Ind.

A. S53.031A	B.	C.	D.
E.	F.	G.	H.
I.	J.	K.	L.

24. A. DATE(S) OF SERVICE From MM DD YY	To MM DD YY	B. PLACE OF SERVICE	C. EMG	D. PROCEDURES, SERVICES, OR SUPPLIES (Explain Unusual Circumstances) CPT/HCPCS	MODIFIER	E. DIAGNOSIS POINTER
				24640	RT	A

Case Study 5.3

1. Skin lesions with abnormal cell structure, with a potential to become malignant.

2. Mole, right foot

3. ICD-10-CM code(s): D22.71, Melanocytic nevi of right lower limb, including hip

4. 3-mm punch biopsy of skin

5. CPT code(s): 11104, Punch biopsy of skin (including simple closure, when performed); single lesion

6.

21. DIAGNOSIS OR NATURE OF ILLNESS OR INJURY Relate A-L to service line below (24E) ICD Ind.

A. D22.71	B.	C.	D.
E.	F.	G.	H.
I.	J.	K.	L.

24. A. DATE(S) OF SERVICE From MM DD YY	To MM DD YY	B. PLACE OF SERVICE	C. EMG	D. PROCEDURES, SERVICES, OR SUPPLIES (Explain Unusual Circumstances) CPT/HCPCS	MODIFIER	E. DIAGNOSIS POINTER
				11104		A

Case Study 5.5

1. Bloody nose; nasal bleeding
2. Epistaxis
3. ICD-10-CM code(s): R04.0, Epistaxis
4. Control anterior nasal hemorrhage, simple
5. CPT code(s): 30901, Control nasal hemorrhage, anterior, simple (limited cautery and/or packing) any method
6.

21. DIAGNOSIS OR NATURE OF ILLNESS OR INJURY Relate A-L to service line below (24E) ICD Ind.

A. R04.0	B.	C.	D.
E.	F.	G.	H.
I.	J.	K.	L.

24. A. DATE(S) OF SERVICE From MM DD YY	To MM DD YY	B. PLACE OF SERVICE	C. EMG	D. PROCEDURES, SERVICES, OR SUPPLIES (Explain Unusual Circumstances) CPT/HCPCS	MODIFIER	E. DIAGNOSIS POINTER
				30901		A

CHAPTER 6

Answers to the vocabulary section should be checked using the Medical Coding in the Real World, *Third Edition, textbook glossary.*

Matching

1. B
3. A
5. E
7. F
9. C

True/False

1. True
3. False. The vehicle used in the ambulance transportation service does impact the code selected.
5. False. Medical necessity does play a part in DMEPOS billing; all services must be considered medically necessary in order to receive reimbursement for the service.
7. True
9. True

Coding

1. HCPCS code(s): A0425 × 15
3. HCPCS code(s): A0430, A0435 × 43
5. Transportation Indicator: C3
7. HCPCS code(s): A0427–RH, A0425 × 12
   ICD-10-CM code(s): R06.02, R07.9
9. HCPCS code(s): A4266
   ICD-10-CM code(s): Z30.09
11. HCPCS code(s): E2100
    ICD-10-CM code(s): E11.9
13. HCPCS code(s): E0601, A7037
    ICD-10-CM code(s): G47.33
15. HCPCS code(s): E0141
    ICD-10-CM code(s): R26.0
17. HCPCS code(s): J0744
19. HCPCS code(s): J3490
21. HCPCS code(s): Q4108 × 5
    ICD-10-CM code(s): L97.429
23. HCPCS code(s): J8560
25. HCPCS code(s): E2100
    ICD-10-CM code(s): H54.8, E11.65
27. HCPCS code(s): L5100
    ICD-10-CM code(s): Z89.511
29. HCPCS code(s): A5112, A5113
    ICD-10-CM code(s): R32

Case Studies

Case Study 6.1

HCPCS code(s): E0627, Seat lift mechanism, electric, any type

DEPARTMENT OF HEALTH AND HUMAN SERVICES
CENTERS FOR MEDICARE & MEDICAID SERVICES

Form Approved OMB
No. 0938-0679
Expires 02/2020

CERTIFICATE OF MEDICAL NECESSITY CMS-849 — SEAT LIFT MECHANISMS

DME 07.03A

SECTION A: Certification Type/Date: INITIAL ___/___/___ REVISED ___/___/___ RECERTIFICATION___/___/___

PATIENT NAME, ADDRESS, TELEPHONE and MEDICARE ID		SUPPLIER NAME, ADDRESS, TELEPHONE and NSC or NPI #
Sally B. Good, 1234 Pleasant Road Pleasantville, TX 12345 (555) 987 - 6543 Medicare ID ______		National Medical Equipment and Supplies 12345 Medical Lane Pleasantville, TX 12345 (555) 576 - 8542 NSC or NPI # 123456789
PLACE OF SERVICE ______	Supply Item/Service Procedure Code(s):	PT DOB 02/17/65 Sex F (M/F) Ht 61.5 (in) Wt ___
NAME and ADDRESS of FACILITY *if applicable (see reverse)*	E0627 ______ ______ ______	PHYSICIAN NAME, ADDRESS, TELEPHONE and UPIN or NPI # (___) ___-____ UPIN or NPI #______

SECTION B: Information in this Section May Not Be Completed by the Supplier of the Items/Supplies.

EST. LENGTH OF NEED (# OF MONTHS): ______ 1-99 *(99=LIFETIME)* | DIAGNOSIS CODES: ______ ______ ______ ______

ANSWERS	ANSWER QUESTIONS 1-5 FOR SEAT LIFT MECHANISM (Check Y for Yes, N for No, or D for Does Not Apply)
☐Y ☐N ☐D	1. Does the patient have severe arthritis of the hip or knee?
☐Y ☐N ☐D	2. Does the patient have a severe neuromuscular disease?
☐Y ☐N ☐D	3. Is the patient completely incapable of standing up from a regular armchair or any chair in his/her home?
☐Y ☐N ☐D	4. Once standing, does the patient have the ability to ambulate?
☐Y ☐N ☐D	5. Have all appropriate therapeutic modalities to enable the patient to transfer from a chair to a standing position (e.g., medication, physical therapy) been tried and failed? If YES, this is documented in the patient's medical records.

NAME OF PERSON ANSWERING SECTION B QUESTIONS, IF OTHER THAN PHYSICIAN (Please Print):
NAME: ____________ TITLE: ____________ EMPLOYER: ____________

SECTION C: Narrative Description of Equipment and Cost

(1) Narrative description of all items, accessories and options ordered; (2) Supplier's charge; and (3) Medicare Fee Schedule Allowance for each item, accessory, and option. (see instructions on back)

Seat lift mechanism, electric, any type

SECTION D: PHYSICIAN Attestation and Signature/Date

I certify that I am the treating physician identified in Section A of this form. I have received Sections A, B and C of the Certificate of Medical Necessity (including charges for items ordered). Any statement on my letterhead attached hereto, has been reviewed and signed by me. I certify that the medical necessity information in Section B is true, accurate and complete, to the best of my knowledge, and I understand that any falsification, omission, or concealment of material fact in that section may subject me to civil or criminal liability.

PHYSICIAN'S SIGNATURE ______________________ DATE ____/____/____

Signature and Date Stamps Are Not Acceptable.

Form CMS-849 (02/17)

Case Study 6.3

HCPCS code(s): E0430, Portable gaseous oxygen system, purchase; includes regulator, flowmeter, humidifier, cannula or mask, and tubing

DEPARTMENT OF HEALTH AND HUMAN SERVICES
CENTERS FOR MEDICARE & MEDICAID SERVICES

Form Approved OMB
No. 0938-0679
Expires 02/2020

CERTIFICATE OF MEDICAL NECESSITY CMS-484— OXYGEN

DME 484.5

SECTION A: Certification Type/Date: INITIAL ___/___/___ REVISED ___/___/___ RECERTIFICATION ___/___/___

PATIENT NAME, ADDRESS, TELEPHONE and MEDICARE ID	SUPPLIER NAME, ADDRESS, TELEPHONE and NSC or NPI #
Javier Gomez, 9232 University Drive Pleasantville, TX 12345 (555) 635 - 9847 Medicare ID	National Medical Equipment and Supplies 12345 Medical Lane Pleasantville, TX 12345 (555) 576 - 8542 NSC or NPI # 123456789

PLACE OF SERVICE ______	Supply Item/Service Procedure Code(s):	PT DOB 01/21/53 Sex M (M/F) Ht. 69 (in) Wt ____
NAME and ADDRESS of FACILITY if applicable (see reverse)	E0430	PHYSICIAN NAME, ADDRESS, TELEPHONE and UPIN or NIP # (___) ___ - ____ UPIN or NPI # ______

SECTION B: Information in this Section May Not Be Completed by the Supplier of the Item Supplies.

EST. LENGTH OF NEED (# OF MONTHS): ____ 1–99 (99=LIFETIME) | DIAGNOSIS CODES: ____ ____ ____ ____

ANSWERS	ANSWER QUESTIONS 1–9. (Check Y for Yes, N for No, or D for Does Not Apply, unless otherwise noted.)
a)____mm Hg b)____% c)___/___/___	1. Enter the result of recent test taken on or before the certification date listed in Section A. Enter (a) arterial blood gas PO2 and/or (b) oxygen saturation test; (c) date of test.
❑ 1 ❑ 2 ❑ 3	2. Was the test in Question 1 performed (1) with the patient in a chronic stable state as an outpatient, (2) within two days prior to discharge from an inpatient facility to home, or (3) under other circumstances?
❑ 1 ❑ 2 ❑ 3	3. Check the one number for the condition of the test in Question 1: (1) At Rest; (2) During Exercise; (3) During Sleep
❑ Y ❑ N ❑ D	4. If you are ordering portable oxygen, is the patient mobile within the home? If you are not ordering portable oxygen, check D.
____LPM	5. Enter the highest oxygen flow rate ordered for this patient in liters per minute. If less than 1 LPM, enter an "X".
a)____mm Hg b)____% c)___/___/___	6. If greater than 4 LPM is prescribed, enter results of recent test taken on 4 LPM. This may be an (a) arterial blood gas PO2 and/or (b) oxygen saturation test with patient in a chronic stable state. Enter date of test (c).

ANSWER QUESTIONS 7-9 ONLY IF PO2 = 56–59 OR OXYGEN SATURATION = 89 IN QUESTION 1

❑ Y ❑ N	7. Does the patient have dependent edema due to congestive heart failure?
❑ Y ❑ N	8. Does the patient have cor pulmonale or pulmonary hypertension documented by P pulmonale on an EKG or by an echocardiogram, gated blood pool scan or direct pulmonary artery pressure measurement.
❑ Y ❑ N	9. Does the patient have a hematocrit greater than 56%?

NAME OF PERSON ANSWERING SECTION B QUESTIONS, IF OTHER THAN PHYSICIAN (Please Print):
NAME________ TITLE________ EMPLOYER________

SECTION C: Narrative Description of Equipment and Cost

(1) Narrative description of all items, accessories and option ordered; (2) Suppliers charge; and (3) Medicare Fee Schedule Allowance for each item, accessory, and option (see instructions on back)

Portable gaseous oxygen system, purchase; includes regulator, flowmeter, humidifier, cannula or mask, and tubing

SECTION D: PHYSICIAN Attestation and Signature/Date

I certify that I am the treating physician identified in Section A of this form. I have received Sections A, B and C of the Certificate of Medical Necessity (including charges for items ordered). Any statement on my letterhead attached hereto, has been reviewed and signed by me. I certify that the medical necessity information in Section B is true, accurate and complete, to the best of my knowledge, and I understand that any falsification, omission, or concealment of material fact in that section may subject me to civil or criminal liability.

PHYSICIAN'S SIGNATURE____________ DATE ___/___/___

Signature and Date Stamps Are Not Acceptable.

Form CMS–484 (12/18)

Case Study 6.5

HCPCS code(s): E0652, Pneumatic compressor, segmental home model with calibrated gradient pressure

Form Approved OMB No. 0938-0679 Expires 02/2020

DEPARTMENT OF HEALTH AND HUMAN SERVICES
CENTERS FOR MEDICARE & MEDICAID SERVICES

CERTIFICATE OF MEDICAL NECESSITY
CMS-846 — PNEUMATIC COMPRESSION DEVICES

DME 04.04B

SECTION A: Certification Type/Date: INITIAL __/__/__ REVISED __/__/__ RECERTIFICATION __/__/__

PATIENT NAME, ADDRESS, TELEPHONE and MEDICARE ID		SUPPLIER NAME, ADDRESS, TELEPHONE and NSC or NPI #
Edith Jackson, 1005 Parkway Drive Pleasantville, TX 12345 (555) 635 - 4587 Medicare ID ____		National Medical Equipment and Supplies 12345 Medical Lane Pleasantville, TX 12345 (555) 576 - 8542 NSC or NPI # 123456789
PLACE OF SERVICE ____	Supply Item/Service Procedure Code(s):	PT DOB 10/02/45 Sex F (M/F) Ht. 61 (in) Wt ___ (lbs)
NAME and ADDRESS of FACILITY *if applicable (see reverse)*	E0652	PHYSICIAN NAME, ADDRESS, TELEPHONE and UPIN or NPI # (___) ___ - ____ UPIN or NPI # ____

SECTION B: Information in this Section May Not Be Completed by the Supplier of the Items/Supplies.

EST. LENGTH OF NEED (# OF MONTHS): ____ 1–99 *(99=LIFETIME)* DIAGNOSIS CODE(S): ____ ____ ____ ____

ANSWERS	ANSWER QUESTIONS 1–5 FOR PNEUMATIC COMPRESSION DEVICES (Check Y for Yes, N for No, Unless Otherwise Noted)
❑ Y ❑ N	1. Does the patient have chronic venous insufficiency with venous stasis ulcers?
❑ Y ❑ N	2. If the patient has venous stasis ulcers, have you seen the patient regularly over the past six months and treated the ulcers with a compression bandage system or compression garment?
❑ Y ❑ N	3. Has the patient had radical cancer surgery or radiation for cancer that interrupted normal lymphatic drainage of the extremity?
❑ Y ❑ N	4. Does the patient have a malignant tumor with obstruction of the lymphatic drainage of an extremity?
❑ Y ❑ N	5. Has the patient had lymphedema since childhood or adolescence?

NAME OF PERSON ANSWERING SECTION B QUESTIONS, IF OTHER THAN PHYSICIAN (Please Print):
NAME: ____ TITLE: ____ EMPLOYER: ____

SECTION C: Narrative Description of Equipment and Cost

(1) Narrative description of all items, accessories and options ordered; (2) Supplier's charge; and (3) Medicare Fee Schedule Allowance for each item, accessory, and option. (see instructions on back)

Pneumatic compressor, segmental home model with calibrated gradient pressure

SECTION D: PHYSICIAN Attestation and Signature/Date

I certify that I am the treating physician identified in Section A of this form. I have received Sections A, B and C of the Certificate of Medical Necessity (including charges for items ordered). Any statement on my letterhead attached hereto, has been reviewed and signed by me. I certify that the medical necessity information in Section B is true, accurate and complete, to the best of my knowledge, and I understand that any falsification, omission, or concealment of material fact in that section may subject me to civil or criminal liability.

PHYSICIAN'S SIGNATURE ____ DATE ___/___/___

Signature and Date Stamps Are Not Acceptable.

Form CMS-846 (02/17)

CHAPTER 7

Answers to the vocabulary section should be checked using the Medical Coding in the Real World, *Third Edition, textbook glossary.*

Multiple Choice

1. A

3. B

5. B

7. A

9. B

11. D

13. C

15. C

Fill in the Blank

1. Problem focused, expanded problem focused, detailed, comprehensive

3. Straightforward, low, moderate, high

Coding

1. ICD-10-CM code(s): F68.12

3. ICD-10-CM code(s): F65.52

5. ICD-10-CM code(s): F07.81, G44.301

7. CPT code(s): 90839, 90840 × 2

9. CPT code(s): 90791, 90785

11. CPT code(s): 99204
ICD-10-CM code(s): F40.02

13. CPT code(s): 90791
ICD-10-CM code(s): F11.251

15. CPT code(s): 99284
ICD-10-CM code(s): F31.12, F41.0

17. CPT code(s): 99406
ICD-10-CM code(s): F17.210

19. CPT code(s): 90845
ICD-10-CM code(s): F91.3

21. ICD-10-CM code(s): F12.23

23. ICD-10-CM code(s): F44.4

25. CPT code(s): 99214

27. CPT code(s): 99204

29. CPT code(s): 99215

Case Studies

Case Study 7.1

1. Headache, depression, insomnia

2. ICD-10-CM code(s): R51, F33.0, G47.00

3. Office visit (evaluation and management encounter)

4. CPT code(s): 99214 (detailed history, problem-focused examination, moderate MDM for an established patient)

5.

21. DIAGNOSIS OR NATURE OF ILLNESS OR INJURY Relate A-L to service line below (24E) ICD Ind.

A. R51	B. F33.0	C. G47.00	D.
E.	F.	G.	H.
I.	J.	K.	L.

24. A. DATE(S) OF SERVICE From MM DD YY	To MM DD YY	B. PLACE OF SERVICE	C. EMG	D. PROCEDURES, SERVICES, OR SUPPLIES (Explain Unusual Circumstances) CPT/HCPCS	MODIFIER	E. DIAGNOSIS POINTER
				99214		ABC

Case Study 7.3

1. Agoraphobia, social anxiety

2. F40.00, F40.10

3. Psychotherapy via telemedicine platform

4. 90832-95

5.

21. DIAGNOSIS OR NATURE OF ILLNESS OR INJURY Relate A-L to service line below (24E)			ICD Ind.
A. R40.00	B. F40.10	C.	D.
E.	F.	G.	H.
I.	J.	K.	L.

24. A. DATE(S) OF SERVICE From MM DD YY	To MM DD YY	B. PLACE OF SERVICE	C. EMG	D. PROCEDURES, SERVICES, OR SUPPLIES (Explain Unusual Circumstances) CPT/HCPCS	MODIFIER	E. DIAGNOSIS POINTER
				90832	95	AB

CHAPTER 8

Answers to the vocabulary section should be checked using the Medical Coding in the Real World, *Third Edition, textbook glossary.*

Multiple Choice

1. A

3. B

5. D

7. A

9. D

Completion

1. *Location.* Where on the body the signs or symptoms are present
Example: throat

3. *Severity.* The intensity of the signs or symptoms, often identified on a scale of 1 to 10
Example: pain level at a 9/10

5. *Timing.* When the signs or symptoms occur
Example: every evening or all day long

7. *Modifying factors.* Under what circumstances do the signs or symptoms improve or worsen
Example: when taking a deep breath

9. *Constitutional.* General constitutional signs or symptoms, such as feeling fatigued or weak

11. *Ears, nose, and throat.* Signs or symptoms involving the ears (such as ringing or pain), the nose (such as rhinorrhea or nose bleeds), and the throat and mouth (such as difficulty swallowing or bleeding gums)

13. *Respiratory.* Signs or symptoms involving the respiratory system, such as shortness of breath, cough, or wheezing

15. *Genitourinary.* Signs or symptoms involving the genitourinary system, such as bedwetting, painful urination, or erectile dysfunction

17. *Integumentary.* Signs or symptoms involving the skin (such as itching or rash) and the breasts (such as breast tenderness or lumps)

19. *Psychiatric.* Signs or symptoms involving the psychiatric system, such as depression or mood swings

21. *Hematologic/lymphatic.* Signs or symptoms involving the hematologic and lymphatic systems, such as bruising easily and swollen glands

Coding

1. Level of HPI: Extended (duration, associated signs and symptoms, timing, modifying factors, context)

3. Level of PFSH: Complete (this is an established patient, which requires one element from each type of history—in this case past allergies and family history of menopause)

5. Level of Examination: Expanded problem focused

7. Amount and/or complexity of data: Minimal

9. Level of MDM: Low

11. ICD-10-CM code(s): E10.9 (long term use of insulin is not reported for Type 1 diabetes mellitus)

13. ICD-10-CM code(s): E11.621, E11.65, L97.421, Z79.4

15. CPT code(s): 99214
ICD-10-CM code(s): J44.1, J45.41

17. CPT code(s): 99396
ICD-10-CM code(s): Z00.00

19. CPT code(s): 81025
ICD-10-CM code(s): N91.2

21. CPT code(s): 99215
ICD-10-CM code(s): J44.0, J44.1, J20.9, Z87.891

23. CPT code(s): 99305
ICD-10-CM code(s): J43.9, Z99.81

25. CPT code(s): G0008, 90658
ICD-10-CM code(s): Z23

27. CPT code(s): 99394
Note: Even though the MDM is high, the patient was not seen within seven days of discharge, so the lower code, 99394, must be assigned.
ICD-10-CM code(s): I82.402, I26.99

29. CPT code(s): 99214, 96127
ICD-10-CM code(s): F90.2

Case Studies

Case Study 8.1

1. ICD-10-CM code(s): R21, M79.644, M79.645

2. CPT code(s): 99213 (Low MDM for established patient)

3.

21. DIAGNOSIS OR NATURE OF ILLNESS OR INJURY Relate A-L to service line below (24E)			ICD Ind.
A. R21	B. M79.644	C. M79.645	D.
E.	F.	G.	H.
I.	J.	K.	L.

24. A. DATE(S) OF SERVICE From MM DD YY	To MM DD YY	B. PLACE OF SERVICE	C. EMG	D. PROCEDURES, SERVICES, OR SUPPLIES (Explain Unusual Circumstances) CPT/HCPCS	MODIFIER	E. DIAGNOSIS POINTER
				99213		ABC

Case Study 8.3

1. ICD-10-CM code(s): I10

2. CPT code(s): 99213 (Low MDM for established patient)

3.

21. DIAGNOSIS OR NATURE OF ILLNESS OR INJURY Relate A-L to service line below (24E)			ICD Ind.
A. I10	B.	C.	D.
E.	F.	G.	H.
I.	J.	K.	L.

24. A. DATE(S) OF SERVICE From MM DD YY	To MM DD YY	B. PLACE OF SERVICE	C. EMG	D. PROCEDURES, SERVICES, OR SUPPLIES (Explain Unusual Circumstances) CPT/HCPCS	MODIFIER	E. DIAGNOSIS POINTER
				99213		A

Case Study 8.5

1. ICD-10-CM code(s): Z00.00, E03.9, D64.9, R73.01, Z23

2. CPT code(s): 99397, 90471, 90653

3.

21. DIAGNOSIS OR NATURE OF ILLNESS OR INJURY Relate A-L to service line below (24E)			ICD Ind.
A. Z00.00	B. E03.9	C. D64.9	D. R73.01
E. Z23	F.	G.	H.
I.	J.	K.	L.

	24. A. DATE(S) OF SERVICE From MM	DD	YY	To MM	DD	YY	B. PLACE OF SERVICE	C. EMG	D. PROCEDURES, SERVICES, OR SUPPLIES (Explain Unusual Circumstances) CPT/HCPCS	MODIFIER	E. DIAGNOSIS POINTER
1									99397		ABCD
2									90471		E
3									90653		E

CHAPTER 9

Answers to the vocabulary section should be checked using the Medical Coding in the Real World, *Third Edition, textbook glossary.*

Multiple Choice

1. C

3. A

5. D

7. B

9. A

Labeling

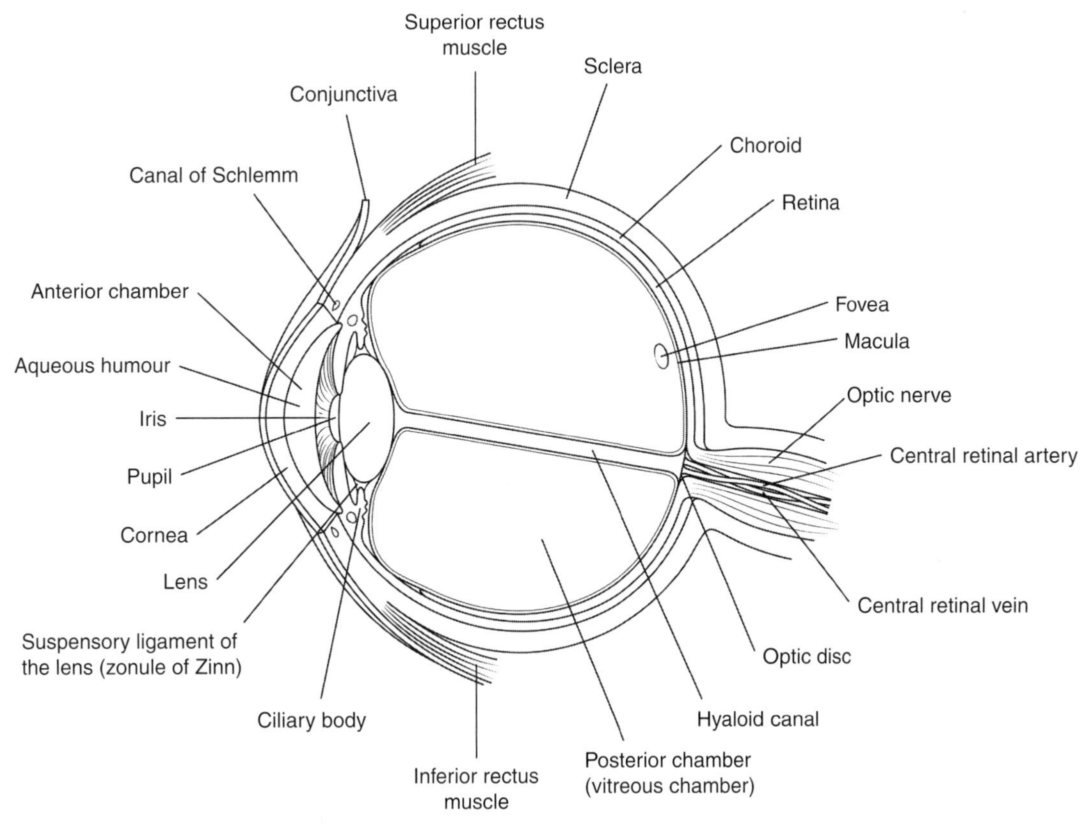

Source: ©AHIMA

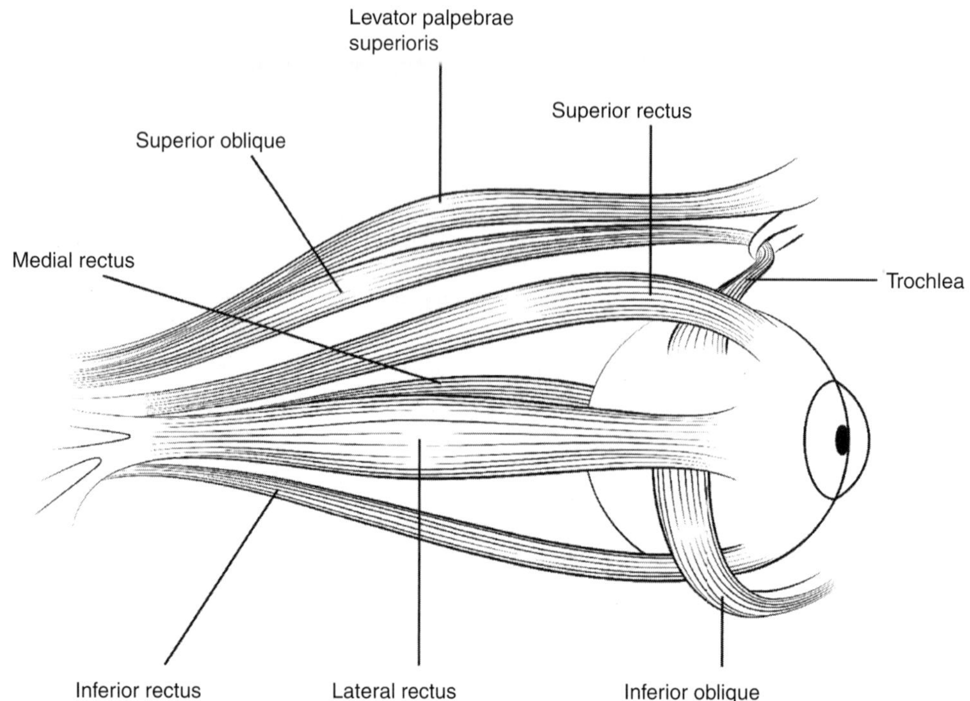

Source: ©AHIMA

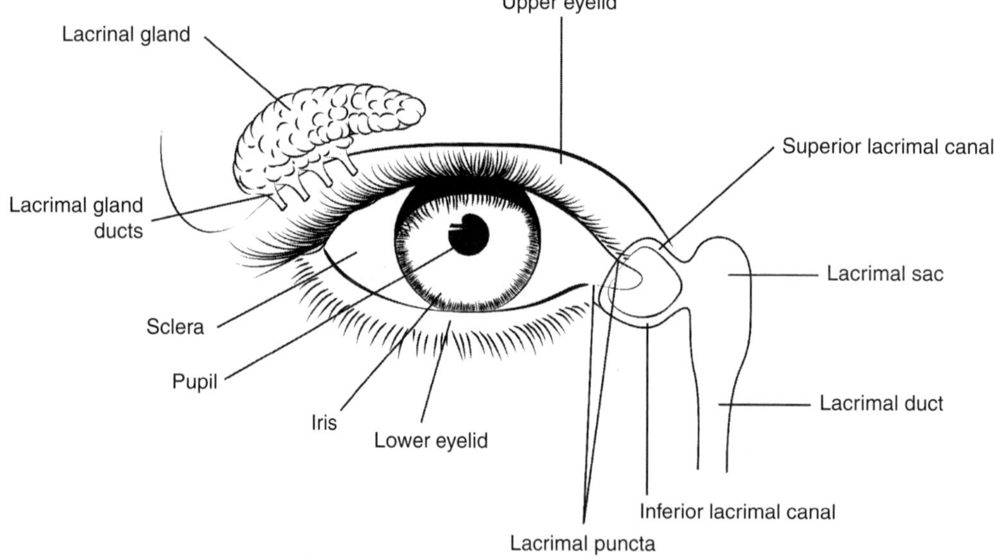

Source: ©AHIMA

Coding

1. CPT code(s): 65091-RT
ICD-10-CM code(s): H44.021

3. CPT code(s): 67825-E2, 67825-E4
ICD-10-CM code(s): H02.052, H02.055

5. CPT code(s): 67105-RT
ICD-10-CM code(s): H33.011

7. CPT code(s): 92002
ICD-10-CM code(s): H52.4

9. HCPCS code(s): V2020, V2300-RT, V2301-LT
ICD-10-CM code(s): H52.4

11. ICD-10-CM code(s): E10.3293, E10.36, L93.0, Z79.4

13. CPT code(s): 99213
ICD-10-CM code(s): H10.223

15. ICD-10-CM code(s): H53.2, I10, T46.6X5A

Case Studies

Case Study 9.1

1. ICD-10-CM code(s): H40.1133, E11.36, H25.13

2. CPT code(s): 99214-25, 92133

3.

21. DIAGNOSIS OR NATURE OF ILLNESS OR INJURY Relate A-L to service line below (24E)			ICD Ind.
A. H40.1133	B. E11.36	C. H25.13	D.
E.	F.	G.	H.
I.	J.	K.	L.

	24. A. DATE(S) OF SERVICE From MM DD YY	To MM DD YY	B. PLACE OF SERVICE	C. EMG	D. PROCEDURES, SERVICES, OR SUPPLIES (Explain Unusual Circumstances) CPT/HCPCS	MODIFIER	E. DIAGNOSIS POINTER
1					99214	25	ABC
2					92133		ABC
3							

Case Study 9.3

1. ICD-10-CM code(s): H40.1133

2. CPT code(s): 92083

3.

21. DIAGNOSIS OR NATURE OF ILLNESS OR INJURY Relate A-L to service line below (24E)			ICD Ind.
A. H40.1133	B.	C.	D.
E.	F.	G.	H.
I.	J.	K.	L.

24. A. DATE(S) OF SERVICE From MM DD YY	To MM DD YY	B. PLACE OF SERVICE	C. EMG	D. PROCEDURES, SERVICES, OR SUPPLIES (Explain Unusual Circumstances) CPT/HCPCS	MODIFIER	E. DIAGNOSIS POINTER
				92083		A

Case Study 9.5

1. ICD-10-CM code(s): H40.1123

2. CPT code(s): 99024

Note: The patient is still within the global period for the procedure performed the day prior.

3.

21. DIAGNOSIS OR NATURE OF ILLNESS OR INJURY Relate A-L to service line below (24E)			ICD Ind.
A. H40.1123	B.	C.	D.
E.	F.	G.	H.
I.	J.	K.	L.

24. A. DATE(S) OF SERVICE From MM DD YY	To MM DD YY	B. PLACE OF SERVICE	C. EMG	D. PROCEDURES, SERVICES, OR SUPPLIES (Explain Unusual Circumstances) CPT/HCPCS	MODIFIER	E. DIAGNOSIS POINTER
				99024		A

CHAPTER 10

Answers to the vocabulary section should be checked using the Medical Coding in the Real World, *Third Edition, textbook glossary.*

Multiple Choice

1. C

3. B

5. D

7. A

9. A

Completion

1. Additional unrelated signs and symptoms?

3. Code for the definitive diagnosis and signs and symptoms

Coding

1. CPT code(s): 99284
ICD-10-CM code(s): A41.9, R65.20, J96.00

3. ICD-10-CM code(s): I21.4, I48.91

5. ICD-10-CM code(s): F41.0, I25.2

7. CPT code(s): 13100, 12034-59, 12001-59
ICD-10-CM code(s): S31.131A, S21.111A, S51.812A, S61.412A

9. CPT code(s): 99213-25, 90473, 90660, S9088
ICD-10-CM code(s): K52.9

11. CPT code(s): 12002
ICD-10-CM code(s): S51.811A

13. ICD-10-CM code(s): T25.222A, T25.221A, T31.0, Y92.014, Y93.H9, X12.XXXA, Y99.8

15. CPT code(s): 99214, 87635
ICD-10-CM code(s): R50.9, R51, R11.0, Z11.52

Case Studies

Case Study 10.1

1. ICD-10-CM code(s): L03.115, Z88.0

2. CPT code(s): 99282

3.

21. DIAGNOSIS OR NATURE OF ILLNESS OR INJURY Relate A-L to service line below (24E) ICD Ind.

A. L03.115	B. Z88.0	C.	D.
E.	F.	G.	H.
I.	J.	K.	L.

24. A. DATE(S) OF SERVICE From MM DD YY	To MM DD YY	B. PLACE OF SERVICE	C. EMG	D. PROCEDURES, SERVICES, OR SUPPLIES (Explain Unusual Circumstances) CPT/HCPCS	MODIFIER	E. DIAGNOSIS POINTER
				99282		AB

Case Study 10.3

1. ICD-10-CM code(s): T22.212A, T22.211A, T20.19XA, T31.0, X03.0XXA, Y99.0

2. CPT code(s): 99282

3.

21. DIAGNOSIS OR NATURE OF ILLNESS OR INJURY Relate A-L to service line below (24E) ICD Ind.

A. T22.212A	B. T22.211A	C. T20.19XA	D. T31.0
E. X03.0XXA	F. Y99.0	G.	H.
I.	J.	K.	L.

24. A. DATE(S) OF SERVICE From MM DD YY	To MM DD YY	B. PLACE OF SERVICE	C. EMG	D. PROCEDURES, SERVICES, OR SUPPLIES (Explain Unusual Circumstances) CPT/HCPCS	MODIFIER	E. DIAGNOSIS POINTER
				99282		A–F

Case Study 10.5

1. ICD-10-CM code(s): S61.011D, W25.XXXD

2. CPT code(s): 99212
Note: This patient is not within the global period for the prior procedure.

3.

21. DIAGNOSIS OR NATURE OF ILLNESS OR INJURY Relate A-L to service line below (24E)			ICD Ind.
A. S61.011D	B. W25.XXXD	C.	D.
E.	F.	G.	H.
I.	J.	K.	L.

24. A. DATE(S) OF SERVICE From MM DD YY	To MM DD YY	B. PLACE OF SERVICE	C. EMG	D. PROCEDURES, SERVICES, OR SUPPLIES (Explain Unusual Circumstances) CPT/HCPCS	MODIFIER	E. DIAGNOSIS POINTER
				99212		AB

CHAPTER 11

Answers to the vocabulary section should be checked using the Medical Coding in the Real World, *Third Edition, textbook glossary.*

Word Bank

	Zero Day Global Period	10-Day Global Period	90-Day Global Period
Procedure type	Simple procedure	Minor surgical procedure	Major surgical procedure
Example of procedure	Diagnostic endoscopy	Wound repair	Pacemaker insertion

Matching

1. F
3. C
5. K
7. J
9. A
11. L
13. M
15. B

Completion

1. Approach. When coding for an endoscopy, it is necessary to select the code for the correct approach to the procedure. For example, an open approach or through a colostomy.

3. Surgical versus diagnostic procedure. When an endoscopy is done to determine a diagnosis and a surgical procedure is performed during the same endoscopy, then the coder should only report the surgical endoscopy code. For example, a diagnostic bronchoscopy that found polyps and then removed the polyps—then the coder would report only the surgical bronchoscopy, not the diagnostic bronchoscopy.

Coding

1. Modifier: -47
3. Modifier: -66
5. Modifier: -54
7. Modifier: -52
9. Modifier: -23
11. Modifier: -80
13. Modifier: -81
15. Modifier: -56
17. CPT code(s): 60225
ICD-10-CM code(s): C73, E27.40, E23.0
19. CPT code(s): 42100
ICD-10-CM code(s): D37.09
21. CPT code(s): 54690-RT
ICD-10-CM code(s): C62.11
23. CPT code(s): 31299
25. CPT code(s): 31625, 31624-51
ICD-10-CM code(s): J84.09
27. CPT code(s): 44950-52-PB
29. CPT code(s): 69632-LT
ICD-10-CM code(s): S09.22XA

Case Studies

Case Study 11.1

1. ICD-10-CM code(s): D22.5, D22.62
2. CPT code(s): 11106, 11105 × 3

3.

21. DIAGNOSIS OR NATURE OF ILLNESS OR INJURY Relate A-L to service line below (24E) ICD Ind.

A. D22.62	B. D22.5	C.	D.
E.	F.	G.	H.
I.	J.	K.	L.

22. RESUBMISSION CODE

23. PRIOR AUTHORIZATION NU

	24. A. DATE(S) OF SERVICE From MM DD YY	To MM DD YY	B. PLACE OF SERVICE	C. EMG	D. PROCEDURES, SERVICES, OR SUPPLIES (Explain Unusual Circumstances) CPT/HCPCS	MODIFIER	E. DIAGNOSIS POINTER	F. $ CHARGES	G. DAYS OR UNITS
1					11106		A		
2					11105		B		3
3									
4									

Case Study 11.3

1. ICD-10-CM code(s): M27.40

2. CPT code(s): 21046

3.

21. DIAGNOSIS OR NATURE OF ILLNESS OR INJURY Relate A-L to service line below (24E) ICD Ind.

A. M27.40	B.	C.	D.
E.	F.	G.	H.
I.	J.	K.	L.

24. A. DATE(S) OF SERVICE From MM DD YY	To MM DD YY	B. PLACE OF SERVICE	C. EMG	D. PROCEDURES, SERVICES, OR SUPPLIES (Explain Unusual Circumstances) CPT/HCPCS	MODIFIER	E. DIAGNOSIS POINTER
				21046		A

CHAPTER 12

Answers to the vocabulary section should be checked using the Medical Coding in the Real World, *Third Edition, textbook glossary.*

Multiple Choice

1. C

3. B

5. D

7. D

9. B

Fill in the Blank

1. Base

3. Modifying factors

5. Qualifying circumstances

7. (Base + Time + Modifying factors) × Conversion factor = Total charge amount

Matching

1. C

3. B

Labeling

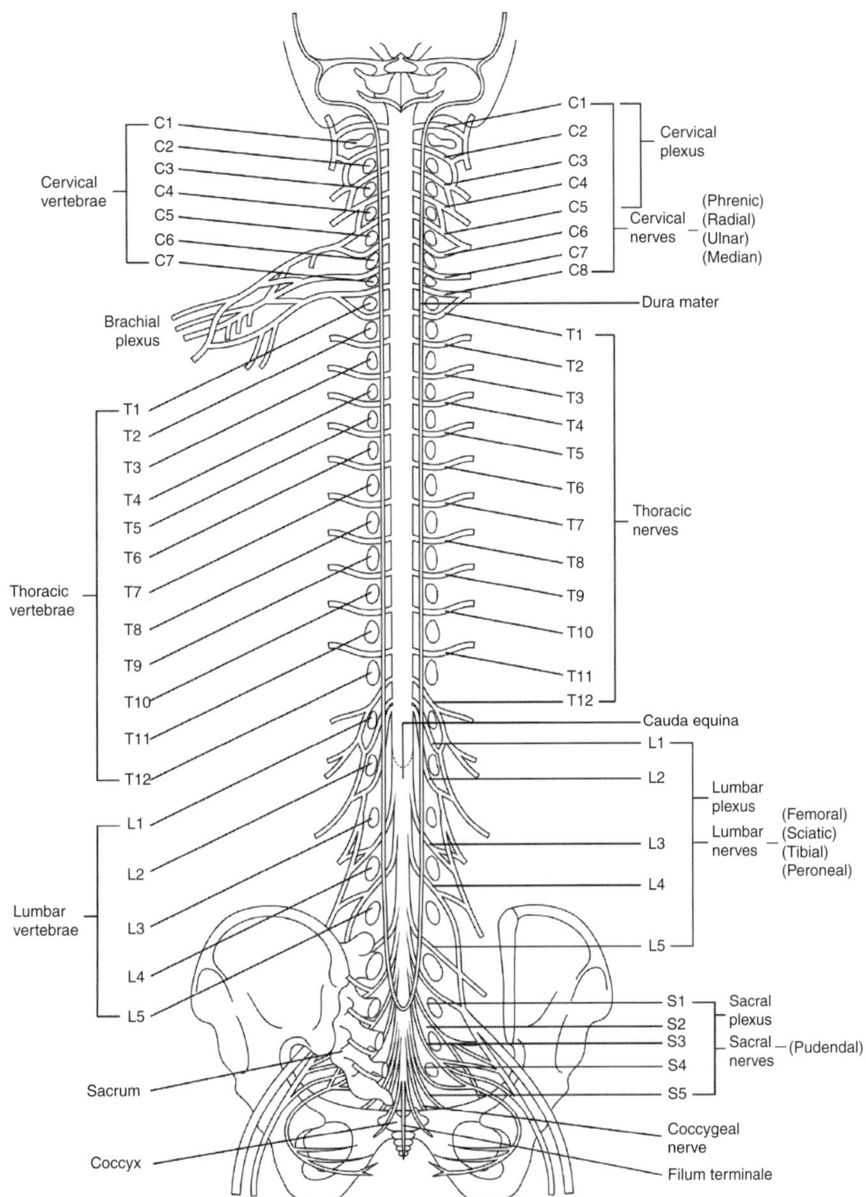

Source: ©AHIMA

Coding

1. CPT code(s): 00546-P1

3. CPT code(s): 00172-P1
ICD-10-CM code(s): Q35.1

5. CPT code(s): 97813, 97814
ICD-10-CM code(s): M54.41, M54.42

7. CPT code(s): 00921-P1
ICD-10-CM code(s): Z30.2

9. CPT code(s): 64635-50, 64636-50 (× 2)
ICD-10-CM code(s): M54.16

11. CPT code(s): 00566
ICD-10-CM code(s): I25.10

13. ICD-10-CM code(s): C61
CPT code(s): 00865

15. CPT code(s): 95971

Case Studies

Case Study 12.1

1. ICD-10-CM code(s): M27.40

2. CPT code(s): 00190-P1 × 4

3.

21. DIAGNOSIS OR NATURE OF ILLNESS OR INJURY Relate A-L to service line below (24E) ICD Ind.

A.	M27.40	B.		C.		D.	
E.		F.		G.		H.	
I.		J.		K.		L.	

22. RESUBMISSION CODE

23. PRIOR AUTHORIZATION NU

	24. A. DATE(S) OF SERVICE From MM	DD	YY	To MM	DD	YY	B. PLACE OF SERVICE	C. EMG	D. PROCEDURES, SERVICES, OR SUPPLIES (Explain Unusual Circumstances) CPT/HCPCS	MODIFIER	E. DIAGNOSIS POINTER	F. $ CHARGES	G. DAYS OR UNITS
1									00190	P1	A		4
2													
3													
4													

Case Study 12.3

1. ICD-10-CM code(s): M48.061, M54.16

2. CPT code(s): 62323, 99152
HCPCS code(s): J3301 × 8

3.

21. DIAGNOSIS OR NATURE OF ILLNESS OR INJURY Relate A-L to service line below (24E) ICD Ind.

A.	M48.061	B.	M54.16	C.		D.	
E.		F.		G.		H.	
I.		J.		K.		L.	

22. RESUBMISSION CODE

23. PRIOR AUTHORIZATION NU

	24. A. DATE(S) OF SERVICE From MM	DD	YY	To MM	DD	YY	B. PLACE OF SERVICE	C. EMG	D. PROCEDURES, SERVICES, OR SUPPLIES (Explain Unusual Circumstances) CPT/HCPCS	MODIFIER	E. DIAGNOSIS POINTER	F. $ CHARGES	G. DAYS OR UNITS
1									62323		AB		
2									99152		AB		
3									J3301		AB		8
4													

Case Study 12.5

1. ICD-10-CM code(s): Q36.9

2. CPT code(s): 00790-P2 × 3

3.

21. DIAGNOSIS OR NATURE OF ILLNESS OR INJURY Relate A-L to service line below (24E) ICD Ind.

A.	K82.8	B.		C.		D.	
E.		F.		G.		H.	
I.		J.		K.		L.	

22. RESUBMISSION CODE

23. PRIOR AUTHORIZATION NU

	24. A. DATE(S) OF SERVICE From MM	DD	YY	To MM	DD	YY	B. PLACE OF SERVICE	C. EMG	D. PROCEDURES, SERVICES, OR SUPPLIES (Explain Unusual Circumstances) CPT/HCPCS	MODIFIER	E. DIAGNOSIS POINTER	F. $ CHARGES	G. DAYS OR UNITS
1									00790	P2	A		3
2													
3													
4													

CHAPTER 13

Answers to the vocabulary section should be checked using the Medical Coding in the Real World, *Third Edition, textbook glossary.*

Multiple Choice

1. C

3. D

5. D

7. B

9. A

Matching

1. E

3. H

5. A

7. I

9. F

Coding

1. CPT code(s): 74182
HCPCS code(s): Q9956 × 4
ICD-10-CM code(s): R16.0, N19

3. CPT code(s): 76872
ICD-10-CM code(s): N40.0

5. CPT code(s): 78305
ICD-10-CM code(s): M86.161, M86.162

7. CPT code(s): 76770
ICD-10-CM code(s): N20.0

9. CPT code(s): 76819
ICD-10-CM code(s): O99.112

Case Studies

Case Study 13.1

1. ICD-10-CM code(s): S89.201D

2. CPT code(s): 73564-RT

3.

21. DIAGNOSIS OR NATURE OF ILLNESS OR INJURY Relate A-L to service line below (24E) ICD Ind.
A. S89.201D B. C. D.
E. F. G. H.
I. J. K. L.
22. RESUBMISSION CODE
23. PRIOR AUTHORIZATION NU

	24. A. DATE(S) OF SERVICE From MM DD YY	To MM DD YY	B. PLACE OF SERVICE	C. EMG	D. PROCEDURES, SERVICES, OR SUPPLIES (Explain Unusual Circumstances) CPT/HCPCS	MODIFIER	E. DIAGNOSIS POINTER	F. $ CHARGES	G. DAYS OR UNITS
1					73564	RT	A		
2									
3									
4									

Case Study 13.3

1. ICD-10-CM code(s): R97.2

2. CPT code(s): 76872

3.

21. DIAGNOSIS OR NATURE OF ILLNESS OR INJURY Relate A-L to service line below (24E) ICD Ind.
A. R97.2 B. C. D.
E. F. G. H.
I. J. K. L.
22. RESUBMISSION CODE
23. PRIOR AUTHORIZATION NU

	24. A. DATE(S) OF SERVICE From MM DD YY	To MM DD YY	B. PLACE OF SERVICE	C. EMG	D. PROCEDURES, SERVICES, OR SUPPLIES (Explain Unusual Circumstances) CPT/HCPCS	MODIFIER	E. DIAGNOSIS POINTER	F. $ CHARGES	G. DAYS OR UNITS
1					76872		A		
2									
3									
4									

Case Study 13.5

1. ICD-10-CM code(s): K40.90

2. CPT code(s): 76705

3.

21. DIAGNOSIS OR NATURE OF ILLNESS OR INJURY Relate A-L to service line below (24E) ICD Ind.

A. K40.90	B.	C.	D.
E.	F.	G.	H.
I.	J.	K.	L.

22. RESUBMISSION CODE

23. PRIOR AUTHORIZATION NU

	24. A. DATE(S) OF SERVICE From MM DD YY	To MM DD YY	B. PLACE OF SERVICE	C. EMG	D. PROCEDURES, SERVICES, OR SUPPLIES (Explain Unusual Circumstances) CPT/HCPCS	MODIFIER	E. DIAGNOSIS POINTER	F. $ CHARGES	G. DAYS OR UNITS
1					76705		A		
2									
3									
4									

CHAPTER 14

Answers to the vocabulary section should be checked using the Medical Coding in the Real World, *Third Edition, textbook glossary.*

Multiple Choice

1. A

3. B

5. A

7. A

9. C

Fill in the Blank

1.1 81, Independent lab

1.2 20

1.3 90

1.4 Laboratory CPT code/service

3.1 gross examination

3.2 microscopic examination

3.3 smear

3.4 frozen section

3.5 permanent section

Coding

1. CPT code(s): 36415, 85025
ICD-10-CM code(s): J06.9

3. CPT code(s): 86689
ICD-10-CM code(s): Z21

5. CPT code(s): 88305
ICD-10-CM code(s): N40.0

7. CPT code(s): 86603
ICD-10-CM code(s): J06.9, R19.7

9. CPT code(s): 87110
ICD-10-CM code(s): A56.02, Z72.51

11. CPT code(s): 80420

13. CPT code(s): 84630

15. CPT code(s): 80337

Case Studies

Case Study 14.1

1. ICD-10-CM code(s): P59.9

2. CPT code(s): 82247

3.

21. DIAGNOSIS OR NATURE OF ILLNESS OR INJURY Relate A-L to service line below (24E) ICD Ind.

A. P59.9	B.	C.	D.
E.	F.	G.	H.
I.	J.	K.	L.

22. RESUBMISSION CODE

23. PRIOR AUTHORIZATION NU

	24. A. DATE(S) OF SERVICE From MM DD YY	To MM DD YY	B. PLACE OF SERVICE	C. EMG	D. PROCEDURES, SERVICES, OR SUPPLIES (Explain Unusual Circumstances) CPT/HCPCS	MODIFIER	E. DIAGNOSIS POINTER	F. $ CHARGES	G. DAYS OR UNITS
1					82247		A		
2									
3									
4									

Case Study 14.3

1. ICD-10-CM code(s): Z13.1

2. CPT code(s): 83036

3.

21. DIAGNOSIS OR NATURE OF ILLNESS OR INJURY Relate A-L to service line below (24E) ICD Ind.

A. Z13.1	B.	C.	D.
E.	F.	G.	H.
I.	J.	K.	L.

22. RESUBMISSION CODE

23. PRIOR AUTHORIZATION NU

	24. A. DATE(S) OF SERVICE From MM	DD	YY	To MM	DD	YY	B. PLACE OF SERVICE	C. EMG	D. PROCEDURES, SERVICES, OR SUPPLIES (Explain Unusual Circumstances) CPT/HCPCS	MODIFIER	E. DIAGNOSIS POINTER	F. $ CHARGES	G. DAYS OR UNITS
1									83036		A		
2													
3													
4													

Case Study 14.5

1. ICD-10-CM code(s): Z13.220

2. CPT code(s): 80061

3.

21. DIAGNOSIS OR NATURE OF ILLNESS OR INJURY Relate A-L to service line below (24E) ICD Ind.

A. Z13.220	B.	C.	D.
E.	F.	G.	H.
I.	J.	K.	L.

22. RESUBMISSION CODE

23. PRIOR AUTHORIZATION NU

	24. A. DATE(S) OF SERVICE From MM	DD	YY	To MM	DD	YY	B. PLACE OF SERVICE	C. EMG	D. PROCEDURES, SERVICES, OR SUPPLIES (Explain Unusual Circumstances) CPT/HCPCS	MODIFIER	E. DIAGNOSIS POINTER	F. $ CHARGES	G. DAYS OR UNITS
1									80061		A		
2													
3													
4													

CHAPTER 15

Answers to the vocabulary section should be checked using the Medical Coding in the Real World, *Third Edition, textbook glossary.*

Multiple Choice

1. A

3. D

5. C

7. A

9. C

Matching

1. F

3. C

5. I

7. H

9. A

Labeling

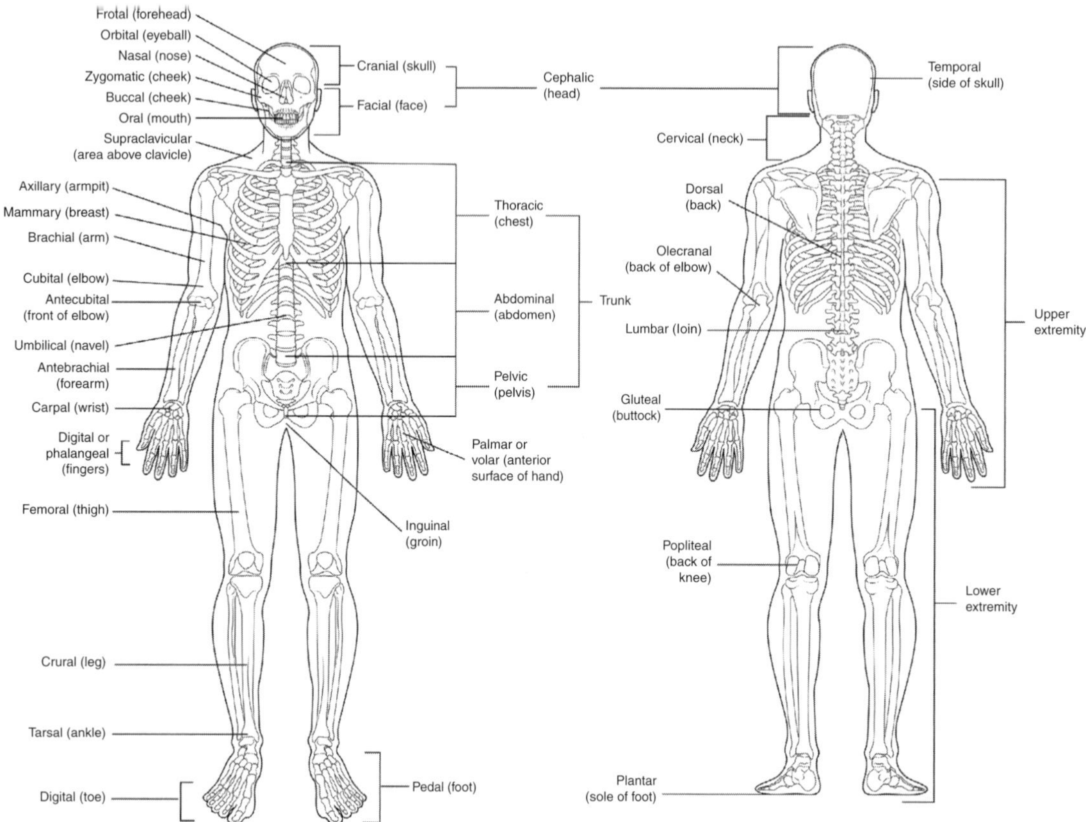

Coding

1. ICD-10-CM code(s): S79.111A
3. CPT code(s): 29125-RT, 73090-RT
   ICD-10-CM code(s): M80.031A
5. CPT code(s): 28810-RT
   ICD-10-CM code(s): I96
7. CPT code(s): 20610-RT
   ICD-10-CM code(s): M00.061, B95.61
9. CPT code(s): 22015
   ICD-10-CM code(s): M46.27
11. ICD-10-CM code(s): M77.11
13. ICD-10-CM code(s): M72.2
15. ICD-10-CM code(s): M75.22
17. ICD-10-CM code(s): M65.4
19. ICD-10-CM code(s): M72.0

Case Studies

Case Study 15.1

1. ICD-10-CM code(s): M25.561
2. CPT code(s): 99203, 73590-RT

3.

21. DIAGNOSIS OR NATURE OF ILLNESS OR INJURY Relate A-L to service line below (24E) ICD Ind.

A. M25.561 B. C. D.
E. F. G. H.
I. J. K. L.

22. RESUBMISSION CODE

23. PRIOR AUTHORIZATION NU

	24. A. DATE(S) OF SERVICE From MM DD YY	To MM DD YY	B. PLACE OF SERVICE	C. EMG	D. PROCEDURES, SERVICES, OR SUPPLIES (Explain Unusual Circumstances) CPT/HCPCS	MODIFIER	E. DIAGNOSIS POINTER	F. $ CHARGES	G. DAYS OR UNITS
1					99203		A		
2					73592	RT	A		
3									
4									

Case Study 15.3

1. ICD-10-CM code(s): S83.231A, S83.271A

2. CPT code(s): 29880

3.

21. DIAGNOSIS OR NATURE OF ILLNESS OR INJURY Relate A-L to service line below (24E) ICD Ind.

A. S83.231A B. S83.271A C. D.
E. F. G. H.
I. J. K. L.

22. RESUBMISSION CODE

23. PRIOR AUTHORIZATION NU

	24. A. DATE(S) OF SERVICE From MM DD YY	To MM DD YY	B. PLACE OF SERVICE	C. EMG	D. PROCEDURES, SERVICES, OR SUPPLIES (Explain Unusual Circumstances) CPT/HCPCS	MODIFIER	E. DIAGNOSIS POINTER	F. $ CHARGES	G. DAYS OR UNITS
1					29880		AB		
2									
3									
4									

CHAPTER 16

Answers to the vocabulary section should be checked using the Medical Coding in the Real World, *Third Edition, textbook glossary.*

Multiple Choice

1. A

3. B

5. B

7. C

9. A

Matching

1. C

3. F

5. B

7. G

Coding

1. CPT code(s): 97161
ICD-10-CM code(s): M17.0

3. HCPCS code(s): V5336
ICD-10-CM code(s): R49.1

5. CPT code(s): 92625
ICD-10-CM code(s): H93.13

7. CPT code(s): 97110-97 (× 2)
ICD-10-CM code(s): S83.511D

9. ICD-10-CM code(s): F84.0, F90.0

11. ICD-10-CM code(s): R48.2

13. CPT code(s): 97164

15. CPT code(s): 97533-96 × 2
ICD-10-CM code(s): F44.6

Case Studies

Case Study 16.1

1. ICD-10-CM code(s): Z96.653

21. DIAGNOSIS OR NATURE OF ILLNESS OR INJURY Relate A-L to service line below (24E) ICD Ind.

A. Z96.653	B.	C.	D.
E.	F.	G.	H.
I.	J.	K.	L.

22. RESUBMISSION CODE

23. PRIOR AUTHORIZATION NU

	24. A. DATE(S) OF SERVICE From MM DD YY	To MM DD YY	B. PLACE OF SERVICE	C. EMG	D. PROCEDURES, SERVICES, OR SUPPLIES (Explain Unusual Circumstances) CPT/HCPCS	MODIFIER	E. DIAGNOSIS POINTER	F. $ CHARGES	G. DAYS OR UNITS
1					97110	97	A		2
2									
3									
4									

2. CPT code(s): 97110-97 × 2

3.

CHAPTER 17

Answers to the vocabulary section should be checked using the Medical Coding in the Real World, *Third Edition, textbook glossary.*

Multiple Choice

1. B
3. A
5. D
7. A
9. C

Matching

1. F
3. D
5. B
7. H
9. G

Labeling

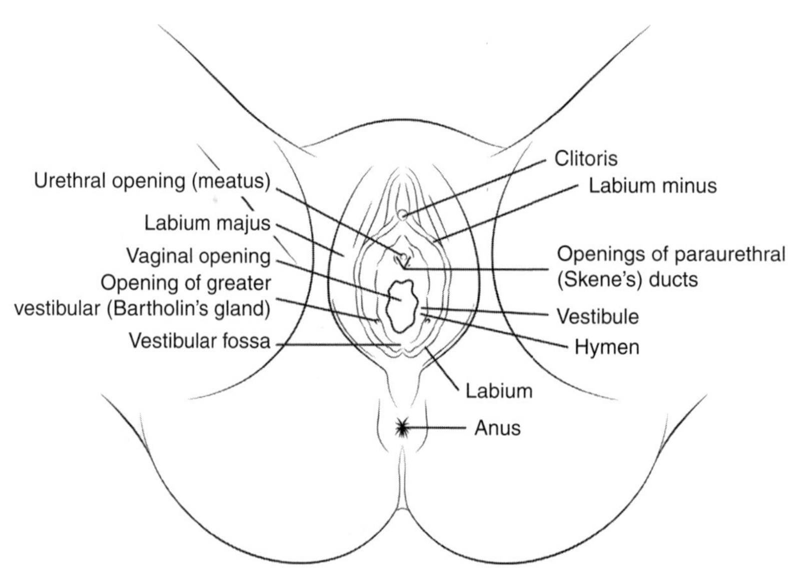

Source: ©AHIMA.

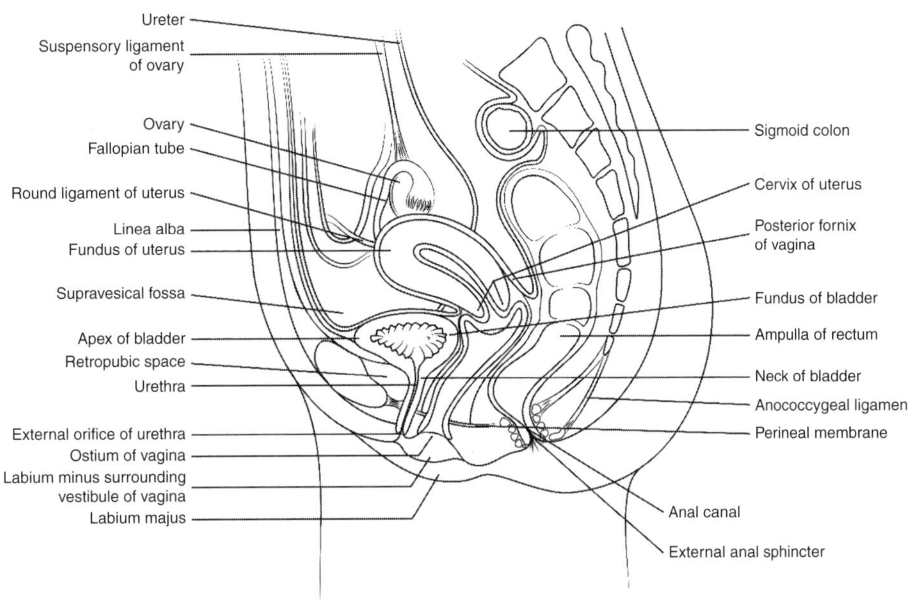

Source: ©AHIMA.

Coding

1. ICD-10-CM code(s): O40.3XX1, O30.003, Z3A.30

3. CPT code(s): 59409
ICD-10-CM code(s): O60.14X0, O32.1XX0, O70.1, Z37.0, Z3A.34

5. CPT code(s): 99203
ICD-10-CM code(s): A54.24, Z72.51, F32.9, F41.9

7. CPT code(s): 59510
ICD-10-CM code(s): O75.82, Z34.40, Z37.0

9. CPT code(s): 59830
ICD-10-CM code(s): O03.87, B95.0

Case Studies

Case Study 17.1

1. ICD-10-CM code(s): D25.9, N80.3, N83.201

2. CPT code(s): 58552, 58662-51

3.

21. DIAGNOSIS OR NATURE OF ILLNESS OR INJURY Relate A-L to service line below (24E) ICD Ind.

A. D25.9	B. N80.3	C. N83.201	D.
E.	F.	G.	H.
I.	J.	K.	L.

22. RESUBMISSION CODE

23. PRIOR AUTHORIZATION NU

	24. A. DATE(S) OF SERVICE From MM DD YY	To MM DD YY	B. PLACE OF SERVICE	C. EMG	D. PROCEDURES, SERVICES, OR SUPPLIES (Explain Unusual Circumstances) CPT/HCPCS	MODIFIER	E. DIAGNOSIS POINTER	F. $ CHARGES	G. DAYS OR UNITS
1					58552		AB		
2					58662	51	C		
3									
4									

Case Study 17.3

1. ICD-10-CM code(s): O80, Z37.0

2. CPT code(s): 99231

3.

21. DIAGNOSIS OR NATURE OF ILLNESS OR INJURY Relate A-L to service line below (24E)			ICD Ind.	22. RESUBMISSION CODE
A. O80	B. Z37.0	C.	D.	23. PRIOR AUTHORIZATION NU
E.	F.	G.	H.	
I.	J.	K.	L.	

	24. A. DATE(S) OF SERVICE From MM DD YY To MM DD YY	B. PLACE OF SERVICE	C. EMG	D. PROCEDURES, SERVICES, OR SUPPLIES (Explain Unusual Circumstances) CPT/HCPCS	MODIFIER	E. DIAGNOSIS POINTER	F. $ CHARGES	G. DAYS OR UNITS
1				99231		AB		
2								
3								
4								

Case Study 17.5

1. ICD-10-CM code(s): N87.1

2. CPT code(s): 57522

3.

21. DIAGNOSIS OR NATURE OF ILLNESS OR INJURY Relate A-L to service line below (24E)			ICD Ind.	22. RESUBMISSION CODE
A. N87.1	B.	C.	D.	23. PRIOR AUTHORIZATION NU
E.	F.	G.	H.	
I.	J.	K.	L.	

	24. A. DATE(S) OF SERVICE From MM DD YY To MM DD YY	B. PLACE OF SERVICE	C. EMG	D. PROCEDURES, SERVICES, OR SUPPLIES (Explain Unusual Circumstances) CPT/HCPCS	MODIFIER	E. DIAGNOSIS POINTER	F. $ CHARGES	G. DAYS OR UNITS
1				57522		A		
2								
3								
4								

CHAPTER 18

Answers to the vocabulary section should be checked using the Medical Coding in the Real World, *Third Edition, textbook glossary.*

Fill in the Blank

1. A. Request: Patient's provider requests the consultation
B. Render: Consultant renders the consultation
C. Report: Consultant sends written report to provider

3. Hematologist

5. Neurologist

7. Nephrologist

9. Central; peripheral

Matching

1. C

3. D

Multiple Choice

1. A

3. C

5. C

7. B

9. A

Labeling

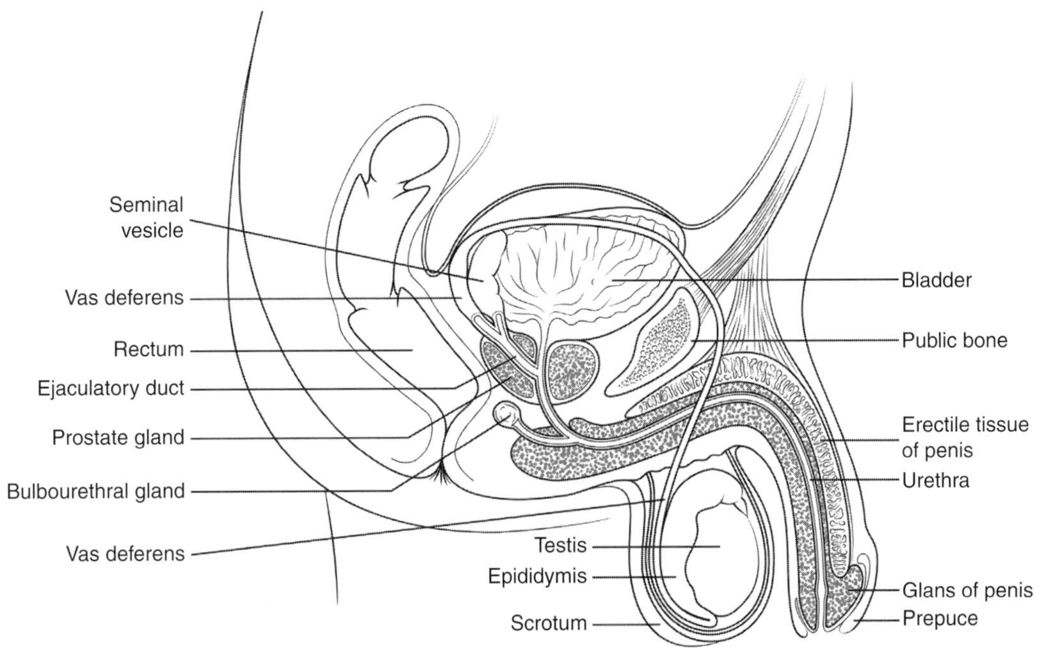

Source: ©AHIMA.

Coding

1. CPT code(s): 77523

3. CPT code(s): 77386

5. CPT code(s): 96360, 96361 × 5

7. ICD-10-CM code(s): Z51.11, C78.7

9. CPT code(s): 63610
ICD-10-CM code(s): D43.4

11. CPT code(s): 95957
ICD-10-CM code(s): G40.A11

13. CPT code(s): 51060
ICD-10-CM code(s): N20.1

15. CPT code(s): 77372

17. CPT code(s): 64865
ICD-10-CM code(s): S04.52XA

19. CPT code(s): 51865
ICD-10-CM code(s): N32.89

Case Studies

Case Study 18.1

1. ICD-10-CM code(s): C61, Z79.818, R35.0, R35.1

2. CPT code(s): 99215, 96372, J9217 × 6

3.

21. DIAGNOSIS OR NATURE OF ILLNESS OR INJURY Relate A-L to service line below (24E) ICD Ind.

A. C61	B. Z79.818	C. R35.0	D. R35.1
E.	F.	G.	H.
I.	J.	K.	L.

22. RESUBMISSION CODE

23. PRIOR AUTHORIZATION NU

	24. A. DATE(S) OF SERVICE From MM DD YY	To MM DD YY	B. PLACE OF SERVICE	C. EMG	D. PROCEDURES, SERVICES, OR SUPPLIES (Explain Unusual Circumstances) CPT/HCPCS	MODIFIER	E. DIAGNOSIS POINTER	F. $ CHARGES	G. DAYS OR UNITS
1					99215		ABCD		
2					96372		A		
3					J9217		A		6
4									

Case Study 18.3

1. ICD-10-CM code(s): N20.1

2. CPT code(s): 52356-LT, 74420

3.

21. DIAGNOSIS OR NATURE OF ILLNESS OR INJURY Relate A-L to service line below (24E) ICD Ind.

A. N20.1	B.	C.	D.
E.	F.	G.	H.
I.	J.	K.	L.

22. RESUBMISSION CODE

23. PRIOR AUTHORIZATION NU

	24. A. DATE(S) OF SERVICE From MM	DD	YY	To MM	DD	YY	B. PLACE OF SERVICE	C. EMG	D. PROCEDURES, SERVICES, OR SUPPLIES (Explain Unusual Circumstances) CPT/HCPCS	MODIFIER	E. DIAGNOSIS POINTER	F. $ CHARGES	G. DAYS OR UNITS
1									52356	LT	A		
2									74420		A		
3													
4													

Case Study 18.5

1. ICD-10-CM code(s): G62.9

2. CPT code(s): 95861

3.

21. DIAGNOSIS OR NATURE OF ILLNESS OR INJURY Relate A-L to service line below (24E) ICD Ind.

A. G62.9	B.	C.	D.
E.	F.	G.	H.
I.	J.	K.	L.

22. RESUBMISSION CODE

23. PRIOR AUTHORIZATION NU

	24. A. DATE(S) OF SERVICE From MM	DD	YY	To MM	DD	YY	B. PLACE OF SERVICE	C. EMG	D. PROCEDURES, SERVICES, OR SUPPLIES (Explain Unusual Circumstances) CPT/HCPCS	MODIFIER	E. DIAGNOSIS POINTER	F. $ CHARGES	G. DAYS OR UNITS
1									95861		A		
2													
3													
4													

CHAPTER 19

Answers to the vocabulary section should be checked using the Medical Coding in the Real World, *Third Edition, textbook glossary.*

Matching

1. C

3. A

5. G

7. H

Multiple Choice

1. C

3. D

5. D

7. C

9. C

Coding

1. CPT code(s): 43020
ICD-10-CM code(s): S11.24XA

3. CPT code(s): 43772
ICD-10-CM code(s): E44.0

5. CPT code(s): 45321
ICD-10-CM code(s): K56.2

7. CPT code(s): 33020
ICD-10-CM code(s): I51.3

9. CPT code(s): 33250
ICD-10-CM code(s): I45.6

11. CPT code(s): 33533

13. CPT code(s): 33533, 33519, 35600
ICD-10-CM code(s): I25.119, F17.210, E66.01, Z68.41

15. CPT code(s): 92920, 92921
ICD-10-CM code(s): I25.811

Case Studies

Case Study 19.1

1. ICD-10-CM code(s): Z12.11, K64.1

2. CPT code(s): 45378

3.

21. DIAGNOSIS OR NATURE OF ILLNESS OR INJURY Relate A-L to service line below (24E) ICD Ind.

A. Z12.11 B. K64.1 C. D.
E. F. G. H.
I. J. K. L.

22. RESUBMISSION CODE

23. PRIOR AUTHORIZATION NU

	24. A. DATE(S) OF SERVICE From MM DD YY	To MM DD YY	B. PLACE OF SERVICE	C. EMG	D. PROCEDURES, SERVICES, OR SUPPLIES (Explain Unusual Circumstances) CPT/HCPCS	MODIFIER	E. DIAGNOSIS POINTER	F. $ CHARGES	G. DAYS OR UNITS
1					45378		AB		
2									
3									
4									

Case Study 19.3

1. ICD-10-CM code(s): Z13.6

2. CPT code(s): 93895

3.

21. DIAGNOSIS OR NATURE OF ILLNESS OR INJURY Relate A-L to service line below (24E) ICD Ind.

A. Z13.6 B. C. D.
E. F. G. H.
I. J. K. L.

22. RESUBMISSION CODE

23. PRIOR AUTHORIZATION NU

	24. A. DATE(S) OF SERVICE From MM DD YY	To MM DD YY	B. PLACE OF SERVICE	C. EMG	D. PROCEDURES, SERVICES, OR SUPPLIES (Explain Unusual Circumstances) CPT/HCPCS	MODIFIER	E. DIAGNOSIS POINTER	F. $ CHARGES	G. DAYS OR UNITS
1					93895		A		
2									
3									
4									

Case Study 19.5

1. ICD-10-CM code(s): I25.10

2. CPT code(s): 93880

3.

21. DIAGNOSIS OR NATURE OF ILLNESS OR INJURY Relate A-L to service line below (24E) ICD Ind.

A. I25.10 B. C. D.
E. F. G. H.
I. J. K. L.

22. RESUBMISSION CODE

23. PRIOR AUTHORIZATION NU

	24. A. DATE(S) OF SERVICE From MM DD YY	To MM DD YY	B. PLACE OF SERVICE	C. EMG	D. PROCEDURES, SERVICES, OR SUPPLIES (Explain Unusual Circumstances) CPT/HCPCS	MODIFIER	E. DIAGNOSIS POINTER	F. $ CHARGES	G. DAYS OR UNITS
1					93880		A		
2									
3									
4									

CHAPTER 20

Answers to the vocabulary section should be checked using the Medical Coding in the Real World, *Third Edition, textbook glossary.*

Matching

1. A

3. P

5. N

7. L

9. J

11. H

13. F

15. D

17. B

Short Answer

1. Approach to the procedure

3. 2; open and percutaneous endoscopic

5. 0DTN0ZZ

Fill in the Blank

1. Section

3. Root Operation or Type

5. Approach

7. Qualifier

Coding

1. ICD-10-PCS code(s): 0JXL0ZC

3. ICD-10-PCS code(s): 04BD3ZX

5. ICD-10-PCS code(s): 0TT00ZZ

7. ICD-10-PCS code(s): 10E0XZZ

9. ICD-10-PCS code(s): 9WB2XKZ, 9WB3XKZ

Case Studies

Case Study 20.1

ICD-10-PCS code(s): 09CKXZZ

Case Study 20.3

ICD-10-PCS code(s): 0XQLXZZ

Case Study 20.5

ICD-10-PCS code(s): BW40ZZZ

Case Study 20.7

ICD-10-PCS code(s): 10E0XZZ

Case Study 20.9

ICD-10-PCS code(s): 0DJD8ZZ

References

American Academy of Orthopaedic Surgeons (AAOS). 2015 (February). Patellofemoral Pain Syndrome. https://orthoinfo.aaos.org/en/diseases--conditions/patellofemoral-pain-syndrome/.

Skin Cancer Foundation. 2019 (May). Actinic Keratosis Overview. https://www.skincancer.org/skin-cancer-information/actinic-keratosis/.

Weiss, J.P. 2012. Nocturia: Focus on Etiology and Consequences. *Reviews in Urology* 14(3-4): 48–55.

Appendix B: Additional Resources

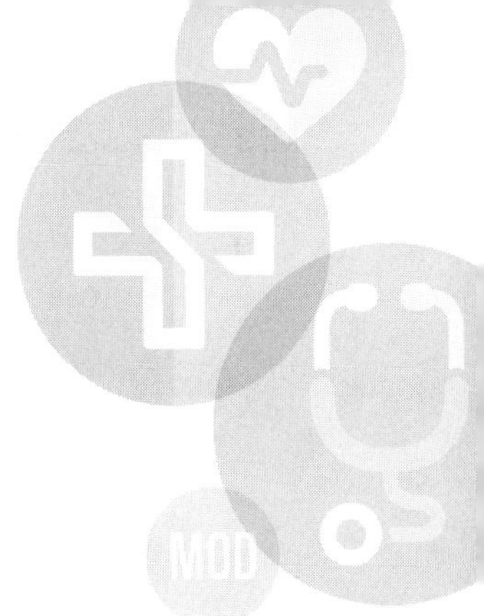

The following is a list of suggested resource materials for medical coding students to be used in addition to the textbook and student workbook.

Code books that are referenced in the textbook:

- ICD-10-CM (current year)
- ICD-10-PCS (current year)
- ICD-9 (as a reference for the legacy system)
- CPT (current year)
- HCPCS (current year)

A medical dictionary for health professionals, such as Mosby. 2021. *Mosby's Medical Dictionary,* Eleventh Edition. St. Louis, MO: Elsevier.

Coding certification study guides:

- American Health Information Management Association (AHIMA). 2022. *CCS Exam Preparation,* Eleventh Edition. Chicago: AHIMA.
- American Health Information Management Association (AHIMA). 2022. *Certified Coding Associate (CCA) Exam Preparation, Eighth Edition.* Chicago: AHIMA.
- National Healthcareer Association (NHA). *Certified Billing & Coding Specialist (CBCS) Printed Study Guide.* Leawood, KS: NHA.
- American Academy of Professional Coders (AAPC). 2019. *Official CPC Certification Study Guide.* Salt Lake City: AAPC.

American Medical Association (AMA). 2017. *Advanced Anatomy and Physiology for ICD-10-CM/PCS 2018.* Chicago: AMA.

American Psychiatric Association (APA). 2013. *Diagnostic and Statistical Manual of Mental Disorders (DSM-5®), Fifth Edition*. Washington, DC: APA.

American Society of Anesthesiologists (ASA). 2020. *Crosswalk 2020.* Schaumburg, IL: ASA.

Appendix C: Blank Forms

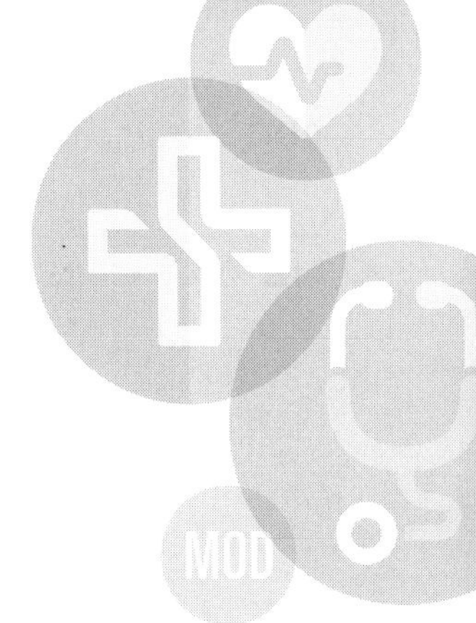

CMS-1500

HEALTH INSURANCE CLAIM FORM

APPROVED BY NATIONAL UNIFORM CLAIM COMMITTEE (NUCC) 02/12

PICA — PICA — CARRIER

1. MEDICARE (Medicare#) — MEDICAID (Medicaid#) — TRICARE (ID#/DoD#) — CHAMPVA (Member ID#) — GROUP HEALTH PLAN (ID#) — FECA BLK LUNG (ID#) — OTHER (ID#)

1a. INSURED'S I.D. NUMBER (For Program in Item 1)

2. PATIENT'S NAME (Last Name, First Name, Middle Initial)

3. PATIENT'S BIRTH DATE MM DD YY — SEX M F

4. INSURED'S NAME (Last Name, First Name, Middle Initial)

5. PATIENT'S ADDRESS (No., Street)

6. PATIENT RELATIONSHIP TO INSURED — Self Spouse Child Other

7. INSURED'S ADDRESS (No., Street)

CITY — STATE

8. RESERVED FOR NUCC USE

CITY — STATE

ZIP CODE — TELEPHONE (Include Area Code) ( )

ZIP CODE — TELEPHONE (Include Area Code) ( )

9. OTHER INSURED'S NAME (Last Name, First Name, Middle Initial)

10. IS PATIENT'S CONDITION RELATED TO:

11. INSURED'S POLICY GROUP OR FECA NUMBER

a. OTHER INSURED'S POLICY OR GROUP NUMBER

a. EMPLOYMENT? (Current or Previous) YES NO

a. INSURED'S DATE OF BIRTH MM DD YY — SEX M F

b. RESERVED FOR NUCC USE

b. AUTO ACCIDENT? YES NO — PLACE (State)

b. OTHER CLAIM ID (Designated by NUCC)

c. RESERVED FOR NUCC USE

c. OTHER ACCIDENT? YES NO

c. INSURANCE PLAN NAME OR PROGRAM NAME

d. INSURANCE PLAN NAME OR PROGRAM NAME

10d. CLAIM CODES (Designated by NUCC)

d. IS THERE ANOTHER HEALTH BENEFIT PLAN? YES NO *If yes*, complete items 9, 9a, and 9d.

READ BACK OF FORM BEFORE COMPLETING & SIGNING THIS FORM.

12. PATIENT'S OR AUTHORIZED PERSON'S SIGNATURE I authorize the release of any medical or other information necessary to process this claim. I also request payment of government benefits either to myself or to the party who accepts assignment below.

SIGNED ______ DATE ______

13. INSURED'S OR AUTHORIZED PERSON'S SIGNATURE I authorize payment of medical benefits to the undersigned physician or supplier for services described below.

SIGNED ______

PATIENT AND INSURED INFORMATION

14. DATE OF CURRENT ILLNESS, INJURY, or PREGNANCY (LMP) MM DD YY — QUAL.

15. OTHER DATE QUAL. MM DD YY

16. DATES PATIENT UNABLE TO WORK IN CURRENT OCCUPATION — FROM MM DD YY — TO MM DD YY

17. NAME OF REFERRING PROVIDER OR OTHER SOURCE — 17a. — 17b. NPI

18. HOSPITALIZATION DATES RELATED TO CURRENT SERVICES — FROM MM DD YY — TO MM DD YY

19. ADDITIONAL CLAIM INFORMATION (Designated by NUCC)

20. OUTSIDE LAB? YES NO — $ CHARGES

21. DIAGNOSIS OR NATURE OF ILLNESS OR INJURY Relate A-L to service line below (24E) — ICD Ind.

A. B. C. D.
E. F. G. H.
I. J. K. L.

22. RESUBMISSION CODE — ORIGINAL REF. NO.

23. PRIOR AUTHORIZATION NUMBER

24. A. DATE(S) OF SERVICE From MM DD YY	To MM DD YY	B. PLACE OF SERVICE	C. EMG	D. PROCEDURES, SERVICES, OR SUPPLIES (Explain Unusual Circumstances) CPT/HCPCS	MODIFIER	E. DIAGNOSIS POINTER	F. $ CHARGES	G. DAYS OR UNITS	H. EPSDT Family Plan	I. ID. QUAL.	J. RENDERING PROVIDER ID. #
1										NPI	
2										NPI	
3										NPI	
4										NPI	
5										NPI	
6										NPI	

25. FEDERAL TAX I.D. NUMBER — SSN EIN

26. PATIENT'S ACCOUNT NO.

27. ACCEPT ASSIGNMENT? (For govt. claims, see back) YES NO

28. TOTAL CHARGE $

29. AMOUNT PAID $

30. Rsvd for NUCC Use

31. SIGNATURE OF PHYSICIAN OR SUPPLIER INCLUDING DEGREES OR CREDENTIALS (I certify that the statements on the reverse apply to this bill and are made a part thereof.)

SIGNED ______ DATE ______

32. SERVICE FACILITY LOCATION INFORMATION — a. NPI b.

33. BILLING PROVIDER INFO & PH # ( ) — a. NPI b.

PHYSICIAN OR SUPPLIER INFORMATION

NUCC Instruction Manual available at: www.nucc.org — ***PLEASE PRINT OR TYPE*** — APPROVED OMB-0938-1197 FORM 1500 (02-12)

UB-04 / CMS-1450

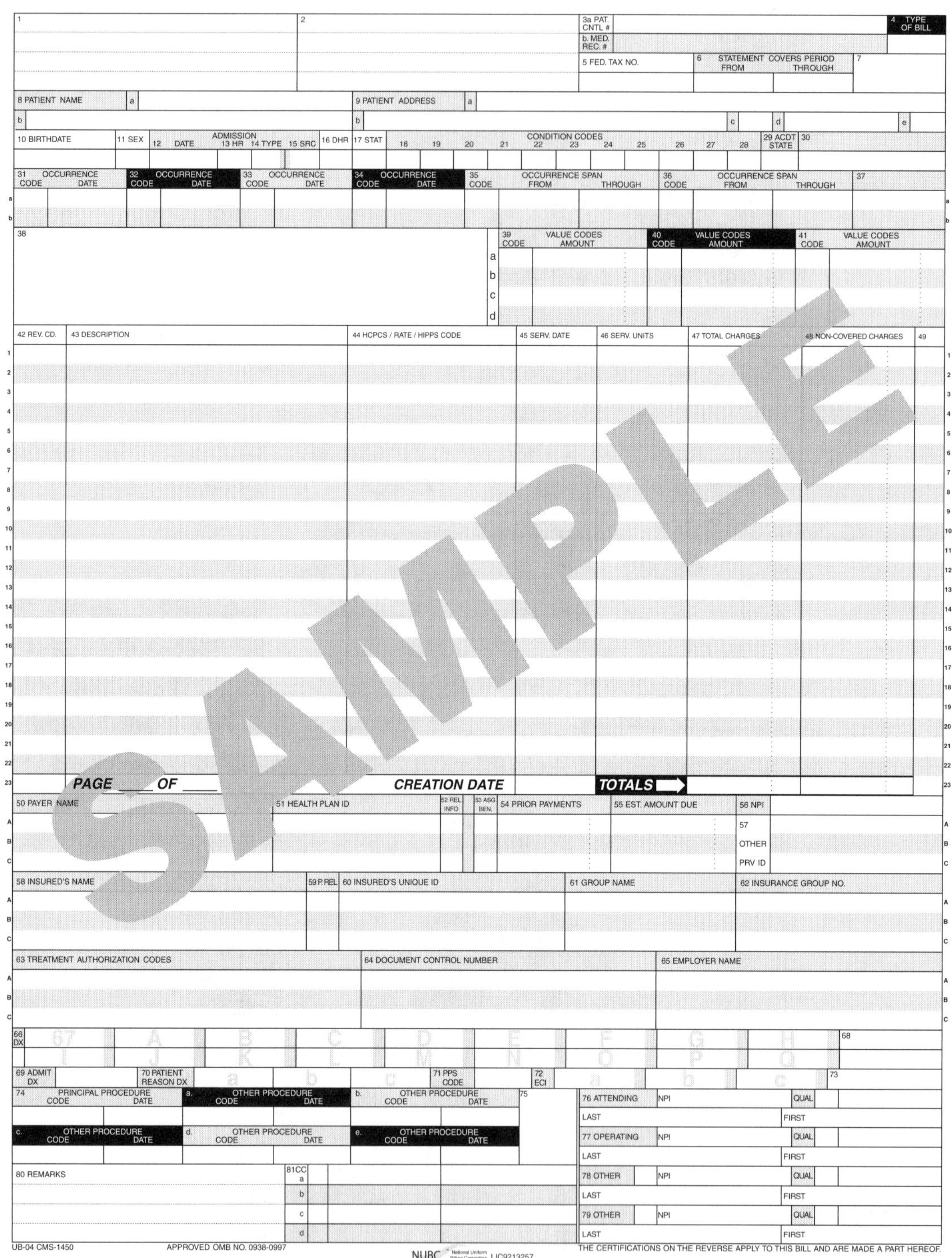

1
2
3a PAT. CNTL #
b. MED. REC. #
4 TYPE OF BILL
5 FED. TAX NO.
6 STATEMENT COVERS PERIOD FROM THROUGH
7
8 PATIENT NAME a b
9 PATIENT ADDRESS a b c d e
10 BIRTHDATE
11 SEX
ADMISSION 12 DATE 13 HR 14 TYPE 15 SRC
16 DHR
17 STAT
CONDITION CODES 18 19 20 21 22 23 24 25 26 27 28
29 ACDT STATE
30
31 OCCURRENCE CODE DATE
32 OCCURRENCE CODE DATE
33 OCCURRENCE CODE DATE
34 OCCURRENCE CODE DATE
35 CODE OCCURRENCE SPAN FROM THROUGH
36 CODE OCCURRENCE SPAN FROM THROUGH
37
38
39 VALUE CODES CODE AMOUNT
40 VALUE CODES CODE AMOUNT
41 VALUE CODES CODE AMOUNT
a b c d
42 REV. CD.
43 DESCRIPTION
44 HCPCS / RATE / HIPPS CODE
45 SERV. DATE
46 SERV. UNITS
47 TOTAL CHARGES
48 NON-COVERED CHARGES
49
1 2 3 4 5 6 7 8 9 10 11 12 13 14 15 16 17 18 19 20 21 22 23
PAGE ____ OF ____
CREATION DATE
TOTALS
50 PAYER NAME
51 HEALTH PLAN ID
52 REL. INFO
53 ASG. BEN.
54 PRIOR PAYMENTS
55 EST. AMOUNT DUE
56 NPI
57 OTHER PRV ID
A B C
58 INSURED'S NAME
59 P.REL
60 INSURED'S UNIQUE ID
61 GROUP NAME
62 INSURANCE GROUP NO.
A B C
63 TREATMENT AUTHORIZATION CODES
64 DOCUMENT CONTROL NUMBER
65 EMPLOYER NAME
A B C
66 DX
67 A B C D E F G H
I J K L M N O P Q
68
69 ADMIT DX
70 PATIENT REASON DX a b c
71 PPS CODE
72 ECI a b c
73
74 PRINCIPAL PROCEDURE CODE DATE
a. OTHER PROCEDURE CODE DATE
b. OTHER PROCEDURE CODE DATE
75
c. OTHER PROCEDURE CODE DATE
d. OTHER PROCEDURE CODE DATE
e. OTHER PROCEDURE CODE DATE
76 ATTENDING NPI QUAL LAST FIRST
77 OPERATING NPI QUAL LAST FIRST
80 REMARKS
81CC a b c d
78 OTHER NPI QUAL LAST FIRST
79 OTHER NPI QUAL LAST FIRST
UB-04 CMS-1450
APPROVED OMB NO. 0938-0997
NUBC National Uniform Billing Committee LIC9213257
THE CERTIFICATIONS ON THE REVERSE APPLY TO THIS BILL AND ARE MADE A PART HEREOF.

SAMPLE